Second Edition

# Pulmonary Function Testing and Cardiopulmonary Stress Testing

PEFR

$FEF_{25\%}$ or $\dot{V}_{max\ 75}$

$FEF_{50\%}$ or $V_{max\ 50}$

$FEF_{75\%}$ or $V_{max\ 25}$

Expiration

Inspiration

2    3    4    5    6

**VOLUME (liters)**

FVC

## Vincent C. Madama

# NORMAL VALUES FOR PULMONARY FUNCTION TESTING

## Normal Values for Pulmonary Mechanics Tests

### Normal Values for *FVC* and Its Components
#### (Based on a 70-inch-tall, 20-year-old caucasian male subject)

$FVC = 5.00$ liters  
$PEFR = 9.10$ l/sec  
$FEV_{0.5} = 3.10$ liters  
$FEV_1 = 4.20$ liters  
$FEV_2 = 4.60$ liters  
$FEV_3 = 4.90$ liters  
$FEF_{200-1200} = 8.70$ l/sec  
$FEF_{25\%-75\%} = 5.20$ l/sec  
$FEF_{75\%-85\%} = 1.70$ l/sec  

$FIVC = 5.00$ liters  
$FIF_{25\%-75\%} = 7.70$ l/sec  
$FEV_{0.5\%} = 50\%-60\%$*  
$FEV_{1\%} = 75\%-85\%$*  
$FEV_{2\%} = 94\%$*  
$FEV_{3\%} = 97\%$*  
$FEF_{25\%} = 8.30$ l/sec  
$FEF_{50\%} = 5.70$ l/sec  
$FEF_{75\%} = 3.20$ l/sec  

*These values for $FEV_{0.5\%}$, $FEV_{1\%}$, $FEV_{2\%}$, and $FEV_{3\%}$ are accepted as being

---

### Approximate Normal (20-year-old subjects of average height and weight) Adult Values for M*VV*

Male = 160 l/min  
Female = 120 l/min

---

### Normal Adult Values for $R_{aw}$
#### Determinations

$R_{aw} = 0.6 - 2.8$ cm $H_2O$/l/sec  
$SR_{aw} = 0.190 - 0.667$ cm $H_2O$/l/sec/l

---

### Normal Adult Values for Elastic Resistance Factors

Elastic Recoil Pressure = 34 cm $H_2O$  
$C_L = 0.2$ l/cm $H_2O$  
$C_r = 0.2$ l/cm $H_2O$  
$C_{LT} = 0.1$ l/cm $H_2O$  
$SC_{LT} = 0.05-0.06$ l/cm $H_2O$/l  
$C_{Dyn} = 0.09-0.07$ l/cm $H_2O$ (at a flow of 0.5 l/sec)

---

### Normal Adult Values for *MIP* and *MEP*

Normal values that are generally accepted as being clinical useful:

$MIP = >-60$ cm $H_2O$  
$MEP = >+80$ to $100$ cm$H_2O$

---

## Normal Values for Lung Volumes, Capacities, and Ventilation Tests

### Normal Values for Lung Volumes, Capacities, and Ventilation

| VOLUME | | NEWBORN INFANT | YOUNG ADULT MALE | APPROX. % OF TLC (YOUNG ADULT MALE) |
|---|---|---|---|---|
| $V_T$ | (ml) | 15 | 500 | 8-10 |
| IRV | (ml) | 85 | 3100 | 50 |
| ERV | (ml) | 40 | 1200 | 20 |
| RV | (ml) | 40 | 1200 | 20 |
| IC | (ml) | 100 | 3600 | 60 |
| FRC | (ml) | 80 | 2400 | 40 |
| VC | (ml) | 140 | 4800 | 80 |
| TLC | (ml) | 180 | 6000 | 100 |
| f | (bpm) | 35–50 | 12–20 | |
| $\dot{V}_E$ | | 525–750 ml/min | 5–6 l/min | |

# PULMONARY FUNCTION TESTING AND CARDIOPULMONARY STRESS TESTING

## SECOND EDITION
## WITHDRAWN

**Vincent C. Madama, M.Ed., RRT**
Associate Professor
Director of Clinical Education
Respiratory Care Program
Rock Valley College
Rockford, Illinois

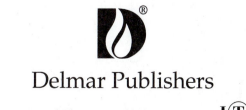

## Delmar Publishers

*an International Thomson Publishing company* I(T)P®

Albany • Bonn • Boston • Cincinnati • Detroit • London • Madrid
Melbourne • Mexico City • New York • Pacific Grove • Paris • San Francisco
Singapore • Tokyo • Toronto • Washington

# NOTICE TO THE READER

Cover Design: Lost Acre Design, Douglas J. Hyldelund

**Delmar Staff:**
Publisher: Susan Simpfenderfer
Acquisitions Editor: Dawn Gerrain
Developmental Editor: Debra Flis
Project Editor: Coreen Rogers
Production Coordinator: John Mickelbank
Art and Design Coordinator: Vincent S. Berger
Editorial Assistant: Donna I. Leto
Marketing Manager: Katherine Slezak

Copyright © 1998
By Delmar Publishers
a division of International Thomson Publishing Inc.

The ITP logo is a trademark under license.

Printed in the United States of America

A service of I(T)P®

For more information, contact:

Delmar Publishers
3 Columbia Circle, Box 15015
Albany, New York 12212-5015

International Thomson Publishing Europe
Berkshire House
168–173 High Holborn
London WC1V 7AA
England

Thomas Nelson Australia
102 Dodds Street
South Melbourne, 3205
Victoria, Australia

Nelson Canada
1120 Birchmount Road
Scarborough, Ontario
Canada, M1K 5G4

International Thomson Editores
Campos Eliseos 385, Piso 7
Cot Polanco
11560 Mexico D F Mexico

International Thomson Publishing GmbH
Königswinterer Strasse 418
53227 Bonn Germany

International Thomson Publishing Asia
221 Henderson Road
#05–10 Henderson Building
Singapore 0315

International Thomson Publishing—Japan
Hirakawacho Kyowa Building, 3F
2-2-1 Hirakawacho
Chiyoda-ku, Tokyo 102 Japan

1 2 3 4 5 6 7 8 9 10 XXX 03 02 01 00 99 98 97

**Library of Congress Cataloging-in-Publication Data**

Madama, Vincent C.
   Pulmonary function testing and cardiopulmonary stress testing/
Vincent C. Madama. — 2nd ed.
      p.      cm.
   Includes bibliographical references and index.
   ISBN 0-8273-8410-6
   1. Pulmonary function tests.   2. Exercise tests.   I. Title.
   [DNLM: 1. Respiratory Function Tests.   2. Exercise Test.   WB 284
M178p 1998]
RC734.P84M33   1998
616.2'40754—dc21
DNLM/DLC
for Library of Congress                              97-37682
                                          CIP

JOIN US ON THE WEB: www.DelmarAlliedHealth.com

**Your Information Resource!**
• What's New from Delmar • Health Science News Headlines
• Web Links to Many Related Sites
• Instructor Forum/Teaching Tips • Give Us Your Feedback
• Online Companions™
• Complete Allied Health Catalog • Software/Media Demos
• And much more!

Visit **www.thomson.com** for information on 35 Thomson publishers and more than 25,000 products! or email: findit@kiosk.thomson.co

# TABLE OF CONTENTS

# PREFACE

## RATIONALE

This book is primarily intended for educating respiratory care practitioners, cardiopulmonary function technologists, and other health care practitioners who must learn about pulmonary function testing, cardiopulmonary stress testing, and indirect calorimetry for nutritional assessment as part of their professional training. Additionally, the book can be used by practitioners and physicians as a general reference on these subjects. It can also serve as a review for the pulmonary function testing specialty examinations of the National Board for Respiratory Care.

## GOALS

Specific goals guided the development and writing of this book:

- To present material organized in a way that effectively guides the learner through the information.
- To use accepted educational techniques for supporting the learning process (i.e., learning objectives, lists of key terms, review questions, a glossary, and appendices) to their greatest effectiveness.
- To maintain a reading level appropriate for the learners who make use of the book.
- To present tables and diagrams that focus the learner's attention on key concepts or groupings of information.
- To supply a study section for the book that reinforces cognitive and psychomotor learning needs.
- To provide appendices of relevant supporting information.

## READING LEVEL

The subjects of pulmonary function testing and cardiopulmonary stress testing must employ medical and highly technical terms. If care is not taken in the writing process, a book on these subjects can have an excessively high reading level, one far beyond the comfort level of students typically enrolled in health care programs.

A deliberate effort has been made to maintain an appropriate reading level for this book. During its writing, very conscious control was maintained over the length and structure of sentences and paragraphs. This was done to establish clear, direct communication of the information a learner needs to master on pulmonary function testing and cardiopulmonary stress testing. Bulleted lists and tables have been used to bring attention to significant points. "Quality Assurance Notes" have been included to clearly identify actions that can be taken to ensure the quality of pulmonary function tests.

The result of all of these features is that the book provides all of the technical information needed for pulmonary function testing and cardiopulmonary stress testing, but at a reading level and with a presentation method that will be comfortable for the typical student in a health care practitioner training program.

## FORMAT OF THE CHAPTERS

The design of a book can have a significant impact on how effective it will be as a tool for learning. Careful thought has been given to the need for chapter elements that facilitate learning. Each chapter in the book contains the following elements:

- A list of related learning topics that are identified as being prerequisite to learning material from the chapter.
- A list of learning objectives that relate specifically to the material in the chapter and identify the learning that is meant to take place.
- A list of key terms that will be found in the chapter. The definitions for all of these terms are provided in the glossary of the book.
- The body of the chapter, in which the information is carefully organized and clearly presented.
- Review questions at the end of each chapter to serve as a benchmark of learning from the chapter.

All of these chapter elements should be reviewed and used by the learner.

## SPECIAL FEATURES OF THE CURRENT EDITION

Input was sought from students and fellow educators who used the first edition of this book and has resulted in some notable changes for this current edition. Their assistance is greatly appreciated.

## ORGANIZATION OF THE BOOK

The current edition reflects a change in the organization of the book's chapters from the first edition. In some ways, the new chapter organization is similar to that of the first edition. For example, as in the first edition,

- Chapters on equipment precede chapters on test procedures. Test equipment operation and use should be learned before the test procedures that require the equipment are learned.
- Chapters on pulmonary function testing procedures precede chapters that discuss normal values, test regimens, and testing for children.
- Chapters on cardiopulmonary stress testing and nutritional assessment procedures are patterned on those describing pulmonary function testing. A chapter on exercise physiology is included to provide a concise background for the chapters on cardiopulmonary stress testing.

The significant changes that have occurred in the current edition are as follows:

- The chapters on equipment are now divided more evenly throughout the book. This provides better correlation between equipment chapters and the tests that make use of the equipment. There are now separate chapters for gas analyzers and for blood gas analyzers instead of the single chapter that combined them in the first edition. The chapter on blood gas analyzers occurs later in the book and now immediately precedes the chapter relating to blood gases.
- The chapter on pulmonary mechanics tests is placed ahead of the chapter on tests for lung volumes and ventilation. It is now the first chapter in which pulmonary function test procedures are described. This is a significant change. Tests for pulmonary mechanics are the least complicated and are the most frequently performed pulmonary function tests. This is true both inside and outside the laboratory setting. Also, pulmonary mechanics tests provide the most broadly applied information acquired from pulmonary function testing. Learning about pulmonary mechanics tests is an effective starting point for learning about other types of test procedures.
- The chapter on quality assurance has now been made the last chapter of the book. This is because it includes information on quality assurance for all types of equipment and forms of testing.

## TABLES AND ILLUSTRATIONS

The tables and illustrations in this edition have been newly formatted to better present information to the learner. A number of new tables have been added to this edition to make the presentation of key points of information even clearer.

## STUDY SECTION

A Study Section is included in this edition of the book. The Study Section is, essentially, material pulled from the workbook that accompanied the first edition of the book. Having this material within the book itself now makes it more accessible to all learners.

The purpose of the Study Section is to provide an additional resource for learning about pulmonary function testing and cardiopulmonary stress testing. The material provided here is too detailed for inclusion in the chapters (i.e., Study Sections I, II, and IV) or relates to material drawn from a variety of chapters in the book (Study Sections III and V).

The Study Sections should be used in the following manner:

- Study Section I, "Evaluation of the Graphic Results of a Forced Vital Capacity Test," should be used in conjunction with Chapter 2 of the book.
- Study Section II, "Sample Calculations for Pulmonary Function Testing," should be used selectively in conjunction with Chapters 2, 4, 5, and 6. This will allow the learner to relate the calculations that are presented in the Study Section to the material in the chapters.
- Study Section III, Case Studies for Pulmonary Function Testing," should be used after Chapters 1 through 8 have been covered. The case studies provided in this study sections will reinforce the learning that occurred from those chapters.
- Study Sections IV and V, "Sample Calculations for Cardiopulmonary Stress Testing" and "Case Studies for Cardiopulmonary Stress Testing," should be used in conjunction with the chapters on cardiopulmonary stress testing.

## APPENDIX PROVIDING REFERENCE SOURCES FOR TESTING STANDARDS AND GUIDELINES

Appendix G has been added to specifically identify the reference source of pulmonary function testing standards from the American Thoracic Society and Clinical Practice Guidelines from the American Association for Respiratory Care. Both organizations have published very concise and effective descriptions for testing. These descriptions have been instrumental in the development of this book and are the basis for a great deal of information provided in the book. Unfortunately, they are too lengthy to be included in original form within the book itself. However, the listing of specific sources for these references in the appendix should help both learners and educators to find them if they are needed in original form.

An additional feature of this appendix is that it provides the Internet addresses of pulmonary medicine–oriented organizations. Although these organizations do not publish standards or guidelines for testing, communication with them through Internet connections may be a source of useful professional information.

# USE OF THE BOOK BY THE STUDENT

The material in this book will provide a strong basis for understanding how pulmonary function tests and cardiopulmonary stress tests are performed. It will also help the learner to understand the interpretation and usefulness of information that pulmonary function testing and cardiopulmonary stress testing can provide.

The learner should have at least a basic knowledge of the following topics before attempting to learn pulmonary function testing and cardiopulmonary stress testing:

- Chemistry, especially as it relates to ions and gas molecules.
- The physics of gas volume, pressure and flow.
- Physics as it relates to the conduction of an electrical current.
- Anatomy and physiology of the pulmonary and cardiovascular systems and the functional relationship between these two systems.
- Typical pathologic and pathophysiologic changes that can occur with the pulmonary and cardiovascular systems.

With this prior knowledge and the effective use of the learning objectives, text materials, and review questions in this book, the subjects of pulmonary function testing and cardiopulmonary stress testing and nutritional assessment should be made understandable.

# ACKNOWLEDGMENTS

I want to offer my thanks to the following individuals and organizations who were helpful to me in producing this book. My thanks to Bob Conboy, a chemist who led me to the references that were used in the developing a correct explanation of how a Sanz pH electrode operates. I offer my appreciation to representatives from the Fisher Scientific Co. and Warren E. Collins, Inc., for their taking time to explain some specific information on the equipment that they supply. My thanks to Joy White, RRT; Ken Scrivano, RRT; and Rita Cantrall for sharing their time and laboratories with me and for providing the patient information that was used in developing the case studies presented in this book.

I want to thank Rene Megan, CRTT, a coordinator for SwedishAmerican Hospital's Cardiopulmonary Rehabilitation Program, for her help in making arrangements for me to take a photograph for the cover of this book. Additionally, I want to thank Dr. Theodore Davis, a retired dentist, for his willingness to let me photograph him while he was undergoing a stress test and to be pictured on the book cover.

The contribution of reviewers is important to the success of any book. The reviewers with whom I worked in producing this book have been very supportive and have offered useful and constructive input. Reviewers who were instrumental in the development of the second edition of this book include the following individuals as well as additional reviewers who do not wish to be listed at this time.

Sandra J. King, RRT, MEd
Clinical Coordinator
Respiratory Care Department
Springfield Technical Community College
Springfield, Massachusetts

Gayle A. Petersen, MS, RRT
Director of Clinical Education
Illinois Central College
Peoria, Illinois

Douglas L. Roth, RRT, CPFT, RCP
Clinical Respiratory Specialist
Cardiopulmonary Services
Community Hospital of San Bernardino
San Bernardino, California

# DEDICATION

This book is dedicated to

My grandfather, Charles Wallace.
   His life presented him with limited opportunities and education and hard labor in the coal mines of West Virginia. His view of life rose above these limitations, however. For him, life was to be treasured and shared with others. He shared with me the wisdom that education and work toward personal growth are two of the most important keys to success in life. His old kerosene miner's lamp has been beside my computer and thoughts of him have been with me throughout the writing of this book.

My parents, Vincent and Nelda Madama.
   Who gave me the best start a person could have.
My daughters, Danielle and Diana.
   Who have been thinking lately that I haven't been much fun to be around.

And, most importantly,

To my wife, Sheila.
   Who is my friend, my companion in adventure, and my heart's flame. Her patience and support have been a constant during work on this book.

# INTRODUCTION

## PURPOSES OF PULMONARY FUNCTION AND CARDIOPULMONARY STRESS TESTING

### PULMONARY FUNCTION TESTING

The pulmonary system has a large amount of functional reserve. However, injury or illness can result in a significant degree of pulmonary dysfunction. This dysfunction can severely limit the length or quality of an individual's life. In acute forms, pulmonary disorders can cause death within minutes. Chronic disorders can take years before resulting in an individual's death, but many of those years may be spent with serious disability and a poor quality of life. To be best managed, pulmonary disorders must be detected and treated at the earliest possible time.

Pulmonary function testing plays a significant role in modern health care. It is used to assess the integrated function of the structures that comprise the thoracic/pulmonary system. These structures include

- Lungs
  - Parenchyma
  - Vasculature
- Air passages serving the lungs
  - Upper respiratory tract (mouth and nose down to and including the larynx)
  - Lower respiratory tract (trachea, mainstem bronchi, and all of the intrapulmonary airways)
- Thoracic/abdominal structures that surround the lungs
  - Pleura
  - Support structures of the thoracic wall (ribs, sternum, costal cartilages, thoracic vertebrae)
  - Muscles of ventilation and controlling nerves
  - Abdominal contents

Dysfunction of one or more of these structural components can cause measurable abnormalities in pulmonary function.

Disorders of the pulmonary system can affect its function in many ways. The problem may be a reduced ability to move air into and out of the lungs because of airway resistance problems. Conversely, the difficulty may relate to poor compliance of the pulmonary or thoracic structures. Disorders of gas exchange within the lung can be another source of dysfunction. Regardless of the source of dysfunction, pulmonary function testing is a key method used for evaluating and managing pulmonary disorders.

## CARDIOPULMONARY STRESS TESTING

The ability to participate in physical activities is taken for granted to most of us. Unfortunately, there are some individuals who have a limited tolerance for performing even simple activities such as walking. There are three basic factors that can, either individually or in some combination, contribute to a person having a limited tolerance for physical activities:

- Poor conditioning.
- The presence of a pulmonary dysfunction.
- The presence of a cardiovascular dysfunction.

Some limitations, such as those resulting from poor conditioning, may be fully reversible. Limitations caused by pulmonary or cardiovascular dysfunction may be improved, at least to some degree, through the use of therapeutic measures. Cardiopulmonary stress testing can be used both to detect the presence of dysfunction and to monitor a subject's progress in either improving conditioning or benefiting from treatment.

# INDICATIONS FOR TESTING

Pulmonary function testing and cardiopulmonary stress testing can be used to detect and assess dysfunction. This is true both for dysfunctions in the early and in the later stages of development.

The indications for testing include

- Medical diagnosis
  - Determination of the presence of a disorder.
  - Assessment of the degree to which pulmonary function or exercise tolerance is affected by injury or disease.
  - Determination of the pathologic nature of a disorder.
  - Planning of therapy required for treating and managing a disorder.
  - Evaluation of the therapeutic effectiveness of medical intervention for a disorder (bronchodilator therapy).
  - Monitoring the progression of a disorder (primary pulmonary disorders, neuromuscular disorders).

- Surgery-related evaluation
  - Preoperative risk assessment (anesthesia/surgical procedure).
  - Postoperative assessment of the effects of thoracic surgery.

- Disability evaluation
  - Rehabilitation (to monitor the effects of a rehabilitation program on the progress of a disorder).
  - Insurance (documentation of baseline function or changes in function).
  - Legal (documentation for Social Security, personal injury lawsuits, etc.).

- Public health/research
  - Epidemiologic survey.
  - General or specific data accumulation.

## SETTINGS IN WHICH TESTING IS PERFORMED

The most extensive studies of pulmonary function and exercise tolerance are performed in hospitals in a laboratory setting. In this setting, all of the previously stated indications for testing may be satisfied. However, the laboratory is not the only place where testing may be performed. Other settings include

- The bedside, either in a general patient-care setting or in an critical-care area.
- A physician's clinic.
- The workplace or other non–health care setting such as a shopping mall, school, etc.

Tests performed in non–health care settings often provide the first indication that an individual is experiencing some degree of dysfunction.

# CHAPTER ONE

# EQUIPMENT FOR VOLUME AND FLOW MEASUREMENT

## RELATED LEARNING

Prior knowledge of the following related information will facilitate understanding and learning of the material in this chapter. The learner will be aided by being able to

1. Explain the effects of ATPS/BTPS conversions as they relate to the measurement of gas volumes.
2. Explain the relationship between flow, drive pressure, and resistance to flow as expressed by Poiseuille's equation.
3. Explain the relationship between volume and pressure changes as expressed by Boyle's law.

## LEARNING OBJECTIVES

Upon successful completion of this chapter, the learner should be able to

1. Describe the operation and use of the following primary volume measuring spirometers:
   a. water-sealed spirometers
   b. dry-sealed spirometers
   c. bellows spirometers
   d. rotor spirometers
2. Describe the operation and use of the following primary flow measuring spirometers:
   a. differential-pressure pneumotachometers
   b. thermal anemometers
   c. ultrasonic sensor spirometers
   d. dedicated peak flow meters

3. Describe the operation and use of the following plethysmographs:
   a. body plethysmographs
   b. respiratory inductive plethysmographs
4. Describe the operation and use of directional breathing valves and directional control valves.
5. Explain how computer interfaces are used for pulmonary function testing.
6. Describe the operation and use of display and recording devices for pulmonary function testing.

## KEY TERMS

A-D (analog/digital) converter
alphanumeric
alternating current
analog electrical signal
anemometer
ATPS
BTPS
Charles' law
D-A (digital/analog) converter
DC analog electrical signal
DC electrical current
digital electronic signal
Hz (Hertz)
inductance

inertia
laminar air flow
light-emitting diode (LED)
linear measurements
liquid crystal display (LCD)
nonlinear measurements
pneumotachometer
potentiometer
soda lime
software
spirogram
subject
ultrasonic

Specialized equipment plays a significant role in the activities of a pulmonary function laboratory. A good working knowledge of laboratory equipment is helpful in understanding how the tests described in later chapters are performed. Equipment for measuring gas volume and/or flow rate are basic to many of the tests performed in a pulmonary function laboratory. This chapter will explain both the broad operating concepts and the specific functional aspects of measuring systems for gas volume and/or flow.

## VOLUME/FLOW MEASURING INSTRUMENTS

*Spirometers* are instruments used to measure the volumes of air that are inhaled and exhaled during breathing. The measurements can relate directly to either the volume or the flow rate of the air that is breathed. In 1846 a researcher named John Hutchinson published a paper on the use of a water-sealed spirometer to measure vital capacities. His work formed a basis for identifying pulmonary tuberculosis before it was clinically symptomatic. Today spirometers still play a significant role in the pulmonary function laboratory.

Spirometers can be classified as functioning by one of two possible operating principles: *primary volume measuring* (PVM) *spirometers* or *primary flow measuring* (PFM) *spirometers.* With the PVM spirometer, the *volume* of air moving into and/or out of the **subject's** lungs is measured directly. Air flow rates must be determined indirectly. The determination is a function of the volume measured and the time over which the volume change occurred. Note that volume is measured in liters.

$$\text{Flow Rate (l/sec)} = \frac{\text{Volume (liters)}}{\text{Time (sec)}}$$

With some PVM spirometers, air flow rates may be determined by measurements on a graphic tracing of the spirometer's movement during the breathing maneuver. Air flow rates can also be determined by electronic systems linked to the spirometer.

PFM spirometers directly measure the *flow rate* of the inhaled and/or exhaled air. Volume must be determined indirectly as a function of the flow rate and the time over which the flow continued.

$$\text{Volume (liters)} = \text{Flow Rate (l/sec)} \times \text{Time (sec)}$$

This calculation is complicated by the fact that air flow rates can change significantly during a single breathing maneuver. As a result, volume determinations cannot easily be performed manually. Electronic systems are generally used to calculate volumes from the flow measurements.

## PRIMARY VOLUME MEASURING (PVM) SPIROMETERS

PVM spirometers are of two categories: volume-collecting/volume-displacement spirometers and flow-through spirometers. PVM spirometers used in the laboratory are generally *volume-collecting* or *volume-displacement* devices. This means that the subject's expiratory air moves into the spirometer, and his or her inspiratory air moves back out from it. The volume, or size, of the spirometer increases and decreases proportionally with subject breathing. Volume-collecting or volume-displacement spirometers may be of the water-sealed, dry-sealed, or bellows type. The other category of PVM spirometer is a *flow-through* device that measures air as it passes completely through. Volumes are not collected within the device. The only spirometer of this category is the rotor/turbine spirometer.

## Water-Sealed Spirometers

Water-sealed spirometers consist of a double-walled, stationary cylinder that has water between the double walls (Figure 1–1). A freely moving cylindrical bell is suspended above and inside the stationary cylinder. It moves up and down freely within the cylinder's double walls. The water serves as an airtight, low-friction seal for the bell. It ensures that spirometer movement is in exact proportion to subject breathing volumes. The spirometer bell moves downward as the subject inhales and upward as the subject exhales.

Water-sealed spirometers can be simple or very complex. Simple systems may have only a single breathing tube connected to the spirometer. Their use is limited to single-breath volume/flow studies. More complex systems (with a double tube, one-way breathing arrangement) can be used for studies that involve prolonged breathing on the spirometer.

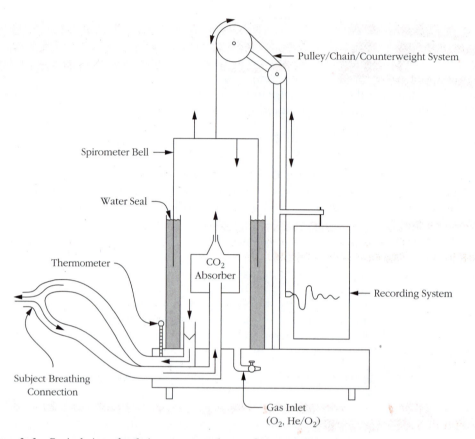

**Figure 1–1** *Basic design of a chain-compensated type of water-sealed spirometer.*

Spirometer bells are available in different sizes, ranging from 7 to 14 liters of volume. The difference in size is the diameter of the bell—smaller volume bells having smaller diameters. Bell diameter also determines the distance that the bell will need to move in response to a given breathing volume. For the same breathing volume, small-diameter bells travel a greater distance than do larger bells. When volume determinations are made from a direct spirometer tracing, this *bell factor* must be included in the calculations.

The bell factor can be demonstrated with the example of a 13.5 liter spirometer bell that has a bell factor of 41.27 ml volume displacement for each millimeter of vertical movement (.04127 l/mm). If a spirometer bell movement of 86 mm is measured on a tracing of a breathing maneuver, the following equation shows how the bell factor is used to calculate the volume breathed by the subject:

Measured Volume = 86 mm × .04127 l/mm

Measured Volume = 3.55 liters

Traditionally, there have been two configurations for water-sealed spirometers: the chain-compensated spirometer and the Stead-Wells spirometer. The *chain-compensated* spirometer was the first to be used (see Figure 1–1). It was originally designed with a lightweight metal bell, although today it is available with a plastic bell. The weight of the bell is balanced by a counterweight. The counterweight is suspended from a chain that is looped over a pulley. In simple models, a pen attached to the counterweight may be used to make **spirograms**.

The chain-compensated type of spirometer is very accurate for simple volume measurement. Unfortunately, with breathing maneuvers that include rapid respiratory rates or rapid changes in air flow rates, some accuracy is lost. This is due to the mass of the bell and counterweight and their resulting **inertia**. Spirometer movement may not change in immediate response to changes in the subject's breathing. The use of plastic bells on more modern units somewhat reduces this problem.

The *Stead-Wells* type of spirometer (Figure 1–2) was developed in response to the inertia problems exhibited by the chain-compensated configuration. A lightweight plastic

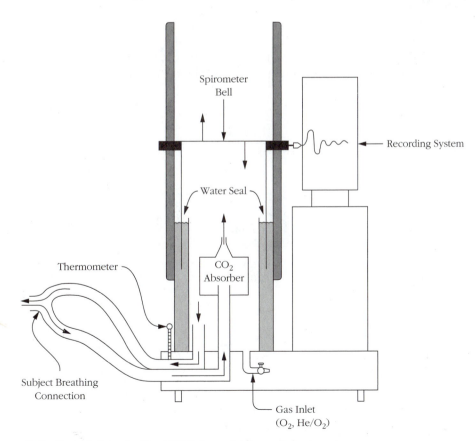

**Figure 1–2**  *Basic design of a Stead-Wells type of water-sealed spirometer.*

bell was used from the beginning. This meant that the counterweight/chain/pulley assembly was not required. The result is a system with better frequency response and better response to rapid flow-rate changes. With simple systems, spirograms can be made with a pen attached directly to the spirometer bell. The tracings produced by the chain-compensated and Stead-Wells spirometers are the same, except that they are inverted in relation to each other (Figure 1–3).

*Summary for Water-Sealed Spirometers.*   Water-sealed spirometers of both types are very rugged and dependable. However, because of their size, weight, and design, they must be used primarily as stationary laboratory systems. Either mechanical recording systems, as described earlier, or electronic recording systems may be used to make spirograms. Some volume measurement error can occur if there are leaks in the system. Damage to the tubing system or bell or inadequate water levels in the spirometer can produce system leaks. With the chain-compensated type of spirometer, volume measurement error can also result when mechanical problems cause resistance to movement of the chain.

## Dry-Sealed Spirometers

Dry-sealed spirometers have an entirely different configuration (Figure 1–4). They consist of a rod-mounted piston within a cylinder. The piston is made of plastic or a lightweight metal. Because it is designed to move horizontally, the piston does not require a counterweight mechanism. It has a larger diameter than the bell on a water-sealed spirom-

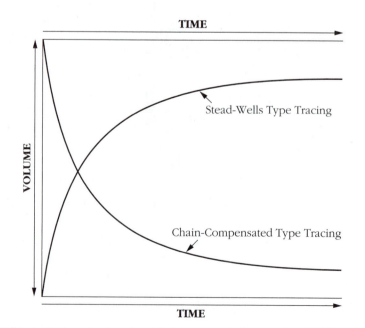

**Figure 1–3**  *Difference between tracings from chain-compensated versus Stead-Wells type spirometers.*

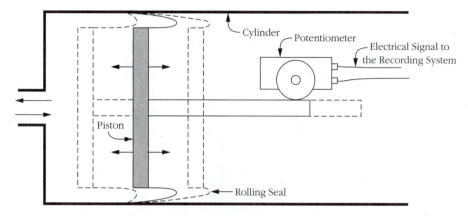

**Figure 1–4** *Basic design of a dry-sealed spirometer.*

eter. As a result, the piston does not need to travel as far with the same volume change. A pen for spirogram tracings can be attached to the piston rod. Generally, however, electronic systems are used to record spirometer movements.

A silicone plastic (silastic) *rolling seal* is used to make the system airtight. The seal consists of a tube that is approximately the same diameter as the piston/cylinder. This tube is turned within itself to form a double-walled cylindrical structure with a closed, U-shaped seal at one end. The "outside" free end of the seal is fastened to the inner wall of the cylinder. The "inside" free end is attached to the edge of the piston. With piston movement in response to volume changes, the lengths of the inside and outside walls of the rolling seal change. The U-shaped end of the seal rolls forward and then back in with piston movement.

*Summary for Dry-Sealed Spirometers.*   Maintenance of dry-sealed spirometers is less of a problem than it is for water-sealed spirometers. Mechanical malfunctions, however, may cause resistance to piston movement. This resistance can be a source of measurement error. Dry-sealed spirometers are more portable than water-sealed spirometers but are nevertheless used primarily in laboratory settings.

## Bellows Spirometers

Bellows spirometers are constructed of a flexible plastic material that is designed to collapse in folds. The bellows unfolds and expands with the subject's expiration and collapses with his or her inspiration. There are two possible bellows designs. A *fully expanding bellows* opens and closes like an accordion. A *wedge-shaped bellows* fully expands only along one edge, similar to the opening and closing of a book (Figure 1–5).

Smaller, more portable units generally make use of a bellows that expands up and down vertically. Larger, primarily laboratory-based systems use bellows that expand back and forth horizontally. This configuration offers very little resistance to movement.

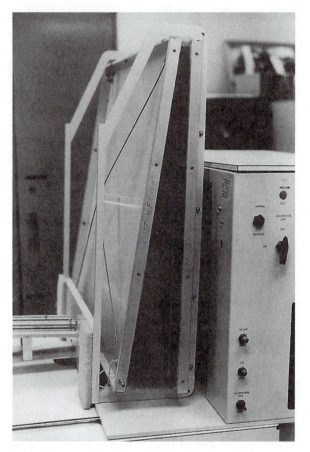

**Figure 1–5** *Wedge-shaped bellows spirometer.*

*Summary for Bellows Spirometers.* Large, horizontally expanding bellows systems can offer the same accuracy as other PVM spirometers. Little routine maintenance is required. Difficulties may arise over time, however. Collection of dirt and moisture within the bellows or aging of the bellows material can cause the folds to be more resistant to expanding. This resistance could affect measurement accuracy. Furthermore, cracks and tears can occur in the bellows over time. Because of these potential problems, periodic inspection of the bellows is necessary to ensure that spirometer accuracy is maintained. Sometimes it is necessary to replace the bellows.

## Summary for Volume-Collecting, Volume-Displacement Primary Volume Measuring Spirometers

Volume-collecting/volume-displacement devices provide an excellent measure of breathing volumes. However, inertia of their moving physical components may be a source of error with rapid changes in air flow rates or subject respiratory rates. Fortunately, modern materials and designs minimize this problem.

Laboratory-based systems of this type are generally used to perform complex tests that involve prolonged subject breathing on the spirometer. Such tests require the addition of peripheral equipment to the spirometer such as **soda lime** absorbers, connections for the input of oxygen or other gases, gas analyzers, and other devices.

Recording systems for PVM spirometers can be either mechanical or electronic. Mechanical systems involve the movement of a pen along one axis and paper movement along the perpendicular axis. The pen is attached to the bell/piston/bellows. The paper can be fastened to a rotating drum or may be moved linearly. Electronic recording systems use a **potentiometer** that is positioned to rotate in response to movement of the bell/piston/bellows. The resulting electrical signal can be used to produce tracings by means of an electronic recorder. (Recorders will be discussed later in the chapter.)

ATPS/BTPS conversions are necessary for accurate volume determination. The air that leaves the subject is at **BTPS**. Once it is exhaled, especially after it has entered the spirometer, the air must be considered to be at **ATPS**. Based on the effects of temperature on gas volume (**Charles' law**) and the fact that the ambient temperature is less than body temperature, the volume of air measured by the spirometer at ATPS is slightly less than the volume actually exhaled by the subject at BTPS. For this reason, measurements made by the system must be converted back to BTPS for accurate subject volume determination. Test results recorded directly by use of a mechanical recorder must be converted to BTPS.

This conversion can be demonstrated by adding to the example equation shown earlier where the bell factor was used to calculate a measured volume. Assuming a room temperature of 20°C and using Table 1 from Study Section II toward the rear of this book, a BTPS conversion factor of 1.102 must be used. Given this information, the following equations demonstrate BTPS volume conversion:

Measured Volume = 86 mm × 0.04127 l/mm

Measured Volume = 3.55 liters

Converted Volume = 3.55 liters × 1.102

Converted Volume = 3.91 liters

The conversion can be built into the mechanism of the recorder so that it is performed automatically. With electronic recording systems, the conversion can be made electronically prior to display of the data. Appendix B provides an explanation of volume conversions.

## Rotor Spirometers

Rotor spirometers are the only type of PVM spirometer that allow the measured air to pass completely through the device as the volume is measured. The most frequently used configuration is the *Wright-type* spirometer. Measurement is based on the rotation of a rectangular, vanelike rotor (Figure 1–6). The rotor consists of a very thin, lightweight metal blade. It spins as a result of the air being directed toward it through tangentially oriented slots. As the rotor spins, it operates a mechanical clocklike gear mechanism. The gears turn hands on the face of the instrument to indicate the measured volume. The face displays volume in units of liters and tenths of a liter. Measurement through the device is unidirectional because of how the slots and rotor blade are arranged.

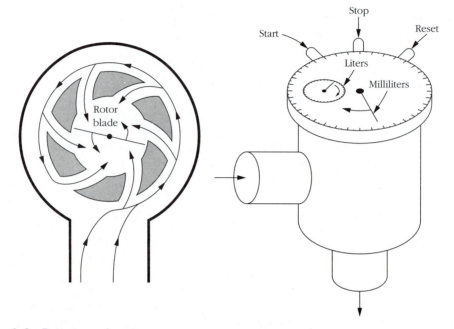

**Figure 1–6** *Rotor-type spirometer.*

Volume measurement by rotor spirometers is similar to the operation of a turnstile. Given that a turnstile is designed for an adult-sized body, the passage of one adult through the turnstile can be "measured" accurately. When an individual passes through a turnstile, it rotates a predetermined, proportional amount and one person is counted. Rotor spirometers use a rotor chamber of fixed volume. As a given quantity of air passes through the chamber, the rotor moves proportionally and the volume is "counted" by the gear mechanism. The instruction manual of one spirometer states that the rotor makes 150 revolutions for each liter of air passing through the chamber.

Measurement error can result from inertia of the mechanical components in rotor spirometers. This error is most likely with very slow or fast air flow rates or during rapid changes in flow rate. Rotor spirometers are generally accurate at flow rates between 3 l/min and 200–300 l/min. Damage to the rotor can occur when flow rates exceed 300 l/min.

There are other spirometers that operate on this basic principle. One type involves use of rotating cogs that operate a gear system. Another uses a rotating turbine that causes interruption of a photoelectric beam. Electronic monitoring of the light beam is used to determine volumes with this type of device.

*Summary for Rotor Spirometers.* Rotor spirometers are limited primarily to handheld use at the bedside for measurement of unforced breathing maneuvers. This is because of their small, portable size and the fact that they are reasonably accurate for this type of measurement. Measurement of a forced expiratory maneuver with a rotor spirometer can result in damage to the rotor. The accuracy of these instruments may be affected by gas density. This is generally not a problem, however, for simple bedside spirometry.

## PRIMARY FLOW MEASURING (PFM) SPIROMETERS

PFM spirometers provide a direct measurement of air flow rates. The flow-rate measurement can then be integrated electronically, on the basis of time, into a volume measurement. PFM spirometers operate on a variety of principles. The different types of PFM spirometers that will be discussed here are differential-pressure pneumotachometers, thermal anemometers, and ultrasonic sensor spirometers.

### Differential-Pressure Pneumotachometers

Differential-pressure **pneumotachometers** have a flow-resistive structure (element) in the path of the gas stream. They function on the basis of how changes in air flow rates through the element affect upstream/downstream pressure relationships within the device (Figures 1–7 and 1–8). The element causes only a small amount of resistance to air flow. It is

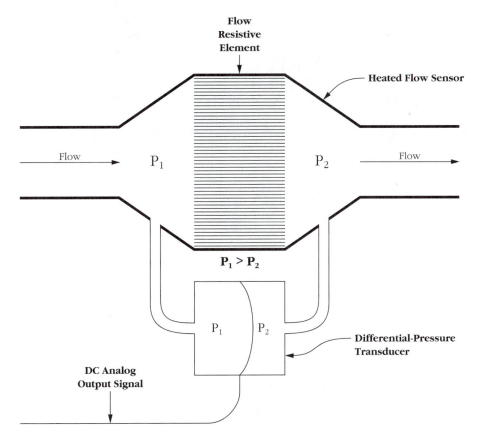

**Figure 1–7**   *Basic design of a differential-pressure pneumotachometer.*

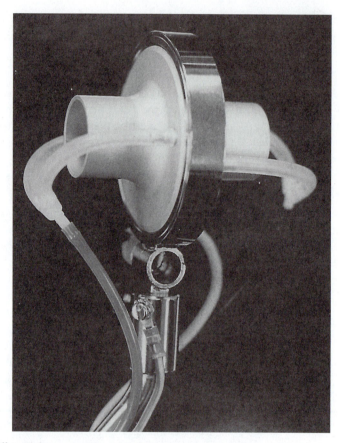

**Figure 1–8** *Differential-pressure pneumotachometer.*

enough, however, to create a measurable difference between upstream ($P_1$) and downstream ($P_2$) pressures. $P_1$ is greater than $P_2$. As air flow rates increase, the difference between $P_1$ and $P_2$ also increases. A differential-pressure strain gauge transducer is used to measure the pressure difference within the device. A **DC analog electrical signal** is produced by the pressure transducer. Changes in the electrical signal are directly proportional to changes in the air flow rate. The electrical signal can be measured and used to indicate air flow rate.

The basis for using pressure to determine flow rates is supplied by Poiseuille's equation. This is a simplified version of the equation:

$$\dot{V} = \Delta P / R$$

It illustrates the relationship between the air flow rate ($\dot{V}$), differential pressure ($\Delta P$), and the resistive element (R). This relationship is true only if air flow through the sensor is **laminar**. If R is fixed and known and $\Delta P$ is measured, then the flow can easily be determined. The spirometer sensor is heated to approximately body temperature. This helps prevent condensation within the device from moisture in the subject's exhaled air. Condensation on the resistive element would increase its resistance and create measurement errors.

The resistive elements used in these spirometers can differ significantly. The *Fleisch-style* sensor makes use of a corrugated metal element. The corrugated metal is folded and bundled to form a series of parallel capillary-like gas channels. Other sensor designs include the use of a screenlike mesh or a flexible diaphragm with a variable-sized orifice at its center.

## Summary for Differential Pressure Pneumotachometers

When well designed and constructed, differential-pressure devices can be very accurate. They are the most widely used PFM spirometers.

The physical characteristics (primarily viscosity) of various gas compositions can affect instrument accuracy. Electronic or computer **software** compensations for viscosity differences can be made.

## Thermal Anemometers

With thermal **anemometers**, air flow rate is measured on the basis of how it affects the temperature of a heated element (Figure 1–9). The element is generally a platinum wire or small metal bead that produces no resistance to air flow. An electrical current is used to keep the element at a fixed temperature. Gas moving through the sensor carries heat from the element. More electrical current is then required to maintain the temperature of the element. Increases in electrical current are directly proportional to increases in air flow rates within the sensor. The element must have a small mass in order to be sensitive to low air flow rates. A small element also helps to minimize the chance of it creating a resistance to air flow through the device.

*Summary for Thermal Anemometers.*   Flow measurement by anemometers is seriously affected by the humidity and temperature of the gas. Accuracy may also be affected by physical characteristics of the gas, such as density. Anemometers are generally limited to unidirectional air flow measurement with separate inspiratory and expiratory sensors.

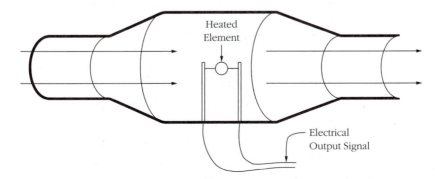

**Figure 1–9**   *Basic design of a thermal anemometer.*

This is done with the sensors placed some distance from the subject by way of a tubing system.

## Ultrasonic Sensor Spirometers

**Ultrasonic** sensor spirometers use a beam of ultrasonic sound waves to measure air flow. The beam detects a special type of gas stream turbulence called a *vortex* (Figure 1–10). Vortices are produced by a baffle in the gas stream with the ultrasonic sensor located downstream from it. Baffle design and the configuration of the sensor chamber both can affect the nature of the vortices produced. The sensor transmits a sound beam across and through the gas stream. The beam is directed from a sending unit on one side to a receiving unit on the other. Each vortex in the gas stream creates a pulse in the sound beam. The receiver produces an electrical signal in response to each pulse. Flow measurement is based on an electronic count of the pulses from the gas stream. The number of detected pulses is directly proportional to the air flow rate.

*Summary for Ultrasonic Sensor Spirometers.*   The accuracy of the ultrasonic sensor spirometer is not affected significantly by gas temperature, humidity, or composition. Collection of condensed water on the baffle or ultrasonic sensor can, however, produce measurement error.

## Summary for Primary Flow Measuring (PFM) Spirometers

Flow through the PFM spirometer sensors must be laminar in order for flow measurement to be accurate. The sensors are carefully designed to achieve the needed laminar flow profile. The manufacturer of a sensor should be consulted prior to any changes being made in mouthpiece size or sensor configuration.

Electronic signals produced by the sensor of a PFM spirometer at very high or low air flow rates may not be accurately proportional (**linear**) to the actual air flow rate. The larger the range of flow rates an instrument must measure, the more likely that **nonlinear** signals will be produced. There are solutions to this problem. The inclusion of more than

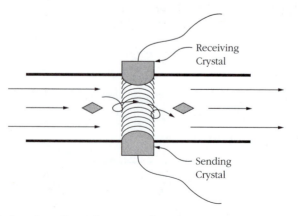

**Figure 1–10**   *Basic design of an ultrasonic sensor spirometer.*

one flow sensor in a spirometer is possible. One sensor would be used to measure low air flow rates, another for higher flow rates. Linearity is more easily assured with each sensor having a smaller range of measurement. Electronic or computer software compensation for nonlinear signals is another possibility. Checks for the accuracy of these compensations are performed as part of the more frequent calibrations required for PFM spirometers.

Because these are flow-through instruments, differences between inspiratory and expiratory gas temperatures can affect volume measurement. Expiratory volumes may be measured to be larger than equal-sized inspiratory volumes. Surprisingly, these differences have been found to be very small (2.5%). This small difference is thought to be due to efficient heat exchange between the gas stream and the sensor walls. Because effectiveness of this exchange varies with air flow rate, a single, simple conversion factor is not possible. It is possible, however, to develop a complex set of ATPS/BTPS computer conversion factors over the full range of flow for a PFM spirometer. If this type of conversion is not available, the measurement error is small enough that it can be ignored. Use of simpler conversions can create more error than exists in the original measurement.

## Dedicated Peak Flow Meters

Dedicated peak flow meters are another type of flow-measuring device. They are designed, however, to measure only the *peak expiratory flow rate* (PEFR) of a subject. For this reason, they are being discussed separately. Peak air flow rates can be measured by use of a variety of similar mechanisms. The main component is generally a movable vane, disk, or sphere. For the purposes of discussion, a vane-type flow meter will be described. The subject exhales with maximal force into the device. The force of the expiratory air flow pushes the vane rapidly forward. As the vane moves, it opens a progressively larger leak in the flow meter. A point is reached where the leak is so large that most of the subject's air flow is lost from the instrument and so can no longer move the vane. At that point, the vane stops moving, and the peak flow is indicated on a scale. The classic version of this device is the *Wright Peak Flow Meter* (Figure 1–11).

*Summary for Dedicated Peak Flow Meters.* The accuracy of dedicated peak flow meters is questionable. Spirometers, as described earlier, can provide a more accurate measurement of PEFR. Yet, dedicated peak flow meters can be useful for periodic tracking of peak flow values, especially in routine assessment of therapies that affect air flow in the lungs.

## SUMMARY FOR VOLUME/FLOW MEASURING (PVM AND PFM) INSTRUMENTS

Primary volume measuring (PVM) spirometers, if well maintained, will provide more accurate, precise, and linear measurements of volume than primary flow measuring (PFM) devices. Their measurements are reproducible with less required calibration than PFM spirometers. PVM spirometers are used for establishing spirometric standards. More frequent calibration may be necessary if a potentiometer is used to convert movement of the spirometer to an electrical signal for recording volumes.

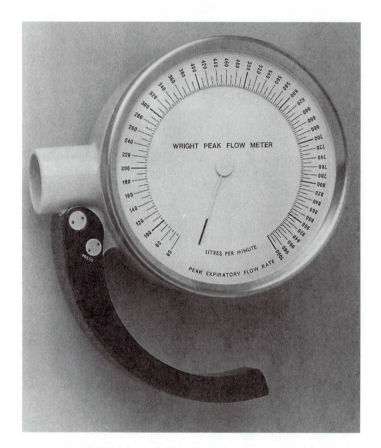

**Figure 1–11** *Professional model Wright Peak Flow Meter.*

Problems of inertia may limit the frequency response of a PVM spirometer and produce an error when rapidly changing flow rates are measured. Some systems, as described earlier, are more prone to this problem than others. Volume-collecting systems have an inherent limit to the volume of air that they can collect and measure. For this reason, they are not practical for exercise testing or for any other continuous or large-volume measurement. The size and weight of these systems greatly limit their portability.

PFM spirometers are designed to serve as lightweight, portable units. They have a better frequency response giving more accurate measurement of rapidly changing flow rates. Because measured air flows through the instrument instead of being collected within, these devices are better suited to situations requiring continuous measurements.

Overall, PFM spirometers are less likely to provide volume measurements that are accurate, precise, and linear than those of PVM spirometers. Quality and accuracy of the units, however, vary considerably depending on the manufacturer. Some of the latest differential-pressure pneumotachometers have excellent accuracy and linearization.

Recommended minimum equipment standards for the performance of spirometers have been published by the American Thoracic Society (ATS). Appendix C provides the ATS standards for spirometer systems. Equipment that is purchased and used should at least meet, and preferably should exceed, these standards. Accuracy of instrument timing mechanisms, whether mechanical or electronic, plays an important role in spirometers. For both PVM spirometers and PFM spirometers, correct timing is necessary for accurate indirect determination of flows or volumes.

# PLETHYSMOGRAPHS

There are two types of plethysmography systems. *Body plethysmography* requires that the subject's entire body be enclosed within a boxlike cabinet during testing. A complex set of components is necessary for system operation and test performance. *Inductive plethysmography* involves the use of sensors strapped around the subject's thorax and abdomen. The equipment is smaller and less complicated.

## BODY PLETHYSMOGRAPHS (BPS)

*Body plethysmographs* (BPs) (Figure 1–12) are used for making two kinds of pulmonary function measurements. The first is *intrathoracic gas volume* ($V_{TG}$). This can be used to determine total lung capacity and will be discussed more fully in Chapter 4. The second measurement is *airway resistance* ($R_{aw}$). Chapter 2 will provide more information on airway resistance measurement.

There are three types of direct measurements made with a BP. These measurements are:

- Inspiratory and/or expiratory air flow rates during the subject's breathing cycle.
- Air volume changes inside the sealed cabinet that result from expansion and contraction of the subject's thorax.
- Changes in air pressure at the subject's mouth.

Cabinet air volume changes are used to reflect changes in lung volume. Mouth pressure changes, when the subject's airway is mechanically obstructed, are interpreted as changes in alveolar pressure. Readings of mouth (alveolar) pressure compared against changes in cabinet air volume are used to determine lung volume. Cabinet air volume changes compared against subject ventilatory air flow rates are used to determine airway resistance.

## Body Plethysmograph Components

The *cabinet* has a volume of approximately 600 liters and is large enough for the subject to sit within (see Figure 1–12). In newer, well-designed models, the cabinet is constructed largely of plexiglass. This allows for good visibility of the subject. It also reduces any claustrophobia that may be experienced by the subject. Cabinets generally include an in-

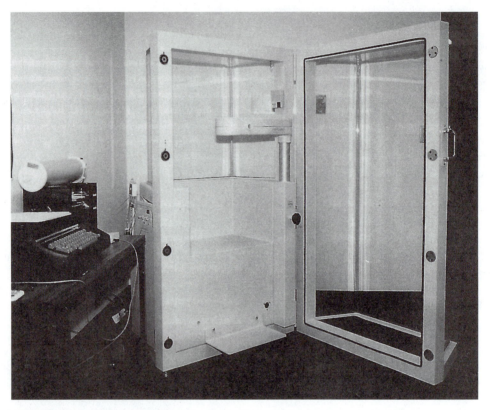

**Figure 1–12** *Body plethysmograph.*

tercom system for easy communication between technologist and subject. The cabinet may have a vent that can be opened or closed by the operator as needed.

Measuring systems are important to BP operation (Figure 1–13). A pneumotachometer/shutter/pressure transducer assembly is located within the cabinet. The type of *pneumotachometer* used for measuring ventilatory air flow rates can vary with the brand of plethysmograph used. The *shutter,* when activated, occludes the mechanical airway of the pneumotachometer. It may be controlled by an electronic solenoid or by a pneumatic system. State-of-the-art BPs have automated shutters that close automatically at predetermined times in a test. The *pressure transducer* is located between the shutter and subject mouthpiece. It is used to measure pressure at the mouth.

The method used for measuring cabinet air volume changes can vary considerably between plethysmograph systems. There are two very different methods for measuring body plethysmograph cabinet volume changes. The two methods are based on using either:

* a nonconstant-volume plethysmograph cabinet, or
* a constant-volume, variable-pressure plethysmograph cabinet.

A body plethysmograph will make use of one or the other type of measuring system. *Nonconstant-volume plethysmographs* use either a primary volume or primary flow measuring

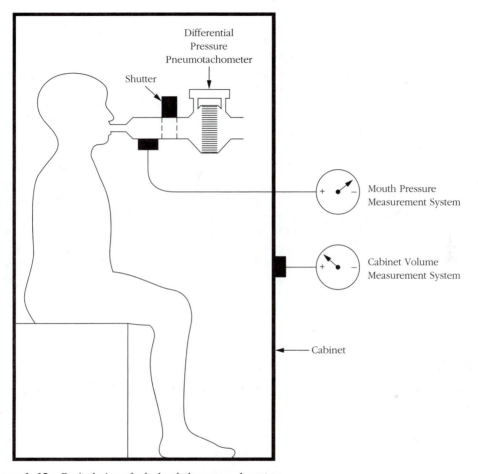

**Figure 1–13** *Basic design of a body plethysmograph system.*

spirometer system attached to the BP's outer wall. They are, as a result, referred to as *volume-* or *flow-type plethysmographs*. These systems directly measure quantities of air that are forced to enter and leave the cabinet. This air movement occurs as a result of the subject's thoracic volume increases and decreases during breathing. Both large and small changes in thoracic volume can be measured.

Conveniently, determination of other nonplethysmographic ventilatory parameters can be made with the subject still within the sealed cabinet. These parameters may include inspiratory capacity and forced expiratory flow rates. Systems of this type are rather complex and expensive.

*Constant-volume, variable-pressure plethysmographs (pressure-type plethysmographs)* have a pressure transducer connected to an opening in the cabinet wall. The transducer directly measures changes in cabinet pressure during subject breathing. The pressure changes can be interpreted as volume changes, as described by Boyle's law ($P_1 V_1 = P_2 V_2$). With the original cabinet volume known (and reduced by the amount of the subject's "volume") and an initial pressure of 0 cm $H_2O$ (atmospheric), pressure changes in the cabinet can be equated with corresponding cabinet volume changes. For accurate assessment of cabinet air volume changes, temperatures within the cabinet must remain stable. Some systems have a small leak built into the cabinet to allow for temperature equilibrium. If panting-type breathing maneuvers are used by the subject, the leak does not present a problem for pressure measurement. These systems provide an excellent frequency response to subject breathing maneuvers. This is the most widely used type of plethysmograph. It is, however, limited strictly to traditional plethysmographic-type determinations.

A *recording system* is an important BP component. It must be a biaxial (X-Y) recorder with a very good frequency response. The recorder is used for plotting pressures measured by the plethysmograph against either ventilatory flow rates or cabinet volume changes. Storage-type oscilloscopes or computer monitors perform well. Real-time electronic recorders can be used, but they may cause distortion of the graphic results at high subject breathing rates. A system for marking and measuring the tracing's tangent angles is also necessary. A clear plastic rotating protractor overlay for the oscilloscope can be used.

Computer use with BPs, compared to computerization of spirometer systems, is a recent development. Computers can enable rapid assessment of the subject's performance and test results. Override capabilities for automated shutters should be included to allow for flexibility in testing difficult subjects. Computers can also allow the operator to control the "best fit" tangent measurement for tracings generated during the tests.

## RESPIRATORY INDUCTIVE PLETHYSMOGRAPHS (RIPS)

*Respiratory inductive plethysmographs* (RIPs) are used to make indirect measurement of ventilatory parameters. They allow the operator to determine breathing volumes without a physical connection to the subject's airway. This is done by evaluating the changes in thoracic and abdominal girth that the subject experiences during breathing. These changes are measured by a *rib-cage strap* (RC) and an *abdominal strap* (AB). Attached to the straps is a unit for producing a high-frequency oscillating (alternating) current through the wires. A small microprocessor unit is also included for storing and processing the data and for use in system calibration.

The straps consist of Teflon-insulated wires that are coiled like a telephone receiver cord. They are enclosed in an elastic material. The girth changes are sensed on the basis of changes in electrical (alternating) current flow through the coiled wires. The **alternating current** produces a magnetic field around the wires. The field, in turn, causes a resistance to the current flow through the wires. This action is called **inductance**. Changes in the number of coils per length of wire changes the inductance of the circuit.

The straps and enclosed coiled wires are stretched by the subject's inspiratory efforts, reducing the number of coils per inch. As a result, the inductance proportionally decreases, and current flow increases. Expiration reverses these events. The resulting increases and decreases in current flow are interpreted as volume changes. When the signal is integrated with input from a timing mechanism, respiratory rate and other time-based measurements can be made.

The RC strap is placed around the subject's chest with its upper border just below the axilla. The AB strap is placed at the umbilical level with its upper border just below the rib cage. In order for an RIP to reflect volume changes accurately, the instrument must be carefully calibrated according to the manufacturer's instructions. Once calibrated, tidal volume, inspiratory and expiratory time, and respiratory rate can then be measured. Also, the percent contribution the subject's ribcage makes during ventilation and the phase relationships between thoracic and abdominal movements during ventilation can also be recorded. With proper calibration of the instrument, it is possible for inspiratory and expiratory flow rates to be determined.

RIPs may be easier to use than a standard spirometer with infants, subjects on mechanical ventilation, sleeping subjects, and small animals. Unfortunately, though, RIPs cannot completely replace direct spirometric measurements. Certain factors reduce their accuracy. Changes in the subject's body position after calibration can result in measurement error. Some studies have shown that errors can also occur when subjects have complex thoracic and abdominal movements. This is because, with RIP, the measurements are made at only two points on the thoracic/abdominal ventilating system. Some complex thoracic/abdominal movements, especially if they begin after calibration, can thus produce inaccurate volume determinations.

There may be a need for frequent calibration to maintain system accuracy. Such frequent calibration can limit usefulness of the device. If used in circumstances that have been documented as effective, however, the RIP can be a beneficial tool for evaluating pulmonary function.

# DIRECTIONAL BREATHING VALVES AND DIRECTIONAL CONTROL VALVES

Directional breathing valves and directional control valves are often used in spirometer systems to control the movement of gas flow through the system.

## DIRECTIONAL BREATHING VALVES

Directional breathing valves are T- or Y-shaped valves that are used at the subject connection of a spirometer breathing circuit. They have three gas flow ports, and the subject's mouthpiece is attached to one of them. The other two ports have one-way valves that permit flow in only one direction through the port breathing valve. One port will only permit gas flow into the valve. The other will only permit flow out of the valve.

The purpose of the valve is to separate the direction of the subject's inspiratory air flow from the direction of the expiratory air flow. As a result of the valve's construction, the subject's inspiratory flow is brought in from one portion of the spirometer breathing circuit. The expiratory flow exits the valve and is directed into a different portion of the breathing circuit.

Well-designed directional breathing valves must

- Have a low resistance to inspiratory and expiratory air flow.
- Have a small deadspace volume to minimize rebreathing of previously exhaled air.
- Be relatively easy to clean after use.

## DIRECTIONAL CONTROL VALVES

Directional control valves in a spirometer breathing circuit are similar in their purpose to traffic signals. They permit control and changes in the direction of gas flow within the breathing circuit. The control valve can be used to direct the flow at different times as needed during a test to different portions of the breathing circuit. Flow may be directed to volume-measuring instruments, gas analysis instruments, and other system components.

Valves of this type are often needed when more complex tests are performed with a spirometer system. In simple systems, the valves may be manually controlled by the technologist performing the test. In more sophisticated systems, the operation of the valves may be controlled by computer.

# COMPUTER INTERFACES

There are two types of computer interfaces. The **A-D (analog/digital) converter** changes electrical signals from measuring systems into data that a computer can use. Another type of interface, the **D-A (digital/analog) converter**, converts computer commands into electrical signals that can control pulmonary function testing equipment.

## ANALOG-TO-DIGITAL (A-D) CONVERTERS

Earlier in this chapter it was explained how a primary volume measuring (PVM) spirometer can make use of a potentiometer for creating an electrical data signal. Primary flow measuring (PFM) spirometer systems create a usable electrical signal in their normal operation. In both cases, the signal created by these devices is in the form of an **analog electrical current**. Unfortunately, since computer function is based on a **digital electronic signal**, the two types of signals are not directly compatible.

An A-D converter allows the analog signal from a measuring system to be used for data management by computer. Figure 1–14 demonstrates the relationship of an A-D converter to the rest of a pulmonary function testing system. The converter is a type of computer input device. It takes the input of the measuring system's analog signal and changes it to an equivalent digital signal. As can be seen in Figure 1–14, a *preprocessor* is sometimes needed to prepare the analog signal for conversion by the A-D converter.

A-D converters do not eliminate the need for technologists to be diligent during the test procedure. The subject and, if available, the video display of a graph of the subject's breathing efforts should be observed carefully during a test before a set of test results is accepted. Otherwise, erroneous test data may be processed and reported.

## DIGITAL-TO-ANALOG (D-A) CONVERTERS

Computerization contributes significantly to pulmonary function testing through electronic control over the test system's operation. This is done by using a D-A converter to translate the computer's digital commands to an electrical signal used to control the test system's components (see Figure 1–14). Through use of the converter, the computer can

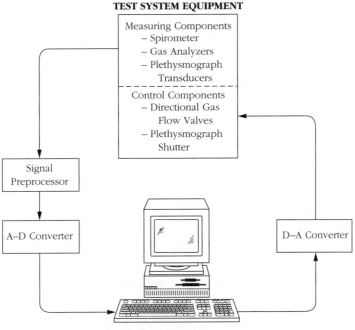

**Figure 1–14** *The function of A-D converters and D-A converters in computerized pulmonary function testing systems.*

operate such items as directional gas flow valves, a plethysmograph's shutter, and other mechanical system components. Related diagnostic software can help a technologist determine whether system malfunctions are due to mechanical failures in the system or to errors made through computer data processing.

Many of the larger laboratory systems make use of D-A converters to control system operations. Table 1-1 provides the positive and negative aspects of automated system control. Often, a system will permit manual override of the automated operations in case the computer becomes inoperable.

**TABLE 1–1  Benefits and Drawbacks of Computer Control of the Measuring System**

| Benefit |
| --- |
| Test procedures are less complicated for the technologist to perform. |

| Drawback |
| --- |
| The technologist may be left with a poor understanding of how the tests are actually performed by the system. |

# DISPLAY/RECORDING INSTRUMENTS

Displays and recording systems are important components of a pulmonary function system. Displays provide an immediate presentation of the test data. This allows the operator to assess patient performance and test results quickly. Recording systems provide a permanent graphic record of the test data. In the past, complex measurements and calculations based on graphic test tracings were used to evaluate the test results. Today, even with computer data management, printed tracings and test data are still important for providing a record of the results of pulmonary function testing.

## DISPLAYS

Display types fall into three categories. They may be designed as analog displays, digital displays, or sophisticated video monitor screen displays (Figure 1–15).

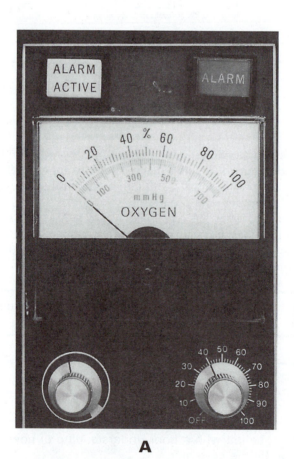

**A**

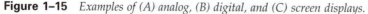

**Figure 1–15**  *Examples of (A) analog, (B) digital, and (C) screen displays.*

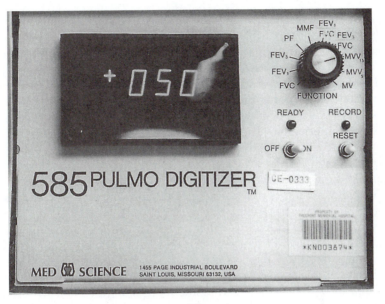

**B**

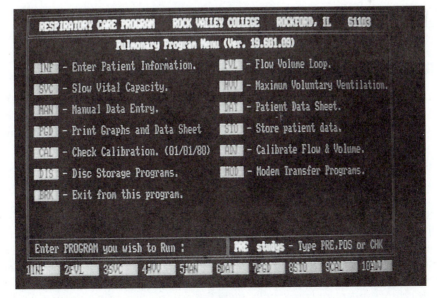

**C**

**Figure 1–15** *Continued.*

*Analog* displays use a moving dial or scale to display changes in data input over a preset range of values. Displays of this type include the traditional car speedometer, radio tuner, compass or clock face, pressure manometer dial face, or Wright spirometer. The display changes can be in response to physical changes in state (pressure, etc.) or changes in a DC electrical signal. These displays are limited primarily to numerical data and are rarely used in modern pulmonary function testing equipment.

*Digital* displays take analog-type input but provide a direct visual representation in the form of **alphanumeric** data. The displays operate in response to a **DC electrical current** input. They are popularly used in electronic calculators. **Light-emitting diodes** (LEDs) or **liquid crystal displays** (LCDs) may be used. The LED displays rely on physically prearranged diodes to present data. As a result, they are limited in what they can display. LCD technology offers much more flexibility in data display. It does not rely as heavily on prearranged visual structures.

*Screen* displays are used today in smaller, portable testing systems as well as in laboratory-based testing systems. With screen displays, alphanumeric data can be presented in a manner similar to digital displays. Additionally, however, screen displays can present graphs, line drawings, and other types of complex visual data. Traditionally, television-type *video monitors* have been used. Some monitors are capable of displaying only monochrome images. Others can display color images. Depending on the quality of color video monitor used, the resolution and ease of viewing of the displayed images can vary considerably. Sophisticated LCD screen-type displays are available with some portable systems. They are capable of providing reasonably good monochrome or color images in a small, lightweight configuration.

A specialized type of videolike screen display is the *oscilloscope*. Although similar to video monitors, oscilloscopes provide simpler images. They are limited to displaying electrical signals in two axial dimensions. The screen display of an ECG monitor is a common application of oscilloscope technology.

## RECORDERS

Recorders, as described earlier, provide a hard copy of a subject's test results. The data recorded may be alphanumeric and/or graphic. The ATS has given a recommendation that all test reports include a volume versus time graphic presentation of test results.

### Mechanical Chart Recorders

Mechanical chart recorders require the movement of both the paper and the recording pen (Figure 1–16). They are used with volume-collecting PVMS systems. Generally, the chart recorder paper moves along a time axis (the X axis). The pen motion is on an axis perpendicular to the motion of the paper motion (the Y axis). Pen movement along the Y axis is proportional to the spirometer's volume changes. The two types of mechanical chart recorders that will be discussed are the rotating chart recorders and linear chart recorders.

*Rotating chart recorders*, or *kymographs*, were the original recording systems used in pulmonary function testing. With these recorders, the paper is attached to a drum that ro-

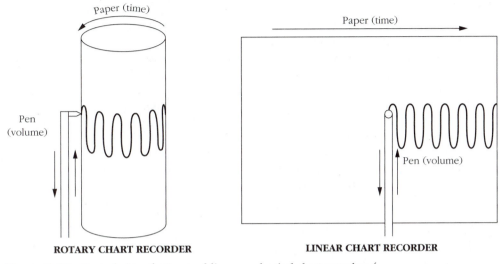

**Figure 1–16** *Basic design of rotary and linear mechanical chart recorders.*

tates at a constant speed and establishes the X axis. It is possible to set different rotation speeds. Slower speeds are used for simple volume spirometry. The faster speeds are for the recording of forced expiratory maneuvers. Pen movement is in some way linked to movement of the spirometer. This can be done, as described earlier, in a chain-compensated or a Stead-Wells configuration.

With *linear chart recorders*, the paper moves along one axis in a straight line. The pen is, again, linked to spirometer movement along a perpendicular axis. These recording systems were used with some older, smaller, portable spirometers. They are still used in some spirometer systems.

*Summary for Mechanical Chart Recorders.* Mechanical chart recorders are generally simple in design and are inexpensive to purchase and maintain. They are limited to making volume-versus-time recordings from volume-collecting PVM spirometers. It is important for the paper to reach a constant speed prior to the recording of spirometer movements. Its failure to do so will cause inaccurate flow calculations from the tracings. It is questionable whether all mechanical recording systems are capable of performing to this standard.

## Electronic Chart Recorders

Any measuring system that can produce an electrical signal can use an electronic chart recorder. Volume-collecting PVM spirometers can create a signal through use of a potentiometer linked to spirometer movement. PFM spirometers provide their data directly as an electrical signal. Regardless of the measuring system, the DC signal is used to control movements of the recording system. The analog input to the recorder is directly proportional to the volumes, times, flow rates, gas concentrations, and so forth, that have been measured. The types of electronic chart recorders that will be discussed are the strip chart recorders, X-Y plotters, and computer-style printers.

*Strip chart recorders* use paper that is stored on a roll and is more narrow than the paper used on other recording systems. ECG machines use similar recording systems. The recording method is generally a heated stylus used on special heat-sensitive paper or an ink-and-pen system. The frequency response of strip chart recorders is excellent, up to approximately 200 **Hz**. A two-channel recorder provides the ability to display parallel volume/time and flow/time tracings on the same strip of paper. A benefit of strip chart recorders is that they can display tracings accurately in real time.

*X-Y plotters* use DC analog signals to run potentiometer-like servomotors. The paper remains stationary, with the pen capable of moving along both the X axis and Y axis. One servomotor, in the pen-support assembly, can control movement of the pen back and forth along one axis. A second servomotor is used to control movement of the entire pen-support assembly back and forth along the perpendicular axis. With some recorders it is possible to have independent sensitivity adjustment for the pen movement along each axis. Sophisticated models are capable of writing out alphanumeric data in addition to producing graphs. A modest frequency response (up to 20 Hz) is possible with X-Y plotters. Such plotters, however, may demonstrate error when used to produce real-time tracings of high-frequency or forced breathing maneuvers.

A variety of *computer-style printers* are available for pulmonary function testing systems. Dot-matrix printers are a basic form of computer printer. Ink-jet printers and laser printers can offer very clear, high-resolution printed images. The choice of computer printer may depend on such factors as the quality of image required, the need for color printing, the printing speed desired, and/or the expense that can be accepted for a printer. It is beyond the scope of this text to describe these printers in any great detail.

*Summary for X-Y Plotters and Computer-Style Printers.* With software commands, X-Y plotters and computer-style printers can provide complex graphic images. They are capable of adding time marks to tracings that compare flow against volume during a breathing maneuver. Additionally, some systems can produce tracings that demonstrate graphic results in three dimensions. The graphs that are produced have an X, a Y, and a Z axis. Relationships between volume, time, and flow during a single breathing maneuver can be demonstrated. Plotters and printers can easily overlay a series of tracings on top of each other. They can also produce graphs in different colors.

## Optical Chart Recorders

Optical chart recorders use a light-sensitive paper that is moved past an oscilloscope display. The light from the oscilloscope records directly on the paper. This type of recorder provides an outstanding frequency response since it has no mechanical parts in the marking system. Unfortunately, optical recorders are more expensive and complex than mechanical or electronic systems and are not frequently used.

## Review Questions

Please use the following review questions to evaluate your learning of information from this chapter. It might be helpful to write out your answers on a sheet of paper. If you are unsure of the answers to these questions, review the chapter to reinforce your learning.

1. What are the differences between primary volume measuring (PVM) and primary flow measuring (PFM) spirometer systems?
2. Relating to PVM spirometers,
   a. How does each of the following types of PVM spirometer system operate?
      - water-sealed spirometers
      - dry-sealed spirometers
      - bellows spirometers
      - rotary vane spirometers
   b. What are some concerns in regard to the use of PVM spirometers?
3. Relating to PFM spirometers,
   a. How does each of the following types of PFM spirometer system operate?
      - differential-pressure pneumotachometers
      - thermal anemometers
      - ultrasonic sensors
   b. What are some concerns in regard to the use of PFM spirometers?
4. How do dedicated peak flow meters operate?
5. Relating to body plethysmographs (BPs),
   a. How are body plethysmographs constructed, and how do they operate?
   b. What are the different types of body plethysmographs?
6. How do respiratory inductive plethysmographs (RIPs) operate?
7. How do directional breathing valves operate?
8. How do computer interfaces for pulmonary function testing systems operate?
9. What purpose do displays serve for pulmonary function testing systems?
10. How do mechanical, electronic, and optical chart recorders operate?

# CHAPTER TWO

# TESTS FOR PULMONARY MECHANICS

## RELATED LEARNING

Prior knowledge of the following related information will facilitate understanding and learning of the material in this chapter. The learner will be aided by being able to

1. Describe the operation and use of spirometers and recording systems as presented in Chapter 1.
2. State and define the standard volumes and capacities into which the lung is divided.
3. Explain the concept of dynamic airway compression.
4. Describe the relationships between laminar flow, turbulent flow, and gas density.

## LEARNING OBJECTIVES

Upon successful completion of this chapter, the learner should be able to

1. Describe the measurement and assessment of a forced vital capacity maneuver and its components.
2. Describe the measurement and assessment of low-density gas spirometry.
3. Describe the measurement and assessment of peak expiratory flow rate monitoring.
3. Describe the measurement and assessment of maximum voluntary ventilation.
4. Describe the measurement and assessment of airway resistance/conductance.
5. Describe the measurement and assessment of elastic recoil pressure/compliance.
6. Describe the measurement and assessment of maximum inspiratory pressure and maximum expiratory pressure.

--- **KEY TERMS** ---

closed-circuit spirometry
open-circuit spirometry
peristalsis
pulmonary function screening

real-time recordings
syncopal episode
tissue resistance to ventilation
Valsalva maneuver

Tests for pulmonary mechanics are used to assess function of the pulmonary/thoracic system under dynamic conditions. Dynamic testing may be used in conjunction with lung volume tests to confirm suspected pulmonary disorders. Some disorders, such as upper airway obstruction, may exhibit themselves only through this type of study. Pulmonary mechanics tests are used to evaluate a variety of breathing maneuvers and dynamic ventilatory parameters. They include

- Forced vital capacity maneuvers ($FEV_t$, $FEV_{t\%}$, $FEF_{200-1200}$, $FEF_{25\%-75\%}$, $FEF_{75\%-85\%}$, PEFR).
- Volume of isoflow.
- Maximum voluntary ventilation.
- Airway resistance/conductance.
- Elastic recoil pressure/compliance.
- Maximum inspiratory/expiratory pressures.

# FORCED VITAL CAPACITY MANEUVER

## TEST DESCRIPTION

The *forced vital capacity* (FVC) maneuver is the most frequently used method for assessing dynamic pulmonary function. Table 2–1 provides the definition for an FVC maneuver. It is evaluated on the basis of both *volumes* and *flow rates* measured from the maneuver. The volume and flow rate components of FVC evaluation will be discussed later. FVC maneuvers are used for pulmonary function screening as well as for in-laboratory testing.

## EQUIPMENT REQUIRED

Relatively basic equipment is used for measuring and assessing FVC and its components. A spirometer and recording system is required. The spirometer may be either a primary flow measuring (PFM) or primary volume measuring (PVM) system.

A recording system linked to the spirometer for the purpose of making graphic tracings is recommended. This is true unless large-group **pulmonary function screenings** are being performed. With screenings, later testing of questionable subjects from the group can provide hard-copy tracings as needed. **Real-time** chart recorders, if used, should have

**TABLE 2–1  Abbreviations and Definitions for a Forced Vital Capacity Maneuver and Its Components**

### Volume/Time Curve

#### Forced Expiratory Volumes (FEV)

| | |
|---|---|
| Forced Vital Capacity (FVC) | The volume of an expiratory vital capacity maneuver exhaled as rapidly and forcefully as possible. |
| Timed Forced Expiratory Volume ($FEV_t$, or $FEV_{0.5}$, $FEV_1$, $FEV_2$, $FEV_3$) | The volume of air exhaled within a specified time from the start of a FVC maneuver—specifically, within the first 0.5, 1, 2, and 3 second(s). |
| Forced Expiratory Volume Percent ($FEV_{t\%}$, or $FEV_{.5\%}$, $FEV_{1\%}$, $FEV_{2\%}$, $FEV_{3\%}$) | The percent of the total FVC volume that was exhaled within a specified time from the start of the maneuver—specifically, within the first 0.5, 1, 2, and 3 second(s). |

#### Forced Expiratory Flow Rates (FEF)

| | |
|---|---|
| Maximum Expiratory Flow Rate ($FEF_{200-1200}$ or $MEFR_{200-1200}$) | The average expiratory flow rate between the first 0.2 and 1.2 liters of the FVC volume. |
| Maximal Mid-Expiratory Flow Rate ($FEF_{25\%-75\%}$ or MMFR) | The average expiratory flow rate over the middle 50% of the FVC volume. |
| Maximum End-Expiratory Flow Rate ($FEF_{75\%-85\%}$) | The average expiratory flow rate between 75% and 85% of the FVC volume. |

### Flow/Volume Loop

#### Forced Expiratory Volumes (FEV)

FVC and the $FEV_T$s are the same as for volume/time curves. Timing marks must be added to the flow/volume loop in order to identify the $FEV_T$s

#### Forced Expiratory Flow Rates (FEF)

| | |
|---|---|
| Peak Expiratory Flow Rate ($FEF_{max}$ or PEFR) | The maximum expiratory flow rate achieved at any point during the FVC maneuver. |

**TABLE 2–1  (*Continued*)**

| | |
|---|---|
| Instantaneous Forced Expiratory Flow Rate (FEF$_{x\%}$, or FEF$_{25\%}$, FEF$_{50\%}$, and FEF$_{75\%}$) | The expiratory flow rate at a specified point in the FVC maneuver—specifically, when 25%, 50%, or 75% of the FVC volume has been exhaled. |
| Instantaneous Forced Expiratory Flow Rate ($\dot{V}_{max\ x}$, or $\dot{V}_{max\ 75}$, $\dot{V}_{max\ 50}$, and $\dot{V}_{max\ 25}$) | The expiratory flow rate at a specified point in the FVC maneuver—specifically, when there is 75%, 50%, or 25% of the FVC volume remaining to be exhaled. |

| *Forced Inspiratory Volume (FIV)* | |
|---|---|
| Forced Inspiratory Vital Capacity (FIVC) | The volume of an inspiratory vital capacity maneuver inhaled as rapidly and forcefully as possible. |

| *Forced Inspiratory Flow Rates (FIF)* | |
|---|---|
| Peak Inspiratory Flow Rate (FIF$_{max}$ and PIFR) | The maximum inspiratory flow rate achieved at any point during the FIVC maneuver. |
| Maximal Mid-Inspiratory Flow Rate (FIF$_{25\%-75\%}$) | The average inspiratory flow rate over the middle 50% of the FIVC volume. |
| Instantaneous Forced Inspiratory Flow Rate (FIF$_{x\%}$, or FIF$_{75\%}$, FIF$_{50\%}$, and FIF$_{25\%}$) | The inspiratory flow rate at a specified point in the FIVC maneuver—specifically, at 75%, 50%, and 25% of the FVC volume. |

accurate speed regulation. They must be running up to speed prior to actual recording of the FVC maneuver. Both spirometer and recorder should meet the minimum standards established by the American Thoracic Society (ATS). Appendix C provides a synopsis of these standards.

## TEST ADMINISTRATION

The usefulness of a dynamic measurement such as FVC depends primarily on the subject's understanding, cooperation, and effort. The instruction and coaching provided by the technologist are crucial for maximizing subject effort. Instructions should be given to the subject before the procedure is started. An active demonstration of the breathing maneuver by the technologist is recommended. Nose clips are not generally necessary when an **open-circuit spirometer** is used. Nose clips are helpful when a slow vital capacity is to be performed and are required when a **closed-circuit spirometer** is used.

During the procedure, appropriate and directive coaching is needed. The subject must be encouraged strongly to perform a maximal inspiration and to continue the inspiratory effort at the full *total lung capacity* (TLC) level for one to two seconds. A maximally forceful and complete expiration to the *residual volume* (RV) level should then be performed.

The subject's forced expiratory maneuver should conform to ATS recommendations. *The forced expiration should be continued for a minimum of six seconds* unless there is an obvious volume plateau demonstrated on the volume/time curve display. During the testing of children, young adults, and some subjects with restrictive pulmonary disease, shorter exhalation times may occur and be acceptable. Generally, however, an effort of at least six seconds is expected for the test to be acceptable. Once the forced expiration is started and has lasted at least six seconds, the effort may be ended when *one* of the following criteria is met:

- There is a volume plateau in the volume/time curve display with no detectable change in volume *for at least one second*. The minimum detectable volume for the spirometer must be 0.030 liter or less.
- The forced expiratory effort has been continued for a reasonable period of time. Some subjects with obstructive disorders may require expirations of 15 or more seconds. It is recommended that expirations greater than 15 seconds not be encouraged. They do not generally produce data useful for test evaluation. Such prolonged efforts, however, may be excessively stressful to the subject.
- The subject demonstrates clinically significant reasons for not continuing the maneuver. These may include dizziness, light-headedness, or **syncopal episodes**.

After the forced expiratory maneuver is performed, some measuring systems require that the subject perform a maximally forceful inspiration back to the TLC level. This last inspiration provides a full flow/volume loop graph for analysis.

*At least three acceptable FVC maneuvers must be performed by the subject.* Up to eight maneuvers may be performed by the subject to produce the three acceptable tests. Eight is considered the maximum for most subjects to avoid problems with fatigue or effort-induced bronchospasm.

A test is considered acceptable when the criteria shown in Table 2–2 are met. Test maneuvers must be repeated and acceptable results collected until test *reproducibility* is demonstrated according to the criteria shown in Table 2–3. The largest FVC and $FEV_1$ do not have to be from the same maneuver. The second largest FVC and $FEV_1$ also do not. Computer-based spirometer systems can rapidly determine if test results are acceptable and reproducible.

It should be noted that reproducibility criteria are meant only to indicate whether additional testing is needed. They should not be used to eliminate data from being reported from the testing. The criteria for reproducibility can be applied after the first three acceptable tests have been recorded. If two reproducible tests cannot be found from among

---

**TABLE 2–2  Criteria for FVC Test Acceptability**

---

A test for FVC can be considered *acceptable* if there is:
Relating to the start of the expiratory effort—

- No excessive subject hesitation or false start by the subject.
- Not a back-extrapolated volume exceeding 5% of the FVC volume or 0.15 liter, whichever is greater.

Relating to the presence of artifacts during the maneuver—

- No cough during the first second of the maneuver (affecting $FEV_1$) or that, in the technologist's opinion, interferes with the accuracy of the test results.
- No **Valsalva maneuver** performed before or during the forced expiration.
- No variable effort demonstrated by the subject during the maneuver.
- No volume loss because of a leak in the system.
- No obstruction of the spirometer mouthpiece. This can be caused by the subject's tongue or by falling of the subject's dentures.
- No premature termination of the forced expiration.

Relating to the end of the expiratory effort—

- No expiratory test maneuver performed for less than six seconds unless a volume plateau is present on the volume/time curve display.

---

---

**TABLE 2–3  Criteria for FVC Test Reproducibility**

---

After the first three acceptable tests have been recorded, tests are *reproducible* and testing may be ended if both of the following are true:

- The two largest FVC values are within 0.2 liter of each other.
- The two largest $FEV_1$ values are within 0.2 liter of each other.

If both of these criteria are not met, testing must continue until

- Both criteria are met with the performance of additional acceptable test maneuvers.
- A total of eight tests has been performed.
- The patient cannot or should not continue.

At minimum, the best three maneuvers should be saved.

---

---

**TABLE 2–4  Criteria for Selecting FVC Test Data for Reporting**

---

Based on *acceptable* test maneuvers:

- The largest value for VC should be reported, even if it is measured from an FVC maneuver.
- The largest values for FVC and $FEV_1$ should be reported, even if they are not taken from the same test maneuver or from a single test considered the best overall test.
- A single *best test* should be selected. The test maneuver that has the largest combined sum of its values for FVC and $FEV_1$ is considered to be the best test.
- The other FVC components ($FEF_{200-1200}$, $FEF_{25\%-75\%}$, etc.) should be reported from the test identified as the single best test.

---

the first three recorded tests, additional testing must be done, up to a maximum of eight tests. A series of test values should not be rejected if reproducibility is not established. Clinically significant events such as bronchospasm may prevent reproducibility. The best of the available data should nevertheless be reported.

Once acceptable test results have been identified, the data to be used for the final report on the subject should be selected according to the criteria shown in Table 2–4.

## EVALUATION OF FVC AND ITS COMPONENTS

Traditionally, assessment of FVC and its components is based on evaluation of both graphic tracings of the maneuver and numerical test results. In the past, the numerical data were derived from measurements made directly on the tracings. Computers in modern systems can make these calculations based on the input from the spirometer sensor. The unit of measure used for volume determinations is the liter (BTPS). For flow determinations, it is generally l/sec (BTPS), although l/min is also acceptable. Two types of spirometry tracing, or graphs, are used in assessing the volume and flow results of an FVC maneuver. One is the classic *volume/time curve*. This curve may be made directly by use of a volume-displacement spirometer and mechanical recorder. The second is a *flow/volume loop*. Graphing of a flow/volume loop requires use of a spirometer system that can measure and record flow rates directly. Modern electronic spirometers are generally capable of producing both types of tracings.

### Volume/Time Curve

The volume/time curve resulting from an FVC maneuver is traced or plotted with volume indicated on the vertical axis and time on the horizontal axis. It may be subdivided into a number of components. Table 2–1 lists FVC components, abbreviations, and definitions. Figures 2–1, 2–2, and 2–3 provide volume/time curves that illustrate FVC and its components. Flow-rate determination is based on the slope of the line between two points on the curve. Steeper or more vertical lines produce a larger value for slope and indicate faster rates of *forced expiratory flow* (FEF) and *forced inspiratory flow* (FIF). Study Section I

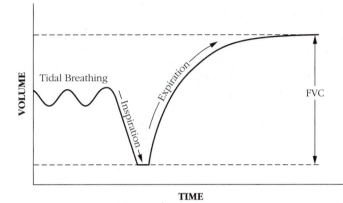

**Figure 2–1**  *Volume/time tracing for an FVC maneuver.*

of this book demonstrates the process used to make measurements and calculations for FVC and its components.

Table 2–5 offers examples of normal FVC values. In general, flow-rate values are less for shorter subjects, for female subjects, and for older subjects. The only exceptions are the $FEF_{200-1200}$ and $FEF_{25\%-75\%}$. Females, for their height, seem to have larger values for these flow parameters.

The FVC of a normal subject should be approximately equal to the vital capacity (VC) measured with an unforced maneuver. A similar maneuver may be performed and mea-

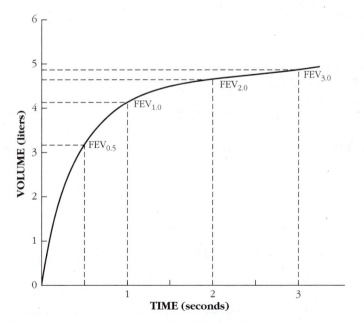

**Figure 2–2**  *Volume/time tracing demonstrating the $FEV_t$ parameters.*

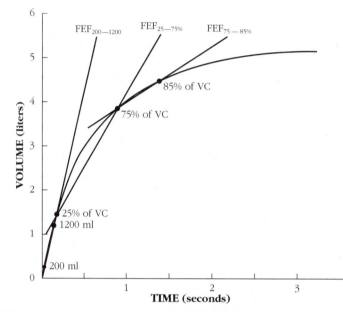

**Figure 2–3** *Volume/time tracing demonstrating the FEF parameters.*

sured by having the subject inhaling forcefully and maximally from the RV level. This is referred to as a *forced inspiratory vital capacity* (FIVC). Values for FVC that are less than the VC value may be the result of obstructive pulmonary disorders or poor patient effort. Direct observation and evaluation of subject effort during the maneuver are important to making accurate volume determinations.

---

**TABLE 2–5    Normal Values for FVC and Its Components (based on a 70-inch-tall, 20-year-old caucasian male)**

| | |
|---|---|
| FVC = 5.00 liters | FIVC = 5.00 liters |
| PEFR = 9.10 l/sec | $FIF_{25\%-75\%}$ = 7.70 l/sec |
| $FEV_{0.5}$ = 3.10 liters | $FEV_{0.5\%}$ = 50%–60%* |
| $FEV_1$ = 4.20 liters | $FEV_{1\%}$ = 75%–85%* |
| $FEV_2$ = 4.60 liters | $FEV_{2\%}$ = 94%* |
| $FEV_3$ = 4.90 liters | $FEV_{3\%}$ = 97%* |
| $FEF_{200-1200}$ = 8.70 l/sec | $FEF_{25\%}$ = 8.30 l/sec |
| $FEF_{25\%-75\%}$ = 5.20 l/sec | $FEF_{50\%}$ = 5.70 l/sec |
| $FEF_{75\%-85\%}$ = 1.70 l/sec | $FEF_{75\%}$ = 3.20 l/sec |

*These values for $FEV_{0.5\%}$, $FEV_{1\%}$, $FEV_{2\%}$, and $FEV_{3\%}$ are accepted as being normal for all subjects, regardless of differences in age, height, gender, etc.*

The results determined for the $FEV_t$ provide an indication of the average flow rate over a time interval. A larger value for $FEV_t$ indicates a faster rate of air flow. As the time interval for the $FEV_t$ becomes longer (e.g., $FEV_2$, $FEV_3$), flow rates later in expiration and through smaller airways are being measured.

The $FEV_1$ has many applications for assessment and is used in a number of clinical circumstances. These include rapid test evaluation during screening procedures, evaluating subject response to bronchodilator therapy or to inhalation challenges for extrinsic asthma, and assessing the existence of exercise-induced bronchospasm.

In order to make accurate determinations of the $FEV_t$, it is important to establish the start of the maneuver (time-zero) correctly. On a volume/time spirometer tracing, this is possible by back-extrapolating the curve. Back-extrapolation is performed by drawing a line tangent to the steep, initial portion of the curve. The line should extend back to intersect with a line indicating the maximal inspiratory volume. The point at which these two lines intersect is the time-zero point. Figure 2–4 demonstrates back-extrapolation. The difference in volume between the maximum inspiratory volume and the volume at the level of the time-zero point is the extrapolated volume. This extrapolated volume must not be more than 5% of the FVC or 0.15 liter, whichever is greater, if the test is to be considered acceptable. Computer systems that use back-extrapolation methods provide adequate time-zero determination for $FEV_t$ measurements.

The $FEV_{t\%}$ are affected directly by the accuracy of the FVC determination. It is important that, in calculating them, the $FEV_t$ be divided by the largest value for FVC demonstrated by the subject.

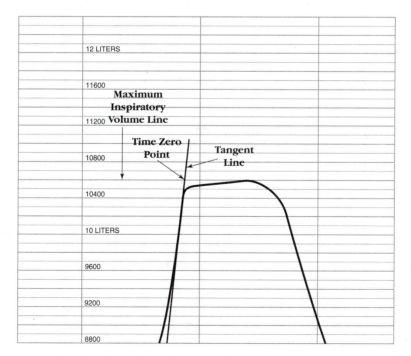

**Figure 2–4** *Back-extrapolation for an FVC tracing.*

**QUALITY ASSURANCE NOTE:** The FVC values may cause serious overestimation of the $FEV_{t\%}$ in situations where the patient performed the FVC maneuvers with poor effort. For this reason, the largest value for a slow VC maneuver is used by some technologists in making $FEV_{t\%}$ determinations. The issue of whether the value for VC was the result of either a forced or a slow maneuver is deemed unimportant.

The $FEF_{200-1200}$ measures flow early in the expiratory maneuver. It intentionally disregards the first 200 ml of the expiratory maneuver. This is because inertia, in both the subject and the spirometer system at the start of the maneuver, may cause the initial volume to be exhaled at a slower rate. Starting flow determination at 200 ml eliminates this artifact. Because the $FEF_{200-1200}$ occurs so early in the expiratory maneuver, it is very dependent on subject effort. Low measured values may be due either to insufficient subject effort or to a poor understanding of the procedure by the subject.

The $FEF_{25\%-75\%}$ measures expiratory flow rates at a later point in the maneuver than the $FEF_{200-1200}$. As a result, its accuracy is slightly less effort-dependent. Poor subject effort can still cause measured values to be less than what the subject is capable of performing, however. Because the $FEF_{25\%-75\%}$ is measured at a later point in the maneuver than for $FEV_{200-1200}$, its normal value is less.

The $FEF_{75\%-85\%}$ measures expiratory flow rates toward the end of the maneuver. Its accuracy is the least effort-dependent. Because it is measured so late in the maneuver, $FEF_{75\%-85\%}$ values will be the smallest of all the FEF values.

The *peak expiratory flow rate* (PEFR) can be determined from a volume/time tracing. It is based on a line drawn tangent to the steepest part of the curve. Use of a PFM spirometer system makes determination of PEFR simpler and more accurate. PEFR is an extremely effort-dependent parameter, and low or inconsistent values may be due to insufficient subject effort. In other words, PEFR values can indicate the quality and/or reproducibility of subject effort.

**QUALITY ASSURANCE NOTE:** Consistent values for PEFR can be used to indicate that the subject's effort has been reasonably reproducible over a series of tests.

## Flow/Volume Loops

The flow/volume loop is plotted with flow indicated on the vertical axis and volume on the horizontal axis. It is possible to plot both a *maximum expiratory flow/volume* (MEFV) curve and a *maximum inspiratory flow/volume* (MIFV) curve. Most spirometer systems allow for plotting of both and produce a complete flow/volume loop.

Flow/volume loops may be subdivided into measured components. Table 2–1 lists the components, abbreviations, and definitions. Table 2–5 offers examples of normal values. Figure 2–5 provides a flow/volume loop that illustrates FVC and its components. One unfortunate point of confusion is the relationship between $FEF_{x\%}$ and $\dot{V}_{max\ x}$ values. Both the $FEF_{50\%}$ and the $\dot{V}_{max\ 50}$ refer to the same data point on a flow/volume loop and will have the same measured value. The $FEF_{25\%}$ and the $\dot{V}_{max\ 75}$ refer to the same data point on a flow/volume loop and will have the same value. The $FEF_{75\%}$ and the $\dot{V}_{max\ 25}$ refer to the same data point and have the same value. The $FEF_{x\%}$ values may be used in relation to either volume/time curves or flow/volume loops. $\dot{V}_{max\ x}$ values are generally given in relation only to flow/volume loops.

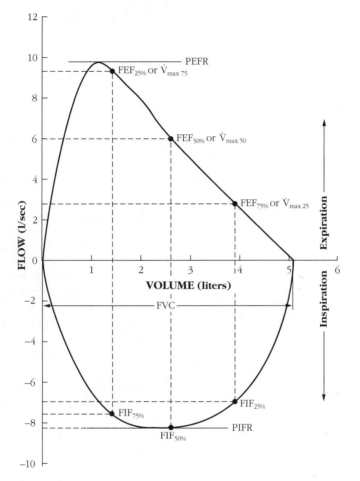

**Figure 2–5** *Flow/volume loop.*

Flow/volume loops are beneficial for a number of reasons. They allow for inspiratory and expiratory peak flow rates to be read directly from the graph. The PEFR is more easily read from a flow/volume loop than it is from a volume/time curve. Instantaneous flow rates at any point in the FVC volume are also easily determined. Some spirometer systems superimpose timing indicators on the flow/volume loop. This allows for determination of the $FEV_t$ from the graph as well.

## INTERPRETATION OF TEST RESULTS

Pulmonary function studies are interpreted by comparing a subject's test values with what are *predicted* to be normal values for that subject. Sources for predicted normal values and their use will be discussed more fully in Chapter 7. It is important to note that diagnostic interpretation for a subject requires the evaluation of data from many different assessment methods. Pulmonary function studies should be evaluated in conjunction with data from the subject's history, physical examination, and other types of clinical assessment. A discussion of the general basis for interpretation of FVC maneuver tests follows.

Interpretation of the test results from a FVC maneuver is based on analysis of a number of factors. Included is evaluation of the volume and the flow-rate components. Restrictive and obstructive pulmonary disorders have both similarities and differences in how they change the FVC test results. Table 2–6 provides the interpretive significance of the FVC maneuver and its components. Table 2–7 shows the patterns of changes in pulmonary function that may result from restrictive, obstructive, and combined disorders. Table 2–8 lists examples of restrictive and obstructive disorders.

**TABLE 2–6  Interpretive Significance of FVC and Its Components**

| Parameter | General Significance |
| --- | --- |
| FVC | Relates directly to changes in VC from volume spirometry. Evaluation of the flow-rate parameters below aids in disorder differentiation. |
| PEFR | Relates to flow rates and disorders in the large, upper airways. Very effort-dependent. Also used to monitor asthma and bronchodilator therapy. |
| $FEV_{0.5}$, $FEV_1$, $FEF_{200-1200}$ | Relate to flow rates and disorders in the large, upper airways. Still may be relatively effort-dependent. |
| $FEF_2$, $FEF_{25\%-75\%}$ | Relate to flow rates and disorders in smaller bronchi and larger bronchioles. Some degree of effort-dependence remains. |
| $FEV_3$, $FEF_{75\%-85\%}$ | Relate to flow rates and disorders in smaller bronchioles. Little or no effort-dependence. |
| $FEV_{t\%}$ | Relates to changes in both flow rates and lung volumes. Generally, opposite results are demonstrated between restrictive and obstructive disorders. |
| $FEF_{x\%}$ | Relates most significantly to flow rates and disorders in the large upper airways. |

TABLE 2–7    **Patterns of Pulmonary Function Changes with Disorders**

| Parameter | Restrictive | Obstructive | Combined |
|---|---|---|---|
| ***FVC Maneuver*** | | | |
| FVC | ↓ | N or ↓ | ↓ |
| $FEV_t$ | ↓ | N or ↓ | ↓ |
| $FEV_{t\%}$ | N or ↑ | ↓ | ↓ |
| $FEV_{x\%}$ | N or ↑ or ↓ | ↓ | ↓ |
| $FIF_{x\%}$ | N | N or ↓ | N or ↓ |
| ***Lung Volume Determination*** | | | |
| TLC | ↓ | N or ↑ | ↓ |
| RV/TLC% | N | ↑ | ↑ |

*N = normal values; ↑ = increased values; ↓ = decreased values.*

TABLE 2–8    **Examples of Restrictive and Obstructive Disorders**

| Restrictive Disorders | Obstructive Disorders |
|---|---|
| ***Pulmonary*** | ***Large Airway Obstruction*** |
| Interstitial fibrosis | *Fixed* |
| Vascular congestion |    Tracheostenosis |
| Pneumoconioses |    Large substernal goiter |
| Sarcoidosis | *Variable intrathoracic* |
| |    Tracheal carcinoma |
| ***Extrapulmonary*** | *Variable extrathoracic* |
| *Thoracic* |    Laryngeal carcinoma |
|    Kyphoscoliosis | |
|    Rheumatoid spondylitis | ***Small Airway Obstruction*** |
| *Abdominal* | Bronchial asthma |
|    Ascites | Emphysema |
|    Peritonitis | Chronic bronchitis |
|    Severe obesity | Bronchiectasis |
| *Neuromuscular defects* | Cystic fibrosis |
|    Poliomyelitis | |
|    Myasthenia gravis | |

*Note: This listing largely ignores acute, traumatic, or surgically related disorders.*

## Restrictive Disorders

Reductions in lung volumes (FVC and $FEV_t$) occur in subjects with restrictive disorders (see Table 2–7). These reductions do not, however, differentiate restrictive from obstructive disorders. Most significant for making restrictive/obstructive differentiations are values for the $FEV_{t\%}$. With restrictive disorders, $FEV_{t\%}$ values will often be larger than predicted. This is because the FVC reductions generally occur to a greater degree than any reductions in expiratory flow rates. Figure 2–6 demonstrates the effects of a restrictive disorder on a volume/time curve. RV, TLC, and RV/TLC% values provide an additional resource for differentiating between restrictive and obstructive disorders. Lung volume determinations, as described in Chapter 4, are a source of this data.

## Obstructive Disorders

Obstructive disorders generally produce decreased values in most of the parameters measured during an FVC maneuver. These decreases are due largely to the air flow limitations that occur with obstructive disorders. Reduction of the FVC value, if it occurs, may be caused by air trapping. The effects of air trapping are more pronounced during a forced expiratory maneuver.

Flow-rate reductions relate primarily to the site of obstructions. As can be seen in Table 2–6, flow rates that are measured early in the maneuver are most affected by large airway obstruction. The flow rates measured later in the maneuver may remain normal in subjects with large airway obstruction. On the other hand, in subjects with small airway obstruction, flow rates later in the FVC maneuver are most affected. Reductions in $FEF_{25\%-75\%}$, $FEF_{75\%-85\%}$, and $FEF_{75\%}$ ($\dot{V}_{max\ 25}$) may serve as an early indicator of small air-

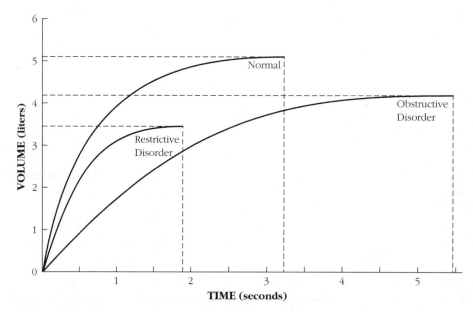

**Figure 2–6**  *Volume/time tracing demonstrating the effects of restrictive and obstructive disorders.*

way disease. Figure 2–6 demonstrates the effects of an obstructive disorder on a volume/time curve.

## Analysis of Flow/Volume Loops

The flow/volume loop has proved a valuable tool in demonstrating pulmonary disorders. It provides a simple graphic representation of the parameters measured with forced expiratory and inspiratory VC maneuvers. More significantly, *it also demonstrates a very characteristic shape in certain disorders.* Some researchers are attempting to provide methods of actually quantifying the shape changes demonstrated by flow/volume curves for subjects with disorders. One proposed method, *angle beta*, quantifies the degree of concavity that the middle portion of the MEFV curve may have toward the volume axis. Figure 2–7 illustrates the shapes that a flow/volume loop may assume in certain disorders. Each overlays a normal flow/volume loop.

With a *restrictive disorder*, the primary change is a decrease in volume. The entire loop is displaced downward to a lower level of lung volume. In Figure 2–7 there is little or no change in flow rates.

In *small airway obstruction* the latter portion of the expiratory loop begins to take on a concave appearance. This concavity is most pronounced in subjects with emphysema because of their greater sensitivity to dynamic airway compression. The entire loop is displaced to a higher lung volume. Air trapping (acute asthma) can produce the same result. It is more pronounced, however, with conditions such as emphysema that cause hyperinflation of the lung.

*Large airway obstructions* also produce characteristic flow/volume loop patterns. A *fixed* large airway obstruction causes relatively equal decreases in both expiratory and inspiratory flow rates. A *variable* large airway obstruction produces different characteristic

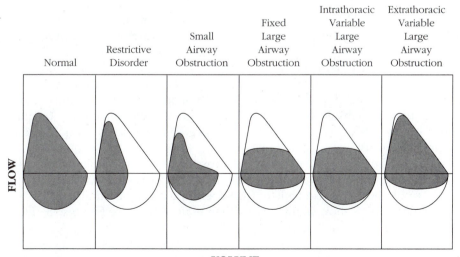

**Figure 2–7**  *Flow/volume loops demonstrating shape changes that may result from pulmonary disorders.*

flow/volume loop patterns depending on whether the obstruction's origin is intrathoracic or extrathoracic.

*Intrathoracic* variable large airway obstructions cause a flattening of the expiratory portion of a flow/volume loop caused by the limitations of expiratory flow. This flattening occurs because obstructions of this type are exposed to the same dynamic forces as the lungs themselves. These are airway-inflating forces during inspiration and airway-collapsing forces (dynamic compression) during expiration. The forced expiration compresses the airway and limits expiratory flow during the effort.

*Extrathoracic* variable large airway obstructions cause a flow limitation on inspiration, with a characteristic flattening of the flow/volume loop's inspiratory portion. The subambient airway pressure that draws air into the lungs during inspiration tends to promote an inward collapse of the large airway structures that precede the airways within the thorax. On expiration, these forces are reversed. Airway collapse is therefore not added as a flow limitation, and flow rates are less affected.

Comparing the $FEF_{50\%}$ and $FIF_{50\%}$ values may be helpful in evaluating upper airway obstruction. These values will be reduced almost equally with a fixed obstruction. A variable intrathoracic obstruction will produce a greater decrease in the $FEF_{50\%}$ value. A variable extrathoracic obstruction will produce a greater decrease in the $FIF_{50\%}$ value.

# LOW-DENSITY GAS SPIROMETRY

## TEST DESCRIPTION

Low-density spirometry involves measuring an FVC maneuver after the subject has breathed a helium/oxygen (80% He/20% $O_2$) mixture. Analysis is based on a flow/volume curve derived from the maneuver. This curve is then compared to a curve derived from a standard FVC maneuver (Figure 2–8). The comparison can serve as a sensitive method for detecting the early stages of small airway disease. It may also help to differentiate the site of an obstruction—between larger versus smaller airways.

The test is based on the relationship between turbulent flow, laminar flow, and gas density. Resistance to turbulent flow changes as gas density changes. In airways where turbulent flow is exhibited, gases with less density than air (He/$O_2$ mixtures) show less resistance to flow. As a result, flow rates are faster with the low-density gas. Laminar flow is independent of gas density. Gas flow resistance and flow rates do not change with changes in gas density.

During an FVC maneuver, the flow rates measured early in the maneuver are limited by the larger, more central airways. A turbulent flow pattern is demonstrated in these airways. As a result, the early segments of the superimposed standard air and He/$O_2$ mixture flow/volume loops show significantly different flow rates (see Figure 2–8). Flow rates are faster with the He/$O_2$ mixture.

Flow through the smaller, peripheral airways (<2 mm in diameter) is measured in the later portion of the expiratory loop. Normally these airways contribute very little to flow resistance through the lungs and limit flow only late in an FVC maneuver. A laminar flow

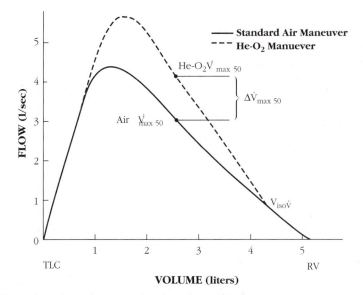

**Figure 2–8** *Flow/volume loops demonstrating the volume of isoflow.*

pattern is demonstrated in these airways. As a result, both the air and He/$O_2$ mixture loops should show the same flow rates and shape in this portion of the maneuver.

The point at which both the standard air and He/$O_2$ mixture loops begin to match is significant. *It indicates the maximum or earliest flow rate that is controlled by density-independent flow through the small, peripheral airways.* The lung volume at which this occurs is referred to as the *volume of isoflow* ($V_{iso\dot{V}}$).

With the development of small airway disorders, resistance in these airways increases. As a result, the air and He/$O_2$ mixture flow rates and curves will match earlier in an FVC maneuver and at a larger lung volume. The resulting larger value for $V_{iso\dot{V}}$ may be used as a sensitive test for evaluating the development of small airway disorders.

## EQUIPMENT REQUIRED

Provided the system can generate a flow/volume loop, the FVC maneuver with the He/$O_2$ mixture may be measured using the same equipment used in standard spirometry. Unfortunately, pneumotachometers are generally unsuitable for the direct measurement of the He/$O_2$ mixture maneuver. The gas content of the expired air changes in its relative concentrations of nitrogen, helium, and oxygen. The resulting gas viscosity changes can produce significant measurement errors. Computer compensation may not always be sufficient to improve accuracy of the spirometer.

A possible solution to this problem is to have the subject's exhaled air collected in a plastic bag that is enclosed in a box. The box is designed with a pneumotachometer mounted in one wall. The bag within the box will expand with the force of the subject's expiration. As the bag expands, the box's air is forced out through the pneumotachometer at an identical flow rate. This way, expiratory flow rates can be measured without the interference of exhaled air viscosity changes.

## TEST ADMINISTRATION

A standard procedure for subject breathing of the He/$O_2$ mixture prior to the FVC maneuver has not been established. Studies have been performed, however, using the three following basic procedures for He/$O_2$ breathing:

1. Breathing the mixture for 10 minutes.
2. Breathing the mixture for three to four VC breaths.
3. Breathing the mixture for one breath prior to the FVC maneuver.

The 10-minute breathing procedure would limit the use of this test for routine screening. It has been found that three to four VC breaths give results comparable to prolonged He/$O_2$ prebreathing. The test actually becomes more sensitive to small airway disorders with less He/$O_2$ prebreathing. Because there is a less than complete equilibrium of both the oxygen and the helium throughout the lungs, a lesser proportion of oxygen may reach the periphery of the lung. The relatively higher concentration of helium would then increase the sensitivity of the test as it relates to flow through the peripheral airways.

At this time, the best choice is probably having the subject take three to four VC breaths of the He/$O_2$ mixture. This is the only method that allows comparison with predicted normal values. With both the standard maneuver and the He/$O_2$ maneuver, at least three acceptable FVCs should be recorded.

## INTERPRETATION OF TEST RESULTS

The standard and He/$O_2$ loops selected for comparison must demonstrate FVC volumes within 2.5%–5% of being the same. The loops may be superimposed at either RV or TLC. It has been suggested that reproducibility of the test results may be increased if the loops are matched at the lower portions of their expiratory limbs instead of at either RV or TLC.

Generally, two points of comparison on the superimposed flow/volume loops are evaluated. These are the *volume of isoflow* ($V_{iso\dot{V}}$) and the *change in flow rate at 50% of vital capacity* ($\Delta\dot{V}_{max\ 50}$) (see Figure 2–8). As stated earlier, the $V_{iso\dot{V}}$ is the volume measured between the point where the two superimposed loops begin to match and the point where the loops share the same RV value. $V_{iso\dot{V}}$ is usually expressed as a percent of the FVC volume. Normally, the value for $V_{iso\dot{V}}$ is 10%–20% of the FVC volume for subjects from young adulthood to middle age. The $V_{iso\dot{V}}$ value appears to increase with increasing age. The value for $V_{iso\dot{V}}$ will increase with the development or worsening of small airway disorders. A larger portion of the FVC maneuver will have flow rates affected by flow limitations in the smaller airways.

The $\Delta\dot{V}_{max\ 50}$ is expressed as a percent of the $\dot{V}_{max\ 50}$ measured from the subject's standard FVC maneuver. It is calculated as follows:

$$\Delta\dot{V}_{max\ 50} = \frac{\dot{V}_{max\ 50}\ (He/O_2) - \dot{V}_{max\ 50}\ (air)}{\dot{V}_{max\ 50}\ (air)} \times 100$$

Normal $\Delta\dot{V}_{max\ 50}$ values for young adult to middle aged subjects have been reported to be approximately 47% ± 14%. The value for $\Delta\dot{V}_{max\ 50}$ will become smaller as small airway disorders develop or worsen. This is because the density-independent flow limitation of the small airways is occurring earlier in the maneuver. As a result, the two loops begin to show similar flow characteristics earlier in the maneuver.

# PEAK EXPIRATORY FLOW MONITORING

## TEST DESCRIPTION

*Peak expiratory flow rate* (PEFR) monitoring generally consists of using a portable, hand-held peak flow meter to evaluate periodically a subject's peak flow capabilities. PEFR is often used for monitoring asthma patients and their management with bronchodilators. The test is done by having the subject perform a maximal inspiration followed by a short, maximally forceful expiration through the PEFR monitoring device. The subject should not cough. The expiratory effort needs to last only one to two seconds.

## EQUIPMENT REQUIRED

PEFR monitoring requires an instrument that can measure with ±10% accuracy or within ±20 l/min of the actual flow rate, whichever is greater. Pediatric PEFR meter measurements typically range from 60 l/min to 100 l/min (no less than 60 l/min), and adult PEFR meter measurements typically range from 100 l/min to 850 l/min (no less than 100 l/min). The upper end of the range should be ≥275 l/min but no greater than 400 l/min for pediatric PEFR meters. For adults, the upper end of the range should be ≥ 700 l/min but no greater than >850 l/min. The device must have a flow resistance of no more than 2.5 cm $H_2O$/l/sec with flows up to 14 l/sec (approximately 850 l/mm). If the device is to be read manually, the reader should be able to resolve units of 5 l/min (with markings of 10 l/min) for pediatric PEFR meters and units of 10 l/min (with markings of 20 l/min) for adult PEFR meters.

Since these devices are often used in the home, data on the instrument's life expectancy and durability must be provided. A package insert should be included with the device that includes the following information:

- Clear instructions on use, with illustration.
- Instructions on cleaning and maintenance of the instrument and methods to recognize its malfunction.
- Appropriate actions to be taken when PEFR readings change significantly (whom to contact).

## TEST ADMINISTRATION

Satisfactory performance of PEFR monitoring by the subject is both volume- and effort-dependent. The forced expiratory effort must be started from a *maximal* inspiratory position, and it must be performed sharply and vigorously. A peak expiratory flow value is generally achieved within the first one tenth of a second of expiratory effort. Proper instruction and coaching of the patient is very important to the success of the testing.

Nose clips are not needed for PEFR monitoring. Testing can be performed with the subject sitting down, but standing is the preferred position. A minimum of three test measurements must be performed. The results should be recorded in the order of their performance. This information can be useful in determining whether test-induced bronchospasm has occurred. The largest value for PEFR should be reported, because it best indicates the subject's current condition.

Results for PEFR may be reported in units of liters per second or liters per minute. Conversion is as follows:

$$\text{Flow in l/sec} = \frac{\text{Flow in l/min}}{60}$$

$$\text{Flow in l/min} = \text{Flow in l/sec} \times 60$$

The measured value must be corrected to BTPS. This may be done automatically by the device or by some conversion method.

If the PEFR monitoring is to be self-administered at home, the subject should be taught

- How to properly use the PEFR meter. Instruction should be by trained personnel and should be repeated on follow-up visits.
- When and how to record test results and other significant information relating to the subject's condition at the time of testing.
- What the standards are for acceptable test results and what should be done if test results are unacceptable.

## INTERPRETATION OF TEST RESULTS

Adult subjects can generally produce peak expiratory flow rates of 400–600 l/min (6.7–10 l/sec). Young adults may generate PEFRs that exceed 600 l/min.

Clinically, decreases in PEFR values are most specifically related to obstruction of the large upper airways. However, a reduction of PEFR is not specific as to where the site of the obstruction may be. If reduced PEFR values are unexpectedly found in a subject, follow-up evaluation for the source of upper airway obstruction can be performed by flow/volume analysis of an FVC maneuver.

Subjects with relatively mild to moderate small airway obstruction often demonstrate normal or near normal PEFR values. This is because they are able to generate a normal PEFR in the fraction of a second of effort before small airway closure occurs and later expiratory flow rates are abnormally slowed. PEFR will correlate well with $FEV_1$ in these subjects.

Subjects with severe small airway obstruction will probably demonstrate definite reductions in PEFRs. However, their reductions in such measurements as $FEF_{25\%-75\%}$ and $FEF_{75\%-85\%}$ will be much more significant than the reductions shown in PEFR. As a result, these later-occurring flow rates are much more useful for diagnosing and evaluating the presence of small airway obstruction.

Monitoring PEFR nevertheless plays an important role in evaluating small airway obstruction. It provides the following advantages:

- PEFR monitoring devices are small and relatively inexpensive.
- Clinically significant worsening of small airway obstruction can cause reductions in PEFRs.
- Subjects can easily be taught to use PEFR monitoring devices for self-performed routine testing.

As a result, routine PEFR monitoring at the bedside in the clinical setting or in the home can be a means for evaluating a subject's response to bronchodilator therapy. Daily monitoring in the home for asthma patients can detect the development of clinically significant increases in small airway obstruction.

The key to PEFR monitoring is serial measurement of PEFR values and a comparison of those values to the subject's past measured values. The subject's best past PEFR values, when he or she is receiving maximally effective bronchodilator therapy, should be used for comparison to identify deterioration of airway function. If both day and night measurements are made, the subject's variations in performance can be used as a basis for devising better treatment to minimize daily fluctuations in lung function.

# MAXIMUM VOLUNTARY VENTILATION

## TEST DESCRIPTION

*Maximum voluntary ventilation* (MVV) is the largest volume that a subject can breathe in and out of the lungs in one minute with maximum voluntary effort. It provides a non-specific overall test of ventilatory function. In the past, the test was referred to as the *maximum breathing capacity* (MBC). The MVV maneuver volume is generally measured for a period of 10–15 seconds. The minimum time period for measurement is five seconds. The volume measured in that time period is then extrapolated to a value for one minute. This is demonstrated by the following equation set up for a 12-second breathing maneuver.

$$\text{MVV} = \text{Measured Volume} \times \frac{60 \text{ Seconds}}{12 \text{ Seconds}}$$

or

$$\text{MVV} = \text{Measured Volume} \times 5$$

Some spirometer systems allow for calculations based on volumes measured for less than 12 seconds. The units used for MVV are l/min.

## EQUIPMENT REQUIRED

MVV may be measured on any spirometer system that is able to measure and record the volumes of breathing. Some older systems are capable only of recording tracings of the volumes of individual breaths (Figure 2–9). The individual volumes then need to be added

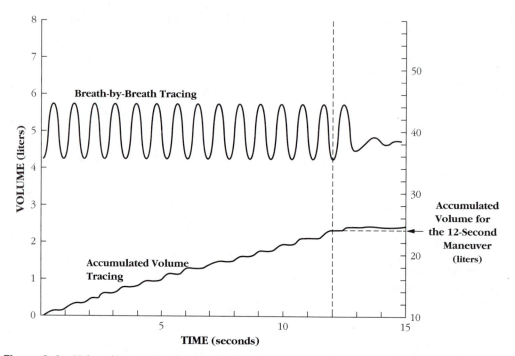

**Figure 2–9** *Volume/time tracing for a maximum voluntary ventilation maneuver.*

together by manual calculation before the MVV can be extrapolated to its one-minute value. Most modern systems record the accumulated volume that is breathed during the measurement time period. These systems can calculate the extrapolated one-minute volume automatically.

## TEST ADMINISTRATION

The subject should be coached to breathe as *rapidly* and as *deeply* as possible during the test. Breathing rates may be between 70 and 120 breaths per minute. Individual volumes should be greater than the subject's tidal volume but less than a vital capacity effort. The pattern is such as one would experience when breathing while running hard. It is important that volume measurement not begin until the subject has achieved and is maintaining a maximum effort. Once begun, the breathing maneuver should continue for at least five seconds. Test durations of 10–15 seconds are generally performed.

Success in measuring a representative MVV value depends greatly on subject effort. For this reason, the technologist plays a significant role in coaching the subject prior to and during the maneuver. Coaching with a cadence of "in—out—in—out" may help the subject maintain a regular, steady rhythm.

Once a value for MVV has been determined, it is possible to judge whether or not subject effort was maximal. An estimated value for any subject's achievable MVV, regardless of the presence of a disorder, may be determined in the following way:

Subject's Measured $FEV_1 \times 35$ = Estimated MVV

---

**TABLE 2–9  Factors That Can Make an MVV Test Unacceptable**

---

A test for MVV may be considered *acceptable* if:

- A volume/time tracing demonstrates the subject's breathing pattern to be regular in volume or breathing rate.
- The end-expiratory baseline on a volume/time tracing remains fairly constant. The only exception to this is if the subject's baseline changes because of air trapping. Air trapping is demonstrated by a baseline that shifts gradually from the FRC level upward toward the TLC level during the time of the maneuver.
- A value for MVV is measured for the subject that is at least as large as the volume determined by multiplying the subject's measured value for $FEV_1$ by 35.

---

**TABLE 2–10  Criteria for MVV Test Reproducibility for Selecting MVV Test Data for Reporting**

---

- *Reproducibility* is achieved when the largest and second largest values measured for MVV are within 10 % of each other.
- The *best test* for MVV is the one that demonstrates the largest MVV value.

---

For example, the estimated MVV value for a young adult male may be calculated by

$$4.27 \text{ liters} \times 35 = 150 \text{ liters}$$

If the measured value for MVV is significantly less than the estimated value, it is likely that subject effort was submaximal.

MVV should be determined from a series of at least two acceptable maneuvers. Maneuvers should be repeated and acceptable results collected until test *reproducibility* is demonstrated. Criteria for MVV test maneuver *acceptability* are stated in Table 2–9. MVV test *reproducibility* criteria are stated in Table 2–10. Most subjects will tolerate performing MVV maneuvers only two or three times and often less. Some subjects who have hyperreactive airways (asthma) may experience bronchospasm from performing an MVV test maneuver. If bronchospasm occurs, the results of following MVV tests will be poorer, and air trapping may be demonstrated in the test tracing.

Once satisfactory results have been accumulated, the data to be reported must be selected. The MVV to be reported is the one from the best MVV test. The criteria for MVV *best test* selection are stated in Table 2–10.

## INTERPRETATION OF TEST RESULTS

Normal values for MVV are directly related to height and are indirectly related to age. Values are greater for taller subjects and become less as subjects become older. Male subjects tend to have greater MVV values than female subjects. Example values for young

**TABLE 2–11   Approximate Normal Adult Values for MVV**

| | |
|---|---|
| Male | = 160 l/min |
| Female | = 120 l/min |

*Note: These values are for 20-year-old subjects of average height and weight.*

adult males and females are shown in Table 2–11. Test results that are within ±30 percent of the predicted value for a subject are considered normal.

The MVV test is useful in interpreting a subject's ventilatory response to exercise during stress testing. It tests the ability to sustain an elevated level of ventilation. Abnormal MVV values are demonstrated when a subject has clinically significant restrictive or, especially, obstructive disease. It is possible for subjects with restrictive pulmonary disorders to have values for MVV that are within normal tolerances. This is because they are able to compensate for the lack of volume increase with significant increases in breathing rate. Moderate to severe obstructive disorders, however, may produce abnormal values for MVV. These abnormal values are largely due to the exaggerated air trapping and ventilatory muscle fatigue that occur with this type of forced breathing pattern.

# AIRWAY RESISTANCE/CONDUCTANCE

## TEST DESCRIPTION

Resistance to air flow ($R_{fl}$) in the pulmonary system is the result of friction between the gas molecules and also between gas molecules and the airway walls. *Airway resistance* ($R_{aw}$) is a measure of the $R_{fl}$ in the pulmonary system. It is the drive pressure required to create a flow of air through a subject's airways. The drive pressure is the difference between atmospheric pressure ($P_{Atm}$) and alveolar pressure ($P_A$) during ventilation. Assuming that the $P_{Atm}$ is constant at zero, changes in $P_A$ create the drive force responsible for ventilation. This relationship can be expressed by the equation,

$$R_{aw} = \frac{P_{Atm-A} \text{ difference}}{\dot{V}} = \frac{P_A}{\dot{V}}$$

Airway passages in the subject that affect $R_{aw}$ with mouth breathing include the mouth; pharynx; larynx; larger, central airways; and smaller, peripheral airways. The diameter of airways within the thorax changes during the breathing cycle. On inspiration, intrathoracic airways are dilated by the more negative intrapleural pressures. Conversely, these airways narrow and return to a resting diameter during expiration. As a result, $R_{aw}$ is less at large lung volumes and is more at small lung volumes. On the same basis, $R_{aw}$ is less during inspiration and is more during expiration. The unit of measure for $R_{aw}$ is cm $H_2O$/l/sec.

*Airway conductance* ($G_{aw}$) is the reciprocal of $R_{aw}$, as demonstrated by the following equation:

$$G_{aw} = \frac{1}{R_{aw}}$$

$G_{aw}$ is a measure of the flow that is generated from the available drive pressure. The unit of measure for $G_{aw}$ is l/sec/cm $H_2O$. As values for $R_{aw}$ increase, the values for $G_{aw}$ in the same subject will decrease.

As described earlier, the values for $R_{aw}$ and $G_{aw}$ vary depending on the lung volume at which they are measured. To allow for standardized, comparable measurements, both are often reported in a way that relates to the lung volume at the time of measurement. This is done by dividing the values for $R_{aw}$ and $G_{aw}$ by the lung volume ($V_L$) at which they were measured.

Since $R_{aw}$ measurement is generally performed at the FRC level, this is the volume that is used. The results are referred to as *specific airway resistance* ($SR_{aw}$) and *specific airway conductance* ($SG_{aw}$). The calculations may be performed as follows:

$$SR_{aw} = \frac{R_{aw}}{V_L} \qquad SG_{aw} = \frac{1/R_{aw}}{V_L}$$

The value of this adjustment is that $R_{aw}$ and $G_{aw}$ comparisons can be made between subjects having different lung volumes and for the same subject at different lung volumes. $SR_{aw}$ is not generally used in the clinical setting.

## EQUIPMENT REQUIRED

A body plethysmograph system is used for the measurement of $R_{aw}$. This is significant because it allows for measurement of both $R_{aw}$ and the subject's lung volume at the same time. Ventilatory flow rates, mouth pressure, and changes in cabinet pressure (with constant-volume/variable-pressure plethysmographs) are measured.

## TEST ADMINISTRATION

$R_{aw}$ is measured with the subject performing a panting-type breathing maneuver. This maneuver is important for three reasons:

- The subject's glottis is open to limit its influence on $R_{aw}$ values.
- The measurement of $R_{aw}$ is performed fairly consistently at the FRC level.
- Artifacts and distortions in the tracing can be minimized.

The subject should be observed during test administration in order to prevent grunting during the panting maneuver. Grunting could artificially increase the measured $R_{aw}$ value.

Separate measurements are made to determine $P_A$ and $\dot{V}$ (Figure 2–10A). $\dot{V}$ is measured while the subject is panting and the plethysmograph shutter is open (SO). $P_A$ is measured while the subject is panting and the shutter is closed (SC). Operation and use of the shutter mechanism of a body plethysmograph will be described in more detail in Chapter 4.

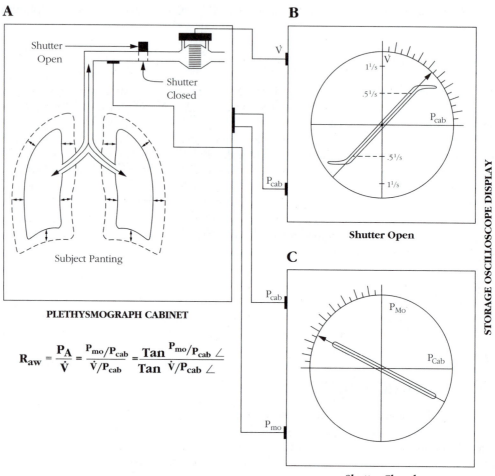

A

Shutter Open

Shutter Closed

Subject Panting

**PLETHYSMOGRAPH CABINET**

B

$\dot{V}$

$1^1/s$

$.5^1/s$

$P_{cab}$

$.5^1/s$

$1^1/s$

**Shutter Open**

C

$P_{cab}$

$P_{Mo}$

$P_{Cab}$

$P_{mo}$

**Shutter Closed**

**STORAGE OSCILLOSCOPE DISPLAY**

$$R_{aw} = \frac{P_A}{\dot{V}} = \frac{P_{mo}/P_{cab}}{\dot{V}/P_{cab}} = \frac{Tan \; P_{mo}/P_{cab} \angle}{Tan \; \dot{V}/P_{cab} \angle}$$

**Figure 2–10**   *Plethysmographic measurement of airway resistance.*

With the airway blocked, changes in $P_{Mo}$ are used to reflect changes in $P_A$. Given these measurements, an equation for determining $R_{aw}$ would be

$$R_{aw} = \frac{P_{Mo}(SC)}{\dot{V}(SO)}$$

In performing the test, the subject first pants with the shutter open. Flow changes are measured. The shutter is then closed at the end-expiratory FRC level while the subject continues to pant. This allows measurement of changes in $P_{Mo}$. Because the $\dot{V}$ and $P_{Mo}$ measurements are made separately and under different conditions (SO and SC), a basis for standardization must be established. This is done by relating changes in both $\dot{V}$ and $P_{Mo}$ to changes in plethysmograph cabinet pressure ($P_{Cab}$) during the panting maneuvers. Figure 2–10 shows the tracings for both $\dot{V}/P_{Cab}$ (2–10B) and $P_{Mo}/P_{Cab}$ (2–10C). In determining $R_{aw}$, the following equation is used:

$$R_{aw} = \frac{P_{Mo}/P_{Cab}}{\dot{V}/P_{Cab}}$$

Calculating $R_{aw}$ in this manner is important for two reasons. First, it allows the determination to be based on measurements made under two different conditions, SO and SC. Second, the $P_{Mo}/P_{Cab}$ tracing may also be used to determine a value for thoracic gas volume ($V_{TG}$). Determination of $V_{TG}$, which is a method for measuring FRC, will be described in Chapter 4. Obtaining a value for $V_{TG}$ (or FRC) at the time $R_{aw}$ is measured enables values for $SR_{aw}$ and $SG_{aw}$ to be obtained.

Average values for both $\dot{V}/P_{Cab}$ and $P_{Mo}/P_{Cab}$ can be determined directly by using the angle tangent value (tan $\angle$) for the slope of each tracing. This allows calculation of an average value for $R_{aw}$ throughout the panting maneuver. The resulting equation for calculating $R_{aw}$ is

$$R_{aw} = \frac{\tan \angle P_{Mo}/P_{Cab}}{\tan \angle \dot{V}/P_{Cab}}$$

Figure 2–10B illustrates that the $\dot{V}/P_{Cab}$ tracing may, in some subjects, assume a sigmoid shape. Considerable hysteresis may be demonstrated because of high air flow rate turbulence in the subject's airways. The turbulence makes establishing a representative slope angle for the tracing difficult. To reduce the problem, a segment of the tracing between 0.5 1/sec above and below the zero flow point is used to establish a slope. This range limit is shown in Figure 2–10B; it provides the best representation of flow during the panting maneuver.

A calibration factor for both $\dot{V}$ ($\dot{V}$ Cal) and $P_{Mo}$ ($P_{Mo}$ Cal) must be included in the $R_{aw}$ equation. Determination of these calibration factors will be discussed in Chapter 16. The flow resistance of the plethysmograph airway system ($R_{sys}$) must also be subtracted. Therefore, the final equation for calculating $R_{aw}$ is as follows:

$$R_{aw} = \left[ \left( \frac{\tan \angle P_{Mo}/P_{Cab}}{\tan \angle \dot{V}/P_{Cab}} \right) \times \left( \frac{P_{Mo}\ Cal}{\dot{V}\ Cal} \right) \right] - R_{sys}$$

The Study Section of this textbook contains a sample calculation for the determination of $R_{aw}$.

Several measurement maneuvers should be performed during the test. The slope tangent values for the maneuvers *should not* be averaged to determine an average $R_{aw}$. Instead, the $R_{aw}$ for each maneuver should be calculated separately. The average value for $R_{aw}$ can then be calculated from the separately calculated $R_{aw}$ values. A value for $V_{TG}$ (FRC), in this case, will need to be calculated separately for each test maneuver.

The mean $R_{aw}$ of several measurement maneuvers can be used as the reported $R_{aw}$ value. Another method is to report the $R_{aw}$ value measured at a lung volume ($V_{TG}$) that is closest to the subject's previously measured FRC. The values for $G_{aw}$, $SR_{aw}$, and $SG_{aw}$ are calculated from the values of $R_{aw}$ and $V_{TG}$ that were selected for reporting.

---

**TABLE 2–12   Normal Adult Values for $R_{aw}$ Determinations**

---

$$R_{aw} = 0.6\text{–}2.8 \text{ cm } H_2O/l/sec$$
$$SR_{aw} = 0.190\text{–}0.667 \text{ cm } H_2O/l/sec/l$$
$$G_{aw} = 0.36\text{–}1.70 \text{ l/sec/cm } H_2O$$
$$SG_{aw} = 0.114\text{–}0.404 \text{ l/sec/cm } H_2O/l$$

---

## INTERPRETATION OF TEST RESULTS

During normal quiet, resting ventilation, the *work of breathing* (WOB) is distributed over elastic and nonelastic sources of resistance to breathing:

1. 65% of the normal WOB is due to *elastic resistance* to ventilation, also referred to as *pulmonary/thoracic compliance*.
2. 35% of the normal WOB is due to *nonelastic resistance* to ventilation. These nonelastic resistances to ventilation include:
   - *Flow resistance*, also referred to as $R_{aw}$, which accounts for 80% of all nonelastic resistance and 28% of the overall resistance to ventilation.
   - *Tissue resistance*, which is the least significant source of resistance to ventilation. It accounts for only 20% of all nonelastic resistance and 7% of the overall resistance to ventilation.

The majority of normal $R_{aw}$ (approximately 90%) is the result of air flow through airways greater than 2.0 mm in diameter. These include the larger, central airways. The airways themselves may be larger in diameter, but their total cross-sectional area at any given level in the tracheobronchial tree is limited. A large airway disorder can rapidly demonstrate itself through increased $R_{aw}$ and WOB.

The smaller, peripheral airways (less than 2.0 mm in diameter) normally contribute very little to $R_{aw}$ because their combined cross-sectional area is so large. This is the reason why a significant amount of small airway disease must occur before the subject's $R_{aw}$ and WOB will be noticeably affected.

The normal values for airway resistance and related parameters are given in Table 2–12. As stated before, a subject's measured $R_{aw}$ is variable, depending on the lung volume at which it is measured. For this reason, it is better to use volume-independent values in making clinical assessments. Determinations of $SR_{aw}$ and $SG_{aw}$ are therefore very useful.

$R_{aw}$ will increase in disorders where the cross-sectional area of the airways has become smaller. These areas can occur in either the larger upper or smaller peripheral airways. Table 2–8 lists obstructive disorders of both the large and small airways. Used in conjunction with flow/volume loops, low-density spirometry, and clinical data, $R_{aw}$ is a valuable tool in evaluating airway disorders. Table 2–13 provides reference values for the degree of severity associated with $R_{aw}$ disorders.

---

TABLE 2–13  **Assignment of Severity for $R_{aw}$ Disorders**

| $R_{aw}$ (cm $H_2O$/l/sec) | Severity |
|---|---|
| 2.8–4.5 | Mild |
| 4.5–8.0 | Moderate |
| >8.0 | Severe |

---

# ELASTIC RECOIL PRESSURE/COMPLIANCE

## TEST DESCRIPTION

The elastic resistance of the lungs can be evaluated by measurements of elastic recoil pressure, compliance, and dynamic compliance. *Elastic recoil pressure* is an indication of the elastic force that is generated by the thoracic/lung system when the lungs are expanded. This force is measured at a specific lung volume. It is generally measured at the TLC level after a maximal inspiration and is referred to as the *maximum elastic recoil pressure*. The units used in reporting elastic recoil pressure are cm $H_2O$, along with the volume at which it was measured.

   *Compliance* is an indication of the elastic resistance ($R_{el}$) to ventilation. It is the amount of transpulmonary pressure ($P_L$) change required to produce a certain change in lung volume. The units used are l/cm $H_2O$ or ml/cm $H_2O$. $R_{el}$ to breathing is the combined result of how *lung compliance* ($C_L$) and *thoracic compliance* ($C_T$) affect the work of breathing. Together, $C_L$ and $C_T$ work to create a total *lung/thoracic compliance* ($C_{LT}$). The mathematical relationship between $C_L$, $C_T$, and $C_{LT}$ is the same as for any other system of resistance, electrical or otherwise:

$$\frac{1}{R_1} + \frac{1}{R_2} = \frac{1}{R_{Total}}$$

or, for the pulmonary system,

$$\frac{1}{C_L} + \frac{1}{C_T} = \frac{1}{C_{LT}}$$

It is significant how this mathematical model expresses the combining of individual sources of resistance to form a system of resistance. Basically, the joining of two resistances to ventilation ($C_L$ and $C_T$) results in a greater combined resistance to ventilation ($C_{LT}$). Said in a different way, with the combined resistance of $C_{LT}$, there is less inspired volume moved per cm $H_2O$ of inspiratory work than would be the case with either $C_L$ or $C_T$ alone. By substituting normal values for $C_L$, $C_T$, and $C_{LT}$, the correctness of this relationship can be demonstrated:

$$\frac{1}{0.2 \text{ l/cm } H_2O} + \frac{1}{0.2 \text{ l/cm } H_2O} = \frac{1}{0.1 \text{ l/cm } H_2O}$$

If each fraction is solved and the units canceled, the math works out as follows:

$5 + 5 = 10$

As will be described, both $C_{LT}$ and $C_L$ can be measured directly through testing procedures. $C_T$ must be calculated from the results of $C_{LT}$ and $C_L$ measurement.

*Dynamic compliance* ($C_{Dyn}$) is a measure of the combined effect of both the $R_{el}$ and $R_{fl}$ that must be overcome during ventilation. It is measured during periods of air flow during breathing. Because the WOB effects of $R_{fl}$ ($R_{aw}$) and $R_{el}$ ($C_{LT}$) are combined in $C_{Dyn}$, the value of $C_{Dyn}$ will be smaller than the value of $C_{LT}$ in the same subject. This means that $C_{Dyn}$ represents the greatest overall WOB; that is, the least inspiratory volume change is measured for a given cm $H_2O$ work of breathing.

## EQUIPMENT REQUIRED

A plethysmograph system generally provides the most convenient arrangement for measuring elastic recoil pressures and compliance. Its components allow the control of subject breathing along with measurement. As will be described, measurement of $C_L$ requires the subject to swallow a special balloon. A pressure-sensing transducer system is linked to the balloon.

## TEST ADMINISTRATION

The subject's lung volume history must be standardized just prior to administration of tests for maximum recoil pressure and compliance. This minimizes the effect that pretest breathing patterns may have on the test results. The lung volume history standardization is done by having the subject perform a maximum inspiration followed by a passive expiration back to the FRC level. Once this standardization maneuver has been completed, the test maneuvers may be performed.

### Elastic Recoil Pressure

Elastic recoil pressure is based on measuring the transpulmonary pressure ($P_L$) required to generate a maximum inspiratory volume. $P_L$ is the difference between alveolar pressure ($P_A$) and intrapleural pressure ($P_{pl}$). The following equation demonstrates this relationship:

$P_L = P_A - P_{pl}$

It may be assumed that $P_A$ is equal to atmospheric pressure (0 mm Hg) during periods of no air flow into or out of the lung. As a result, changes in $P_{pl}$ alone can be used to reflect changes in $P_L$.

During the procedure, $P_{pl}$ changes are measured through changes in esophageal pressure. This is done by having the subject swallow a 10 cm long esophageal balloon. The balloon's length minimizes the effects of esophageal **peristalsis** on balloon pressure. A catheter, with the balloon at its distal end, is passed through one nostril, the nasopharynx, and into the esophagus. When the balloon is positioned in the lower third of the esophagus, esophageal pressure ($P_{eso}$) changes approximate changes in $P_{pl}$. A spirometer system is used at the same time for measuring the lung volume changes during breathing.

For measurement of maximum recoil pressure, the subject performs a maximum inspiratory maneuver and holds the effort at the TLC level for several seconds. The highest initial $P_{pl}$ value, as soon as the TLC level is reached and air flow has stopped, is recorded for the elastic recoil pressure. The initial higher pressure is used because the $P_{pl}$ value decays (decreases) as inspiration is maintained. This pressure decrease is thought to be due to "stress relaxation" of the lung.

## Lung Compliance

$C_L$ is determined by relating $P_L$ changes during breathing to changes in lung volume. Measurements made during lung deflation are the most useful in clinical applications. A body plethysmograph provides components useful for measuring $C_L$. The test procedure begins with the subject inhaling to the TLC level. A slow expiration down to the FRC, or possibly residual volume (RV), level is then performed. During expiration, the shutter in the pneumotachometer circuit is used to intermittently occlude the subject's airway for one to two seconds.

With each occlusion, the subject must hold the expiratory effort at that lung volume (glottis open). After the expiratory hold has caused the expiratory air flow to cease, a value for the subject's $P_{pl}$ is measured and recorded. A value for $P_{pl}$ is determined through measurement of a value for $P_{eso}$ as described previously. The data collected from this test are either manually or electronically plotted on a graph (Figure 2–11). A line is then marked on the curve from the FRC volume to the FRC plus 0.5 liter (FRC 0.5) volume. The value

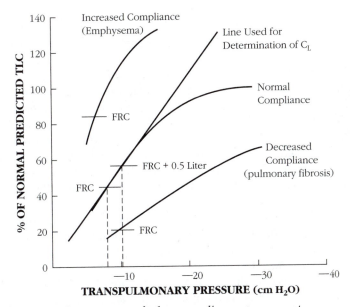

**Figure 2–11** *Static volume/pressure curve for lung compliance measurement.*

for $C_L$ is based on the slope of this line. Using the changes in lung volume ($\Delta V_L$) and $P_{pl}$ ($\Delta P_{pl}$) indicated by the line, $C_L$ can be calculated using the following equation:

$$C_L = \frac{\Delta V_L}{\Delta P_{pl}} = \frac{0.5 \text{ liter}}{P_{pl}FRC\ 0.5 - P_{pl}FRC}$$

The tangent value for the line slope can be used if it is indicated directly by the measuring system. At least three volume-pressure curves should be measured, with separate $C_L$ determinations made for each.

A value for inspiratory $C_L$ may be determined. Airway occlusion and $P_{pl}$ measurements are performed while the subject inhales from the FRC (or RV) level to TLC. If an expiratory $C_L$ value is also desired for the subject, it should be performed with expiration during the same breath. Most subjects find it difficult to perform this full inflation-deflation $C_L$-measurement procedure. If it can be done, however, the results provide information on the amount of hysteresis that exists between the inflation and deflation curves.

## Total Lung/Thoracic Compliance

$C_{LT}$ is based on the change in transthoracic/pulmonary pressure ($P_{TL}$) required to produce a change in $V_L$, or

$$C_{LT} = \frac{\Delta V_L}{\Delta P_{TL}}$$

$P_{TL}$ is the difference between atmospheric pressure ($P_{Atm}$) and $P_A$ when there is no air flow in the lungs. The relationship is

$$P_{TL} = P_{Atm} - P_A$$

The difficulty in determining a value for $C_{LT}$ is that *the $P_{TL}$ measurements must be made with the subject's ventilatory muscles completely relaxed.* Three methods are possible. One method involves having the subject's torso and extremities inside a sealed chamber similar to an iron lung ventilator. As the $P_{Atm}$ of the chamber is made more negative, larger (than at rest) lung volumes are produced and measured with a spirometer. $P_A$, when there is no air flow through the lungs, may be assumed to be atmospheric, or 0.0 mm Hg.

Another method uses an opposite principle. The subject, preferably anesthetized, is intubated with an endotracheal tube. Introduction of larger (than at rest) measured lung volumes into the subject generates higher positive $P_a$ values. Pressures measured at the endotracheal tube may be substituted for $P_A$ when there is no air flow. The $P_{Atm}$ is truly atmospheric and is constant at 0.0 mm Hg.

The final method for $C_{LT}$ determination makes use of the shutter/pneumotachometer system of a body plethysmograph. The subject inspires a series of measured lung volumes through the pneumotachometer. At each lung volume, the shutter is closed so that the subject's inspiratory muscles may be relaxed completely against it. Mouth pressure is measured, and if there is no air flow, it may be assumed to approximate $P_A$. The $P_{Atm}$, again, is truly atmospheric and is constant at 0.0 mm Hg.

Because compliance is affected by the lung volume at which it is measured, it is helpful to standardize $C_{LT}$ to a subject's lung volume. *Specific compliance* ($SC_{LT}$) provides a method based on correlating a subject's $C_{LT}$ value to the value of the subject's FRC:

$$SC_{LT} = \frac{C_{LT}}{FRC}$$

This correlation allows evaluation of a subject's $C_{LT}$ despite changes in her or his FRC as a result of disorders.

## Thoracic Compliance

As stated previously, $C_T$ cannot be measured directly. However, once $C_L$ and $C_{LT}$ have been determined, $C_T$ can then be calculated. Based on the relationship described earlier, the equation for calculating $C_T$ is as follows:

$$\frac{1}{C_T} = \frac{1}{C_{LT}} - \frac{1}{C_L}$$

## Dynamic Compliance

$C_{Dyn}$ can be measured during quiet tidal breathing. The same equipment arrangement as was described for $C_L$ can be used. Determination is based on dividing the measured tidal volume ($V_T$) by the change in $P_{pl}$ ($\Delta P_{pl}$) during breathing. $\Delta P_{pl}$ is the difference between the end-inspiratory ($P_{pl}insp$) and end-expiratory ($P_{pl}exp$) $P_{pl}$ values. The following equation demonstrates determination of $C_{Dyn}$:

$$C_{Dyn} = \frac{V_T}{\Delta P_{pl}} = \frac{V_T}{P_{pl}insp - P_{pl}exp}$$

*Frequency dependence of compliance* can be evaluated by measuring values for $C_{Dyn}$ at different subject respiratory rates. During measurement, it is important for the subject to breathe with a constant $V_T$. Use of a real-time $V_T$ display can help the subject maintain a constant volume. First, the subject must inhale to TLC and exhale back to FRC. Then, with the subject maintaining a constant $V_T$, $P_{pl}$ measurements are made at different subject breathing rates. Afterward, the subject must perform another inspiration to TLC. $C_{Dyn}$ determinations are made based on the $P_{pl}$ value measured at each respiratory rate. The pre- and post-TLC-maneuver measurements allow the technologist to judge whether or not a change in the end-expiratory volume resulted from the procedure.

## INTERPRETATION OF TEST RESULTS

Normal values for factors relating to elastic resistance in the pulmonary system are listed in Table 2–14. Values for maximum elastic recoil pressure decrease slightly with advancing age. Values for $C_L$ are directly proportional to both subject age and height. $C_L$ increases slightly with greater age and height. Male subjects demonstrate slightly greater values for $C_L$ than do females.

---

**TABLE 2–14   Normal Adult Values for Elastic Resistance Factors**

---

Elastic Recoil Pressure = 34 cm $H_2O$

$$C_L = 0.2 \text{ l/cm } H_2O$$

$$C_T = 0.2 \text{ l/cm } H_2O$$

$$C_{LT} = 0.1 \text{ l/cm } H_2O$$

$$SC_{LT} = 0.05\text{–}0.06 \text{ l/cm } H_2O/l$$

$$C_{Dyn} = 0.09\text{–}0.07 \text{ l/cm } H_2O \text{ (at a flow of 0.5 l/sec)}$$

---

Serial determinations of compliance are useful in following the progress of disorders. Restrictive pulmonary disorders produce reductions in $C_L$. Restrictive extrapulmonary disorders can be responsible for reductions in $C_T$. Table 2–8 provides a list of restrictive disorders. Emphysema produces abnormal increases in $C_L$. But the increased lung volumes resulting from emphysema cause $C_T$ values in those subjects to be reduced. Because of the increased $C_L$ and off-setting decrease in $C_T$, subjects with emphysema often demonstrate a normal value for $C_{LT}$.

$C_{Dyn}$ and its relation to breathing frequency provides a sensitive tool for evaluating obstructive airway disorders. Table 2–8 provides a list of obstructive airway disorders. In normal subjects, increased breathing frequencies produce only slight decreases in $C_{Dyn}$. With obstructive pulmonary disorders, however, faster breathing rates can cause very significant reductions in $C_{Dyn}$ values. For example, small airway obstruction may be suspected if a subject's $C_{Dyn}$ while breathing at a rate of 60 breaths per minute is less than 75% of the value measured at a breathing rate of 20. This may be true even if values for $R_{aw}$ and other pulmonary function parameters are within normal ranges.

# MAXIMUM INSPIRATORY AND EXPIRATORY PRESSURES

## TEST DESCRIPTION

Tests for *maximum inspiratory pressure* (MIP) and *maximum expiratory pressure* (MEP) measure a subject's ventilatory muscle strength. Both tests are administered with the subject performing maximum ventilatory maneuvers against an occluded airway. MIP is a measure of the most negative (subatmospheric) pressure that can be generated with an inspiratory effort. Generally the subject initiates the maneuver from the RV volume level. This maneuver provides a strength test for the diaphragm, intercostals, and inspiratory

---

TABLE 2–15   Use of MIP and MEP Tests

---

### Use of MIP Evaluation

---

- Assessment of neuromuscular disorders or injury of the inspiratory muscles.
- Assessment of reduced inspiratory muscle strength resulting from
     *Chronic lung hyperinflation (emphysema)*
     *Severe chest wall deformities*
     *Effects of drugs*
- Assessment of inspiratory muscle strength for monitoring
     *Weaning from continuous mechanical ventilation*
     *Breathing-retraining exercises*

---

### Use of MEP Evaluation

---

- Assessment of neuromuscular disorders or injury of the expiratory muscles.
- Assessment of impaired cough function with retained secretions.
- Assessment of weaning from continuous mechanical ventilation.

---

accessory muscles. It relates to a subject's ability to breathe sufficiently deeply to maintain ventilation and a ventilatory reserve.

MEP is the greatest positive (supra-atmospheric) pressure that a subject can generate. The maneuver for MEP measurement is initiated from the TLC volume level. It provides a test of strength for the abdominal muscles and other accessory muscles for expiration. Lung and thoracic elastic recoil also affect the results of an MEP maneuver. The ability of a subject to cough effectively relates directly to the capacity to generate a sufficient MEP.

Units of either cm $H_2O$ or mm Hg may be used when reporting results for MIP and MEP tests. Neither of these tests is routinely performed as part of pulmonary function assessment in the laboratory. Table 2–15 provides a list of clinical situations where MIP and MEP may be useful.

## EQUIPMENT REQUIRED

A three-way directional breathing valve or a shutter mechanism is required to provide intermittent airway occlusion. An apparatus for measuring airway pressure changes is also needed. Either a direct-reading dial-type manometer or an electronic pressure transducer and recorder may be used. The measurement capabilities for MIP should range from at least −10 cm $H_2O$ to, minimally, −60 cm $H_2O$ or to as much as −120 cm $H_2O$. For MEP, the measurement capabilities should range from 0.0 cm $H_2O$ to, minimally, +100 cm $H_2O$.

Nose clips and a flanged mouthpiece are required to maintain an airtight seal during the procedure. A controlled leak between the occlusion apparatus and the subject is needed to minimize the possible influence of the subject's cheek muscles. The leak may be produced by use of a tube 15 mm long with an inner diameter of 1 mm or similar size. A large-bore needle may be sufficient to allow air to enter the oral cavity in compensation but not affect the accuracy of the measurement.

## TEST ADMINISTRATION

The subject should be connected to the breathing circuit with nose clips on and be allowed a brief adjustment period prior to pressure measurement. For MIP, the subject should be instructed to exhale to the RV level. At end-expiration, the airway is occluded. The subject must then make a maximal inspiratory effort for at least three but not more than five seconds. The most negative pressure *after the first second of effort* should be recorded. With rest periods in between, the test should be repeated two more times for a total of three recorded maneuvers.

For MEP, the subject must inhale to the TLC level prior to airway occlusion. The subject then performs an expiratory maneuver with maximal effort. The most positive pressure (ignoring the transient initial maximum) with two or three seconds of subject effort should be recorded. If a pressure greater than 100 cm $H_2O$ is achieved, repeat tests are not clinically necessary. Results less than this may indicate the need for repeat attempts.

## INTERPRETATION OF TEST RESULTS

Table 2–16 provides approximate normal values for MIP and MEP.

> **QUALITY ASSURANCE NOTE:** Poor patient effort must initially be suspected when less than normal test results are demonstrated. This is because of the very effort-dependent nature of these tests. Normal values are generally greater for males than for females. They become less with advancing age.

Generally, there is not a strong correlation between MIP, MEP, and other pulmonary mechanics tests, especially the ones that are relatively effort-independent. For this reason,

---

**TABLE 2–16  Normal Adult Values for MIP and MEP**

| | |
|---|---|
| Normal values that are generally accepted as being clinical useful: | |
| MIP | $>-60$ cm $H_2O$ |
| MEP | $>+80$ to 100 cm $H_2O$ |

| Examples of normal values using some available predictive equations (based on a 20-year-old subject): | | |
|---|---|---|
| Males | MIP | $-132$ cm $H_2O$ |
| | MEP | $+247$ cm $H_2O$ |
| Females | MIP | $-94$ cm $H_2O$ |
| | MEP | $+160$ cm $H_2O$ |

---

*Note: The values predicted by these equations are often considered to be excessively large. These high values may be due to the special mouthpiece used for the study on which the predictive equations are based.*

it is difficult to assign a series of impairment levels to less than normal MIP and MEP results. Significant reductions of MIP and MEP are required before reductions in VC may be demonstrated. A subject's MVV is more greatly affected by reductions in MIP than by reductions in MEP.

It is generally accepted that an MIP value of $-20$ cm $H_2O$ or smaller indicates a need for mechanical ventilatory support. Subjects with an MEP value of less than $+40$ cm $H_2O$ may have difficulty in coughing effectively and clearing secretions. It has been found that subjects with generalized neuromuscular disorders may demonstrate reductions in both MIP and MEP. Quadriplegic subjects, however, demonstrate a greater loss of MEP than of MIP. Moreover, MIP results may improve significantly as a result of therapy in quadriplegics.

## Review Questions

Please use the following review questions to evaluate your learning of information from this chapter. It might be helpful to write out your answers on a sheet of paper. If you are unsure of the answers to these questions, review the chapter to reinforce your learning.

1. What is an FVC maneuver? How is it measured?
2. What types of tracings can be made from an FVC maneuver?
3. Relating to the measured components of a volume/time tracing from an FVC maneuver:
   a. What are the measured components of a volume/time tracing from an FVC maneuver?
   b. What are normal values for each identified components?
   c. What is the clinical significance of each component?
   d. How do obstructive and restrictive pulmonary disorders affect the values of the identified components?
4. Relating to the measured components of flow/volume loop tracing from an FVC maneuver:
   a. What are the measured components of flow/volume loop tracing from an FVC maneuver?
   b. What are normal values for each identified component?
   c. What is the clinical significance of each identified component?
5. What are criteria for test repetition, acceptability, reproducibility, and data selection for reporting for FVC testing?
6. Relating to low-density gas spirometry:
   a. What is the diagnostic significance of low-density gas spirometry?
   b. How is low-density gas spirometry performed?
   c. How are the results of low-density gas spirometry interpreted?
7. Relating to PEFR monitoring:
   a. How is PEFR monitoring performed?
   b. What key points should be taught for home monitoring of PEFRs?

     c. What is the relationship between PEFR monitoring and the effects of large and small airway obstruction?

     d. How can PEFR monitoring be used for patients receiving bronchodilators?

8. Relating to MVV maneuver testing:
     a. What is an MVV maneuver test?
     b. What instructions should be given to the subject prior to performing an MVV test?
     c. What is the method for determining a target value for MVV?
     d. What are the criteria for test repetition, acceptability, reproducibility, and data selection for reporting for MVV testing?
     e. How do obstructive pulmonary disorders affect MVV values?

9. Relating to the measurement of airway resistance/conductance:
     a. How is airway resistance/conductance measured?
     b. How can these measurements be used to evaluate pulmonary disorders?

10. Relating to the measurement of elastic recoil pressure/compliance:
     a. How is elastic recoil pressure/compliance measured?
     b. What types of measurements are made?
     c. How do restrictive and obstructive disorders affect elastic recoil pressure/compliance measurements?

11. Relating to the measurement of MIP and MEP:
     a. How are MIP and MEP measured?
     b. How can MIP and MEP measurements be used?
     c. What are normal MIP and MEP values, and what are values that indicate clinically significant changes?

# CHAPTER THREE

# EQUIPMENT FOR GAS ANALYSIS

## ———— RELATED LEARNING ————

Prior knowledge of the following related information will facilitate understanding and learning of the material in this chapter. The learner will be aided by being able to

1. Describe the operation and use of display and recording systems as presented in Chapter 1.
2. Relate the information in this chapter to basic concepts of gas chemistry and physics.

## ———— LEARNING OBJECTIVES ————

Upon successful completion of this chapter, the learner should be able to

1. Describe the construction, operation, and use of the following types of oxygen analyzers:
   a. paramagnetic analyzers
   b. thermal conductivity analyzers
   c. electrochemical analyzers
2. Discuss the following general concerns in regard to oxygen analyzers:
   a. sampling characteristics
   b. direct measurement of partial pressure versus concentration of oxygen
   c. effects of humidity on the calibration of oxygen analyzers
3. Describe the operation and use of the following dedicated gas analyzers:
   a. thermoconductivity helium analyzers
   b. photointensity nitrogen analyzers
   c. infrared $CO/CO_2$ analyzers
4. Describe the operation and use of the following spectrum gas analyzers:
   a. gas chromatograph
   b. mass spectrometer

—————————— **KEY TERMS** ——————————

adsorption                                    electrical potential
desiccant                                     galvanometer
diatomaceous earth

Gas and blood gas analyzers play an important role in assessing pulmonary function. Gas analyzers are required for many pulmonary function tests. They are generally included as components in laboratory-based testing systems. Analyzer systems can be divided into two groups. *Dedicated analyzers* are used to analyze a single gas component in a mixed-gas sample. A good example of this type of analyzer is the commonly used oxygen analyzer. The electrodes incorporated in blood gas analyzers are each dedicated to a specific gas. It should be noted that the same basic principle of operation applies to analyzers dedicated for use with different gases. For example, thermal conductivity measuring systems can be used for oxygen analyzers as well as for helium analyzers.

*Spectrum analyzers* are able to analyze a mixed-gas sample and determine the concentration of each of the gases within the sample. With a sample of room air, this type of analyzer could determine the quantities of nitrogen, oxygen, carbon dioxide, and so forth. Specific examples of dedicated analyzers and spectrum analyzers are described in this chapter.

Analyzer systems can have their sample measurements converted to a DC analog electrical signal. This signal can then be used to operate a display of the test results or to provide input to a measurement recording system.

# ANALYZERS FOR USE WITH GASEOUS SAMPLES

## DEDICATED GAS ANALYZERS

### Dedicated Oxygen Analyzers

Oxygen analyzers have very broad applications in health care. As a result, there are many excellent and detailed references describing their operation. An important point to note is the difference in what oxygen analyzers actually measure. All oxygen analyzers display a value for the percentage of oxygen. However, most oxygen analyzers do not in fact measure the concentration, or percentage, of oxygen. Instead, they measure the *partial pressure* of oxygen in the gas sample. These types of analyzers can provide an accurate reading of the percentage of oxygen only if they are properly calibrated at the current barometric pressure. The gases used for calibration should match the humidity level of the gas sample that is going to be analyzed. Only one type of dedicated oxygen analyzer—the thermal conductivity analyzer—is able to directly measure and display the concentration of oxygen in a sample. A review follows of the types of oxygen analyzers that may be used and some concerns for their application in the clinical setting.

*Paramagnetic Oxygen Analyzers.* Paramagnetic oxygen analyzers make use of a unique property of oxygen: its attraction to magnetic fields. Other gases are repelled by magnetic fields. These analyzers use two nitrogen-filled glass spheres in a "dumbbell" arrangement with each sphere suspended in a magnetic field. Larger quantities of oxygen in the sample will cause a greater displacement of the spheres from the magnetic fields. Paramagnetic analyzers directly measure the relative quantity of oxygen molecules attracted to the magnetic field. As a result, this measurement relates more closely to the partial pressure of oxygen in a sample than to its concentration.

Paramagnetic analyzers require a static, dry sample. This is to prevent air currents in the sample chamber from moving the glass spheres and interfering with oxygen measurement. Consequently, continuous analysis of moving gas samples is not possible with these analyzers. The gas sample must pass through a **desiccant** before analysis to prevent condensation on the moving components within the sample chamber. Paramagnetic analyzers must sit level and steady in order to provide accurate measurements. They are not frequently used.

*Thermal Conductivity Oxygen Analyzers.* The actual mechanics of thermal conductivity analyzers will be discussed in connection with their use as helium analyzers. They are useful for intermittent, single-sample analysis. Thermal conductivity oxygen analyzers do not, however, allow for continuous analysis of moving gas samples. As stated earlier, this type of analyzer responds more directly to the concentration (percent) of oxygen in the sample than to its partial pressure.

*Electrochemical Oxygen Analyzers.* With electrochemical analyzers, oxygen enters the sensor by diffusing across a membrane. Once inside, it is consumed in an electrochemical reaction, and the results of analysis appear on a display. (The principles of electrochemistry will be discussed in Chapter 10. Details and illustrations of oxygen electrochemistry will be offered there.) These analyzers directly determine the partial pressure of oxygen in the sample.

There are two types of electrochemical oxygen analyzers. Though both operate on the same basic electrochemical principle, they can differ in the materials used in their construction. There is a more important difference, however. The sensors for *galvanic fuel cell* analyzers (Figure 3–1A) use no outside current in the electrochemical reaction. The chemical consumption of oxygen alone by the sensor is used to produce a measurable electrical current. A battery may be used to operate a digital display, alarms, and so on, for the analyzer unit. This type of analyzer requires a sensor with a large surface area for contact with the gas sample. The large surface area is necessary if the response time for the analyzer is to be acceptably fast. Even with a large sensor, response time is not rapid. Sensor life expectancy is based on total accumulated oxygen consumption. Frequent use of the analyzer at high oxygen concentrations will shorten sensor life. Sensors are generally long-lived and require little maintenance. When they can no longer be calibrated correctly, they are replaced.

With the sensors for *polarographic* analyzers (Figure 3–1B) an electrical current is added to polarize the electrochemical cell. This causes the oxygen-consuming reaction to occur more easily. As a result, a sensor with a smaller membrane surface area can be used. Re-

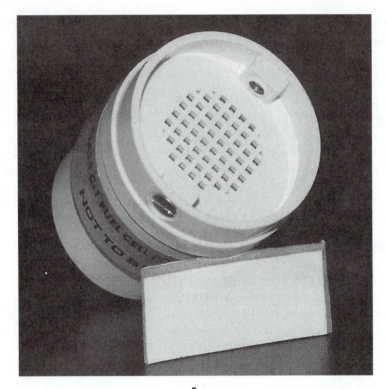

**A**

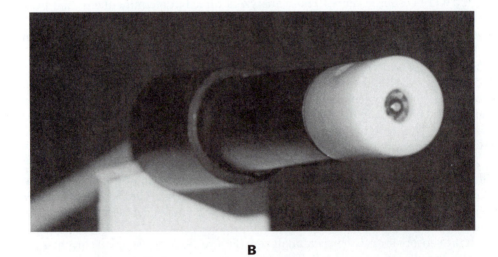

**B**

**Figure 3–1** *Examples of (A) galvanic and (B) polarographic oxygen analyzer sensors.*

sponse time for these analyzers is very rapid. Sensor life is limited, however, unless routine maintenance is performed. Maintenance includes cleaning oxidants from the sensor and replacing the electrolyte solution.

Electrochemical analyzers are the only dedicated oxygen analyzers capable of continuous measurement of moving gas samples. Although measurement is not affected by humidity, once these analyzers are calibrated, they are preferably used for analyzing dry gas samples. Condensation of moisture on the membrane will slow the rate of oxygen diffusion into the sensor. As a result, the measured $FIO_2$ displayed by the analyzer will be less than the actual $FIO_2$ of the gas that has been analyzed.

## Dedicated Helium Analyzers

Dedicated helium analyzers, as stated earlier, operate on the principle of *thermal conductivity*. They are sometimes referred to as *catharometers* or *katharometers*. Thermal conductivity analyzers make use of two significant facts. The first is that gases differ in their ability to dissipate heat. The larger the molecular weight of a gas, the greater will be its ability to dissipate heat. Additionally, as the concentration of a given gas in a mixture changes, so do the heat dissipation properties of the mixture. Second is the fact that electrical circuits operating at higher temperatures are more resistant to a current flow than are cooler circuits.

To analyze gas concentrations, a circuit called a *Wheatstone bridge* is used (Figure 3–2). A Wheatstone bridge has two resistance elements bridged by a **galvanometer**. The gal-

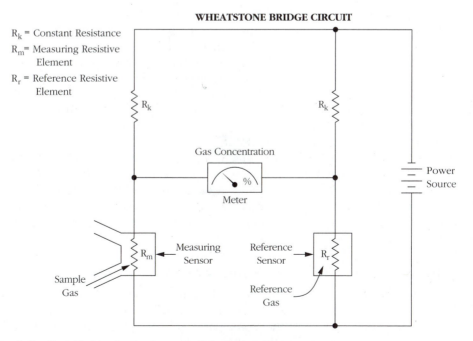

**Figure 3–2**   *Basic design of a thermoconductivity gas analyzer.*

vanometer measures the electrical resistance differences between the two elements. These elements may be thermistor beads or metal filaments. They are heated as the result of a constant current passing through them. One element is used as a measuring sensor and is exposed to the gas sample that will be analyzed. The other is used as a reference sensor. It is constantly exposed to a gas mixture that is similar in composition to the intended test sample. The reference mixture, however, has a known concentration of the gas that the analyzer is designated to measure, in this case helium.

In operation, a sample is placed in the chamber containing the measuring resistance element of the analyzer. When there is a difference in helium concentration between the test sample and the reference mixture, there will be a difference in the electrical resistances of the two elements. The resulting change in current flow through the elements is measured by the galvanometer. This measurement is then displayed as a gas concentration.

Air currents in the measuring chamber can be another source of resistive element cooling. If moving air currents are present in the sampling chamber of a thermal conductivity analyzer, then this added source of element cooling will cause a measurement error. For this reason, thermal conductivity analyzers require intermittent, static samples. They cannot be used for continuous analysis of moving gas samples. The presence of too many gases with similar molecular weights is also a source of error. Carbon dioxide and water vapor are generally removed from the sample prior to analysis in order to reduce their influence. Thermal conductivity analyzers have a relatively slow response time but are very useful in certain applications.

## Dedicated Nitrogen Analyzers

Nitrogen analyzers make their measurements on the basis of photointensity. They may be referred to as *Giesler tube ionizers*. In nitrogen analyzers a photocell is used to measure the light emitted from a sample of ionized gas. This process is called *emission spectroscopy*. A vacuum pump draws the sample gas into a chamber where it is ionized by a high-voltage electrical current (Figure 3–3). The emitted light is filtered to allow only the blue light of ionized nitrogen to pass on to the photocell. The analog electrical output of the photocell is directly proportional to the intensity of the light. Greater quantities of nitrogen in the sample produce a greater photocell output.

The accuracy of this type of analyzer may be affected by fluctuations in the vacuum pump pressure. The presence of helium or excess carbon dioxide and/or water vapor in the sample can also affect measurement accuracy. However, generally such problems do not occur in the situations where this type of analyzer is used. Photointensity nitrogen analyzers can be applied to the continuous, breath-by-breath measurement of respiratory gases.

## Dedicated Carbon Dioxide/Carbon Monoxide Analyzers

Dedicated analyzers for carbon dioxide and carbon monoxide both operate on the same principle, so only carbon monoxide analyzers will be described here. The function of these analyzers is based on the principle that some gases are able to absorb infrared radiation to a greater degree than others. The three main analyzer components are an infrared ra-

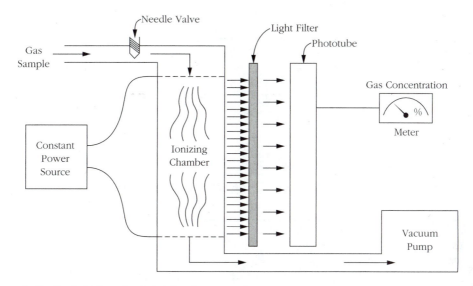

**Figure 3–3** *Basic design of a photointensity gas analyzer.*

diation source, a pair of gas-filled chambers, and a detection system (Figure 3–4). The infrared radiation source contains a filter system that allows emission of radiation selected specifically for the gas—carbon monoxide or carbon dioxide—to be analyzed.

One of the two gas-filled chambers is used to hold the test gas sample. The second is a reference chamber that holds a mixture for use in comparison with the sample. This comparison mixture has a zero concentration of the gas that the analyzer is dedicated to measuring. Radiation from the source passes through both chambers.

If quantities of carbon monoxide are present in the test sample gas, they cause absorption of some of the radiation passing through the sample chamber. Larger concentrations of carbon monoxide in the sample gas cause greater radiation absorption. Consequently, less radiation is able to pass through and out of the sample chamber. Also, less radiation passes out of the sample chamber than out of the reference chamber, since the reference chamber does not contain any carbon monoxide. Greater differences in the amount of radiation transmitted through the two chambers indicate greater amounts of carbon monoxide in the sample. A rotating chopper blade causes the radiation to be transmitted alternately through each cell at a rate of 50 times a minute.

A detector system is the third component of the analyzer system. One configuration uses a photon detector to analyze the differences in the amounts of radiation passing through the two chambers. Another configuration uses a detector system that consists of a chamber divided by a flexible metal diaphragm. A metal plate is situated near the diaphragm on the sample side of the detector. The diaphragm and plate are given opposite electrical charges. Movement of the diaphragm closer to or farther from the plate increases or decreases the **electrical potential** difference between them. Both sides of the chamber contain a quantity of the gas for which the analyzer is dedicated, in this case carbon monoxide. As the gas in one side of the detector receives and absorbs more radiation, it

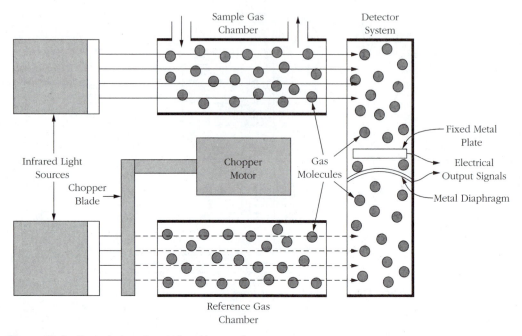

**Figure 3–4** *Basic design of an infrared gas analyzer.*

becomes heated and increases in volume. This moves the diaphragm in relation to the plate and changes the electrical potential of the system.

With a sample in place, radiation is transmitted alternately through the two chambers. This causes alternating increases and decreases in potential in the detector. Larger cyclic changes in potential indicate a greater concentration of carbon monoxide in the sample.

The gas sample for these analyzers is generally passed through a desiccant prior to measurement. Major changes in ambient temperature and/or barometric pressure may require recalibration of the analyzer. A warmup period is needed to ensure that the heat-producing components in the analyzer have reached temperature equilibrium. Such equilibrium is necessary so that heating from the transmitted radiation will be the only factor that affects the temperature and volume of the gases in the detector.

## GAS CHROMATOGRAPHS

Gas chromatographs are a type of spectrum analyzer (Figure 3–5). They operate by first separating out and holding the gas components of a mixed-gas sample. The gases are then released one at a time, and the individual quantities are analyzed. In pulmonary laboratories, thermal conductivity analyzers are generally used.

The separation and holding occurs in columns containing materials with selective **adsorptive** properties. **Diatomaceous earths** are used to adsorb, separate, and hold nitrogen, oxygen, and carbon monoxide in what is called a *molecular sieve column*. Porous polymer columns are used for separating out carbon dioxide and higher hydrocarbons. Gas separation is based on molecular weight, and generally a combination of columns is re-

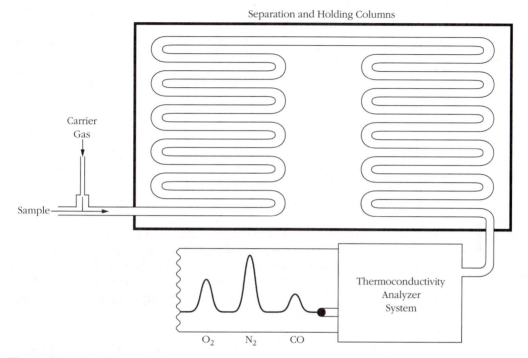

**Figure 3–5** *Basic design of a gas chromatograph.*

quired. A carrier gas such as helium, nitrogen, or hydrogen is used to carry the sample through the columns. The carrier cannot be the same as the gas the system is designed to measure.

Once adsorption has occurred, the gases are released by the columns in a predictable manner. The columns may be heated to accelerate this process. As each individual gas from the sample is discharged, its concentration is determined by the analyzer. The rising and falling of the analyzer output with each gas can be traced as a *chromatogram*. The height of each peak indicates the concentration of that gas.

Gas chromatographs are designed primarily to analyze discrete, individual samples. Analysis time can range from 30 seconds to several minutes. Gas chromatographs are generally used to determine quantities of nitrogen, oxygen, and carbon dioxide in a sample. Desiccants are employed to remove water vapor from the sample prior to analysis. Periodically, the molecular sieve columns need to be reconditioned by baking. Baking removes the carbon dioxide that tends to be trapped within them. Gas chromatographs are available in a wide range of cost and complexity.

## MASS SPECTROMETERS

Mass spectrometers are spectrum analyzers that represent the most sophisticated means for analyzing the concentrations of respiratory gases. They measure by "counting" the relative number of ionized molecules of each gas in the sample (Figure 3–6). A vacuum

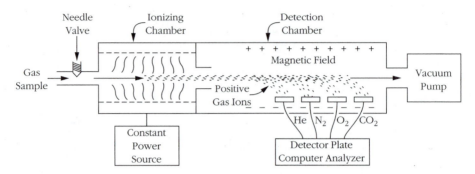

**Figure 3–6** *Basic design of a mass spectrometer.*

pump is used to draw the sample into an ionizing chamber. The gas molecules are converted into positively charged ions. These ions are then drawn into a chamber where they are attracted to a series of detection plates in the negative portion of a magnetic field. The distance an ion travels before being drawn to a detection plate is based on its molecular weight. Gases with greater mass travel farther before being drawn to a plate and counted. Lighter gases travel less far before detection.

The detection systems in mass spectrometers generally have a specific plate to measure the relative concentration of each gas in the sample. The electrical output of a plate is proportional to the concentration of the gas it detects. Because carbon monoxide and nitrogen have the same molecular weight, their separate concentrations cannot be easily measured by this method. Mass spectrometers that can handle these separate measurements are very expensive.

Mass spectrometers provide an extremely rapid response time and are easily integrated into computerized applications. Monitoring of blood gas tensions with these systems is possible through the use of an indwelling catheter. Technical difficulties with the catheters have limited their usefulness. Mass spectrometers are very complex and expensive to purchase and maintain. They do, however, provide for an extremely flexible and quickly responsive gas analysis system.

## Review Questions

Please use the following review questions to evaluate your learning of information from this chapter. It might be helpful to write out your answers on a sheet of paper. If you are unsure of the answers to these questions, review the chapter to reinforce your learning.

1. How does each of the following types of oxygen analyzer operate?
   a. paramagnetic analyzers
   b. thermal conductivity analyzers
   c. electrochemical analyzers
2. How do galvanic and polarographic oxygen analyzers differ from each other?

3. What are some general concerns in regard to oxygen analyzers?
4. How does each of the following types of gas analyzer operate?
    a. helium analyzers
    b. nitrogen analyzers
    c. infrared $CO/CO_2$ analyzers
    d. gas chromatographs
    e. mass spectrometers

# CHAPTER FOUR

# TESTS FOR PULMONARY VOLUMES AND VENTILATION

## RELATED LEARNING

Prior knowledge of the following related information will facilitate understanding and learning of the material in this chapter. The learner will be aided by being able to

1. Describe the operation and use of spirometers and recording systems as presented in Chapter 1.
2. Describe the operation and use of body plethysmographs as presented in Chapter 1.
3. Explain how the respiratory quotient and respiratory exchange ratio describe the exchange rates of oxygen and carbon dioxide in the body.
4. Explain the significance of Boyle's law in regard to the relationship between volume changes and pressure changes ($P_1V_1 = P_2V_2$).
5. Explain in basic terms the pathophysiologic difference between obstructive and restrictive pulmonary disorders.
6. Describe the effects of breathing 100% oxygen on a subject's FRC (absorption atelectasis).
7. Perform pressure unit conversions between mm Hg and cm $H_2O$.
8. Perform weight unit conversions between lb and Kg.
9. Describe the difference in technique and appearance of the films for PA (or AP) and lateral chest X rays.

## LEARNING OBJECTIVES

Upon successful completion of this chapter, the learner should be able to

1. Describe the use of direct spirometry to measure vital capacity and to make determinations of the lung volume and capacities.

2. Describe the use of the following gas dilution techniques for indirect spirometry to determine a value for functional residual capacity:
   a. nitrogen washout method
   b. helium dilution method
3. Describe the use of body plethysmography for indirect spirometry to determine a value for thoracic gas volume (functional residual capacity).
4. Describe the process for nonspirometric/radiologic estimation of lung volume.
5. Interpret the results of lung volume and ventilation tests.

## KEY TERMS

Douglas bag
epidemiologic studies
homeostasis
planimeter

regression equation
tangent of an angle
Tissot spirometer

# PULMONARY VOLUMES AND VENTILATION

The total volume of the lungs can be subdivided into smaller units of volume. These units are based on total lung capacity (TLC), the resting end-expiratory lung volume, and a series of specific breathing maneuvers. They are defined as consisting of four lung volumes and four lung capacities. A capacity is a larger unit which includes two or more of the defined lung volumes. Figure 4–1 shows these traditionally defined lung volumes and capacities. It also provides a spirogram tracing of the related breathing maneuvers. Table 4–1 provides specific definitions for the lung volumes and capacities. Table 4–2 lists normal values at birth and for a young adult male.

Ventilation is the result of tidal breathing over a period of time, generally one minute. The following equation demonstrates this concept.

$$\dot{V}_E = \frac{\text{Liters of Ventilation}}{\text{One Minute}}$$

The expressions "exhaled minute ventilation" and "minute volume" are both traditionally used to describe ventilation. The two factors that determine how much ventilation occurs are the frequency of breathing (f) and the size of the tidal volume ($V_T$). This relationship can be demonstrated in an equation:

$$\dot{V}_E = f \times V_T$$

Normal values for f, $V_T$, and $\dot{V}_E$ are provided in Table 4–2.

Lung volumes, capacities, and ventilation can be measured in one of two ways. *Direct spirometry* is used to measure all volumes and capacities except for RV, FRC, and TLC. It is also used to measure ventilation. *Indirect spirometry* is required for the determination of RV, FRC, and TLC. Both of these measurement categories will be discussed.

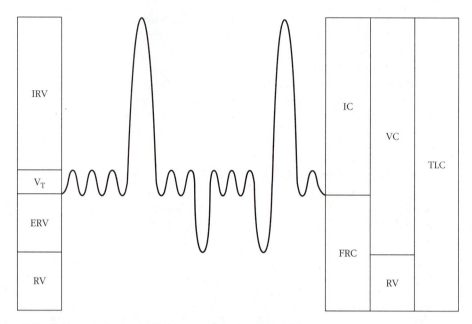

**Figure 4–1** *Spirogram demonstrating lung volumes and capacities.*

# DIRECT SPIROMETRY

Direct spirometry involves use of a spirometer to measure the volumes of air moving into and out of a subject's lungs during breathing. The measurements are given in units of liters or milliliters and are corrected to BTPS. RV is a lung volume that cannot be exhaled and is therefore not measurable by direct spirometry. As a result, FRC and TLC also cannot be determined by direct spirometry.

## LUNG VOLUMES AND CAPACITIES

A consistent point of reference is needed for accurate lung volume measurement. The resting end-expiratory or FRC lung volume provides a reliable, stable reference level. At this point, the expansion properties of the thorax and the collapsing forces of the lung are in balance. Consequently, it is the normal resting volume for the pulmonary system. With proper coaching of a subject, his or her tidal breathing can provide a clearly defined FRC baseline level. Three or more tidal breaths with a volume variance of less than 100 ml acceptably indicates this baseline.

Instructions for lung volume studies must be provided to subjects before they begin breathing on the spirometer. Measurements should begin with the tidal breathing. Once the subject has shown a relaxed, consistent breathing pattern, she or he should be coached to perform a *vital capacity* (VC) maneuver.

## TABLE 4–1  Definitions for Lung Volumes and Capacities

### Volumes

| | |
|---|---|
| Tidal volume ($V_T$) | The volume of air that is inhaled and then exhaled with each normal breath. |
| Inspiratory reserve volume (IRV) | The maximum volume of air that can be inhaled following and above a normal tidal inspiration. |
| Expiratory reserve volume (ERV) | The maximum volume of air that can be exhaled from the resting end-expiratory level. |
| Residual volume (RV) | The volume of air that remains in the lung after a maximum expiration. |

### Capacities

| | |
|---|---|
| Inspiratory capacity (IC)<br>$IC = V_T + IRV$ | The maximum volume of air that can be inhaled from the normal resting end-expiratory level. |
| Functional residual capacity (FRC)<br>$FRC = ERV + RV$ | The volume of air remaining in the lungs at the resting end-expiratory level. |
| Vital capacity (VC)<br>$VC = IRV + V_T + ERV$<br>or<br>$VC = IC + ERV$ | The maximum volume of air that can be exhaled following a maximum inspiration *or* inhaled following a maximum expiration. |
| Total lung capacity (TLC)<br>$TLC = IRV + V_T + ERV + RV$<br>or<br>$TLC = IC + FRC$<br>or<br>$TLC = VC + RV$ | The volume of air contained within the lungs following a maximum inspiration. |

There is some question as to whether the VC maneuver should be performed as an expiration followed by an inspiration or as an inspiration followed by an expiration. There is rarely a significant difference in the test results when both breathing techniques have been compared in the same individual. In some subjects, however, a deep inspiration can trigger bronchospasm and affect the measurement. Therefore, to avoid the effects of bronchospasm, the maneuver should be performed as a maximal expiration followed by a maximal inspiration.

**TABLE 4–2  Normal Values for Lung Volumes, Capacities, and Ventilation**

| Volume | Newborn Infant | Young Adult Male | Approximate Percent of TLC (Young Adult Male) |
|---|---|---|---|
| $V_T$ (ml) | 15 | 500 | 8–10 |
| IRV (ml) | 85 | 3100 | 50 |
| ERV (ml) | 40 | 1200 | 20 |
| RV (ml) | 40 | 1200 | 20 |
| IC (ml) | 100 | 3600 | 60 |
| FRC (ml) | 80 | 2400 | 40 |
| VC (ml) | 140 | 4800 | 80 |
| TLC (ml) | 180 | 6000 | 100 |
| f (bpm) | 35–50 | 12–20 | |
| $\dot{V}_E$ | 525–750 ml/min | 5–6 l/min | |

The subject should breathe on the spirometer using a mouthpiece and with noseclips on. He or she should exhale completely to the RV level and then inhale completely to the TLC level. Once at the TLC level, the subject should exhale back down to the RV level before returning to tidal breathing.

The subject must be observed to ensure that the lips are sealed, nothing obstructs the mouth, and that there are no leaks in the system. Three key points for this test are

1. The breathing by the subject during the maneuver should be relaxed and controlled, not forceful.
2. The inspirations and expirations should be at a relatively constant flow rate.
3. The subject should maintain a brief volume plateau at both the maximal expiratory level and inspiratory level.

The most significant factor affecting test performance is subject effort. Generally, the subject will feel that she or he has reached maximal inspiration or expiration before actually having done so. It is important for the technologist administering the test to recognize this and provide coaching that will produce maximal efforts. Conversely, the technologist should carefully recognize when a maximal effort has been made. Continued coaching after a subject's limits have been reached can have negative effects on the subject. In later tests, the subject may be less willing to cooperate with test instructions and coaching.

A minimum of two acceptable measurements must be made. Acceptable maneuvers should be repeated until reproducibility is demonstrated. No more than four attempts at measuring VC should be made. The criteria for test acceptability and reproducibility and selection of data for reporting are stated in Table 4–3.

---

**TABLE 4–3  Criteria for VC Test Acceptability and Reproducibility and Selection of Data for Reporting**

---

### Acceptability Criteria

---

A test for VC can be considered *acceptable* if:

- The end-expiratory volume of the three tidal breaths that precede the VC maneuver varies by less than 0.1 liter.
- No coughing occurs during the maneuver that, in the technologist's opinion, interferes with the accuracy of the test results.
- No variable effort is demonstrated by the subject during the maneuver.
- No volume loss from a leak in the system is demonstrated.
- No obstruction of the spirometer mouthpiece occurs. Obstruction can be caused by the subject's tongue or by falling of the subject's dentures.
- Maximal expiratory and inspiratory efforts are demonstrated. There should be at least a brief, observable volume plateau at both maximal expiration and inspiration.

---

### Reproducibility Criteria

---

After the first two tests for VC have been performed, *reproducibility* is demonstrated if:

- The largest VC and second largest VC values are within 0.2 liter of each other.

If this criterium is not met after two tests, testing must continue until:

- The criterium is met with the performance of additional acceptable test maneuvers.
- A total of four tests have been performed.
- The patient cannot continue.

---

### Data-reporting Criteria

---

- The largest value for VC from an acceptable test should be selected for reporting.

---

**QUALITY ASSURANCE NOTE:** Measurements of VC should be made before FVC tests are performed. This is recommended to help avoid possible muscle-fatigue and volume-history effects on VC measurement.

Once direct measurements for $V_T$ and VC have been made, the remaining measurable volumes and capacities can be determined. Expiratory reserve volume (ERV) is the volume of air that was exhaled during the VC maneuver from the FRC baseline down to the

RV level. Inspiratory capacity (IC) is the volume of air inhaled from the FRC level up to the TLC level. Inspiratory reserve volume (IRV) is determined by subtracting $V_T$ from IC. (Refer again to Figure 4–1.)

It is possible for the subject to perform separate maneuvers for ERV and IC for volume determination. This is not generally necessary, however. Accurate measurement of IRV as a separate volume is not possible. This is because the tidal end-inspiratory level does not provide a stable baseline from which to initiate and complete the maneuver.

## VENTILATION

Measurement of minute ventilation requires the subject to breathe on the spirometer for at least one minute. A brief period of time should be given for the subject to breathe and to become comfortable on the device prior to the start of measurement. Once begun, the measurement is performed for one minute. The number of breaths taken by the subject during the measurement period should be noted.

The total cumulative exhaled volume of the tidal breathing during the measurement period is used as the value for minute ventilation. The unit of measure is liters per minute (l/min) corrected for BTPS. A value for average tidal volume can be determined if the value for minute volume is divided by the number of breaths measured.

Measurement of minute ventilation can be based on inhaled volumes. This is not generally done, however. The result of an inhaled volume measurement will be slightly greater than for an exhaled volume measurement in the same subject. This is due to the fact that in a normal subject the value for the respiratory quotient and therefore the respiratory exchange ratio is 0.8. The volume of oxygen inhaled is greater than the volume of carbon dioxide that is exhaled. As a result, an exhaled breath will be slightly smaller than an inhaled breath. Consequently, there is a difference between inhaled and exhaled measurement of minute ventilation.

## SUMMARY FOR DIRECT SPIROMETRY

In the past, volume measurements for direct spirometry had to be made by hand from a spirometry tracing. Today volume determinations can be performed by a computer linked to the spirometer system. The operation manual for each spirometer system will describe the procedure required for test performance.

# INDIRECT SPIROMETRY

Indirect spirometry is used to determine lung volumes that are not measurable by direct spirometry. These volumes are RV, FRC, and TLC. Most often, indirect spirometry is performed to measure FRC volume. As stated before, FRC is the most reproducible lung volume, and it provides a consistent baseline for measurement. Once FRC has been determined, the subject's RV and TLC can be calculated. The methods and concerns for this process will be described later.

There are two basic approaches to indirect spirometry. One is the use of *gas dilution techniques*. These techniques involve using either an *open-circuit method* or a *closed-circuit method*. *Body plethysmography* is the second basic approach to indirect spirometry. Each approach will be described in turn. As before, the measurements are given in units of liters or milliliters and are reported at BTPS. Sample calculations for the indirect spirometry methods are presented in the study section of this textbook.

## GAS DILUTION TECHNIQUES

Regardless of the method, gas dilution techniques for determining lung volumes operate on the same basic principle. This principle is similar to Boyle's law except that the fractional concentration of a known gas is used instead of its partial pressure. It may be expressed in the following equation where C is concentration and V is volume.

$$C_1 V_1 = C_2 V_2$$

By having known (or measured) gas concentrations at the start and end of the study and a single known volume, the unknown volume can be determined. For example,

$$V_1 = \frac{C_2 V_2}{C_1}$$

The actual calculations for the two gas dilution methods are fairly complex. They still are based, however, on this simple proportional relationship.

It should be noted that the gas dilution methods can only measure lung volumes in communication with conducting airways. Air trapped within the lung and not in communication with conducting airways cannot experience the required gas dilution. Subjects with obstructive or bullous disease can have trapped, noncommunicating air within their lungs that is not detectable by gas dilution techniques. As a result, the FRC in these subjects may be measured as being less than its actual volume.

> **QUALITY ASSURANCE NOTE:** With gas dilution measurements, system air leaks will produce measurement errors.

Tight system connections, a flanged mouthpiece with a good subject seal, and use of nose clips are all important to accurate measurement. Another potential source of a "system" leak that can affect measurement results is the subject having a perforated eardrum.

## Open-Circuit (Nitrogen Washout) Method

In the classic representation of the open-circuit method, the natural volume of nitrogen in the subject's lungs is washed out and diluted with 100% oxygen (Figure 4–2). The washout procedure must be carefully initiated with the subject breathing in 100% oxygen from the FRC baseline level.

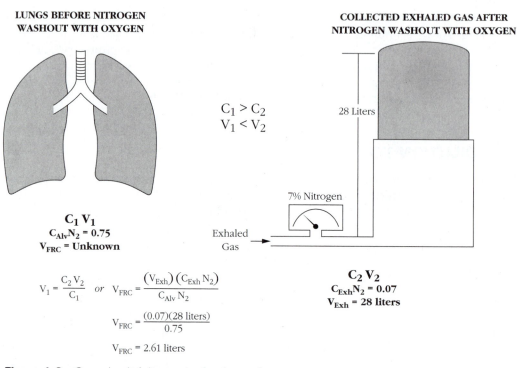

**LUNGS BEFORE NITROGEN
WASHOUT WITH OXYGEN**

**COLLECTED EXHALED GAS AFTER
NITROGEN WASHOUT WITH OXYGEN**

$C_1 > C_2$
$V_1 < V_2$

28 Liters

7% Nitrogen

**$C_1 V_1$**
$C_{Alv}N_2 = 0.75$
$V_{FRC} = $ Unknown

Exhaled
Gas $\longrightarrow$

$$V_1 = \frac{C_2 V_2}{C_1} \quad or \quad V_{FRC} = \frac{(V_{Exh})(C_{Exh} N_2)}{C_{Alv} N_2}$$

**$C_2 V_2$**
$C_{Exh}N_2 = 0.07$
$V_{Exh} = 28$ liters

$$V_{FRC} = \frac{(0.07)(28 \text{ liters})}{0.75}$$

$$V_{FRC} = 2.61 \text{ liters}$$

**Figure 4–2** *Open-circuit (nitrogen washout) procedure.*

**QUALITY ASSURANCE NOTE:** Subjects who use supplemental oxygen (e.g., nasal cannula, etc.) have already "washed out" some nitrogen from their lungs. A measurement error will result if the test is performed during or immediately following the use of supplemental oxygen. Supplemental oxygen should be discontinued for at least a few minutes prior to the test to eliminate this source of error. If the subject cannot tolerate even a short period of time without supplemental oxygen, then a different method for FRC determination should be used.

As the subject continues to breathe the oxygen, all of his or her exhaled gas is collected in a **Tissot spirometer** to allow for measurement of its volume. It is not possible, however, to completely wash out and eliminate nitrogen from the lungs. A nitrogen analyzer in the breathing circuit is used to monitor nitrogen concentrations. Using this method for FRC determination, the test is ended when the criteria shown in Table 4–4 are met.

In most adult subjects, it takes approximately three to seven minutes of breathing 100% oxygen to wash the nitrogen from the lungs. Because prolonged breathing of 100% oxygen may have negative effects on some subjects, tests should generally not extend beyond seven minutes.

Special care should be taken with subjects who have chronic obstructive pulmonary disease (COPD). In some people with COPD, chronic hypercapnia can blunt the normal blood carbon dioxide stimulus that maintains regular breathing. As a result, hypoxemia

---

### TABLE 4–4 Criteria for Ending a Nitrogen Washout Test

---

A nitrogen washout test is successfully completed when the following criterion is met:

- The exhaled nitrogen levels decrease to become less than 1.0% (1.2%–3.0% in some references) for subjects without obstructive disorders.

The test may have to be prematurely discontinued if the following occurs:

- A system leak is signaled by a sudden increase in the expired nitrogen concentration.
- The patient is not able to continue the test.
- The Tissot spirometer, if used, become full.

---

replaces hypercapnia as the physiologic factor that stimulates regular breathing. Prolonged breathing of 100% oxygen may increase the blood oxygen level in these subjects to a point where the stimulus to breathe is lost. Hypoventilation and acidosis may result. Since this risk in subjects with COPD is not predictable, all COPD subjects with chronic hypercapnia should be observed closely during the test for negative response to the oxygen. If oxygen-induced hypoventilation is documented as a problem for a subject, a different method for FRC determination should be used.

Once the nitrogen washout test is completed, a value for FRC is determined in the following way. While in the lung, the unknown FRC volume ($V_{FRC}$) had a known concentration of nitrogen ($C_{Alv}N_2$). The $C_{Alv}N_2$ in the lungs is considered to be approximately 0.75. This is based on the atmospheric nitrogen concentration minus the values for alveolar carbon dioxide and water vapor pressure at BTPS. The final collected volume of exhaled gas ($V_{Exh}$) in the Tissot spirometer has a measurable concentration of nitrogen ($C_{Exh}N_2$). FRC determination is based on the following equation:

$$V_{FRC} = \frac{(C_{Exh}N_2)(V_{Exh})}{C_{Alv}N_2}$$

or

$$V_{FRC} = \frac{V_{Exh}N_2}{C_{Alv}N_2}$$

In actual FVC determination by this method, the calculation is slightly more complex. Two correction factors must be added to the equation. First, as stated before, there is still a small final concentration of alveolar nitrogen remaining at the end of the test ($C_FN_2$). This value must be subtracted from the original $C_{Alv}N_2$ as a correction factor. $C_FN_2$ is determined by having the subject take in a deep breath of oxygen at the end of the test. This volume is then exhaled slowly and for as long as possible. The end-expiratory $CN_2$ for the breath is used as the $C_FN_2$. This final exhaled volume should not be exhaled into the Tissot spirometer. It should be directed elsewhere.

A second correction factor is the volume of nitrogen released from the body tissues during the washout procedure (*body tissue nitrogen* correction factor or $BTN_2$ Factor). This volume is part of the $V_{Exh}$. Its value must be subtracted from the $V_{Exh}$ for accurate FRC determination. Several different equations can be used to estimate the volume of added tissue nitrogen. Depending on the source, values for the $BTN_2$ Factor range from 30 ml to 50 ml per minute of the washout procedure ($T_{Test}$). For our purposes, 40 ml/min (0.04 l/min) will be used.

Given these factors, a more complete equation for $V_{FRC}$ determination can be developed:

$$V_{FRC} = \frac{(C_{Exh}N_2 \times (V_{Exh} + V_D)) - (BTN_2 \text{ Factor} \times T_{Test})}{C_{Alv}N_2 - C_FN_2}$$

The measurements for this calculation are made under ATPS conditions. Before reporting the test results, the result of this calculation must be converted to BTPS conditions. The time taken to complete the nitrogen washout should be reported along with the test results. If for some reason a nitrogen washout test is not acceptably completed, the test can be repeated after a delay of at least 15 minutes. The delay may have to be longer for subjects who have an obstructive pulmonary disorder.

Modern computer-operated pneumotachometer systems do not require collection of the total $V_{Exh}$ or measurement of the final $C_{Exh}N_2$. Instead, simultaneous breath-by-breath $C_{Exh}N_2$ and $V_{Exh}$ measurements are made. These values are integrated automatically into a single value for the $V_{Exh}N_2$ of each breath. The computer adds up a total value for $V_{Exh}N_2$ during the washout period. Necessary corrections can be made by computer software for tissue nitrogen and the other additional variables. $V_{FRC}$ is then determined, as described earlier, by dividing the $V_{Exh}N_2$ by the $C_{Alv}N_2$. Another benefit of using computer-based systems is that the distribution of ventilation (discussed in Chapter 5) can be evaluated at the same time that $V_{FRC}$ is being determined.

## Closed-Circuit (Helium Dilution) Method

During the closed-circuit method, the subject's FRC lung volume is joined with a second, separate gas volume. This second gas volume is prepared to contain helium at a known initial concentration. Tidal breathing mixes the subject's FRC with the second, helium-containing gas volume. As a result, the total combined gas volume has a lower helium concentration. The change in helium concentration is in direct proportion to the amount of the subject's FRC volume added to the original helium-containing gas volume.

In its classic representation, the test is performed in the following way. A measured volume of helium ($V_{Added}He$) is placed into a volume-displacement spirometer, Figure 4–3. Generally, 0.5–2.0 liters of helium gas is used depending on the size of the spirometer. The helium mixes with the spirometer air volume. As a result, the initial helium concentration ($C_IHe$) measured within the system is approximately 0.10–0.15 (10–15% He). After the helium has been added, the total spirometer (tubing, etc.) system gas volume ($V_S$) can be calculated by use of the following equation.

$$V_S = \frac{V_{Added}He}{C_IHe}$$

**SPIROMETER SYSTEM BEFORE HELIUM DILUTION**

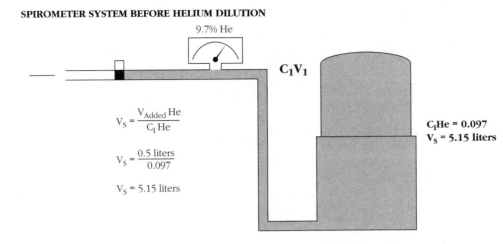

9.7% He

$C_1V_1$

$$V_S = \frac{V_{Added}\, He}{C_I\, He}$$

$$V_S = \frac{0.5\ liters}{0.097}$$

$$V_S = 5.15\ liters$$

$C_I He = 0.097$
$V_S = 5.15$ **liters**

**SUBJECT/SPIROMETER SYSTEM AFTER HELIUM DILUTION**

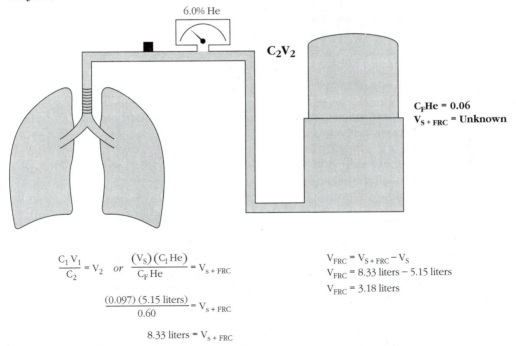

6.0% He

$C_2V_2$

$C_F He = 0.06$
$V_{S+FRC} =$ **Unknown**

$$\frac{C_1 V_1}{C_2} = V_2 \quad or \quad \frac{(V_S)(C_I\, He)}{C_F\, He} = V_{S+FRC}$$

$$\frac{(0.097)(5.15\ liters)}{0.60} = V_{S+FRC}$$

$$8.33\ liters = V_{S+FRC}$$

$V_{FRC} = V_{S+FRC} - V_S$
$V_{FRC} = 8.33\ liters - 5.15\ liters$
$V_{FRC} = 3.18\ liters$

**Figure 4–3**  *Closed-circuit (helium dilution) procedure.*

With the system prepared in this way, the test may then be performed. A valve is opened between the subject and the spirometer. This must be done just as the subject begins to inhale a tidal breath from the FRC level. For a period of time, usually less than seven minutes, the subject rebreathes on the spirometer system. The time required for achieving helium equilibration can be reduced by having the subject periodically (every 30 seconds) perform a slow inspiratory capacity maneuver. Using this method for FRC determination, the test is ended when the criteria shown in Table 4–5 are met.

Once the helium dilution test is completed, a value for FRC is determined in the following way. During the rebreathing time period, the helium mixes and reaches equilibrium throughout the total subject/spirometer gas volume. This volume ($V_{S+FRC}$) consists of the spirometer system volume ($V_S$) and the subject's FRC volume ($V_{FRC}$). At the end of the test, the $V_{S+FRC}$ also has a final helium concentration ($C_F He$) (see Figure 4–3). The following equation demonstrates the proportional relationships between the initial and final helium concentrations and gas volumes.

$$(C_I He)(V_S) = (C_F He)(V_{S+FRC})$$

or

$$\frac{C_I He}{C_F He} \times V_S = V_{S+FRC}$$

A larger value for $V_{S+FRC}$ produces a greater dilution of the helium and a greater proportional difference between the $C_I He$ and $C_F He$. Since the $V_S$ may be assumed to be unchanged during the test, the size of $V_{S+FRC}$ is directly related to the size of the added $V_{FRC}$. Therefore, *the difference between the $C_I He$ and $C_F He$ is directly proportional to the size of the subject's FRC*. Subjects having a larger FRC will demonstrate a greater difference between $C_I He$ and $C_F He$.

This fact allows two simultaneous substitutions that permit the equation to be related directly to the subject's FRC volume:

- The substitution of the difference in He concentrations ($C_I He - C_F He$) for the $F_I He$.
- The substitution of $V_{FRC}$ for the $V_{S+FRC}$.

---

### TABLE 4–5  Criteria for Ending a Helium Dilution Test

---

A helium dilution test is successfully completed when the following criterion is met:

- The helium concentration in the system stabilizes and fluctuates no more than 0.02% during a 30-second period.

The test may have to be prematurely discontinued if the following occurs:

- A system leak is detected by a sudden decrease in the system helium concentration.
- The patient is not able to continue the test.

---

The equation can then be rewritten as:

$$(C_IHe - C_FHe)(V_S) = (C_FHe)(V_{FRC})$$

or

$$\frac{C_IHe - C_FHe}{C_FHe} \times V_S = V_{FRC}$$

The deadspace volume of the mouthpiece must be subtracted from the calculated $V_{FRC}$ as a correction.

Other adjustments can be made to the $V_{FRC}$, although they are not always recommended. Helium absorption into the bloodstream can be compensated for by subtracting 0.06–0.105 liter from $V_{FRC}$. Corrections for the effects of the respiratory exchange ratio and changes in spirometer nitrogen concentration can also be made. These two combined correction factors ($V_{He-N_2}$ Factor) amount to a suggested subtraction of 0.10 liter from the $V_{FRC}$. As a result, the final equation for determining a value for $V_{FRC}$ using the closed-circuit method is

$$V_{FRC} = \left( \frac{C_IHe - C_FHe}{C_FHe} \times V_S \right) - V_{He-N_2} \text{ Factor}$$

Once a value for $V_{FRC}$ is determined, it must be converted from ATPS to BTPS for reporting. If it takes more than seven minutes for the subject to achieve equilibrium, this also should be reported. If the test must be repeated for some reason, it should be delayed for at least four minutes. Four minutes allows time for any residual helium to wash out of the lungs before the next test.

During the test, a blower in the system helps to circulate and effectively distribute the air. A soda lime canister is used to prevent carbon dioxide retention by the subject. Subject hypoxemia during the test is prevented by the addition of oxygen to the closed spirometer system. One technique is the *oxygen-bolus method*. With this method, a large bolus of oxygen is added to the spirometer before the start of the test. The test usually ends when the oxygen bolus is consumed. This method may limit the amount of time available for helium equilibrium.

More frequently used is the *volume-stabilized method*. With this method, oxygen is added to the system continuously during the test. The rate of oxygen addition is titrated to match the rate of consumption by the subject during the test. The duration of the test is not limited by this method.

With either technique, oxygen consumption is monitored by observing the baseline of a spirometer tracing. The baseline moves upward or downward, depending on the type of spirometer, in direct proportion to the rate that oxygen is being consumed from the system. The volume-stabilized method is the one most frequently used and is the one assumed in this description.

Automated systems are available for closed-circuit FRC determination. They may consist of a primary flow measuring spirometer and a **Douglas bag**–like reservoir for the rebreathed helium-containing volume. Operations such as determining system volume can be performed automatically. Computer software can be used to perform the calculations required for determination of FRC.

## Summary for the Gas Dilution Methods

Generally no significant difference exists between the lung volume determinations made from the two gas dilution methods. This is especially true if prolonged nitrogen washout times are given with the open-circuit method for subjects having severe obstructive disorders. The open-circuit method has the disadvantage of requiring a correction for tissue nitrogen contribution. It has an advantage, however. In addition to providing a measurement of FRC, the nitrogen washout test also provides a generally accepted method for assessing the distribution of ventilation. This will be discussed in Chapter 5.

# BODY PLETHYSMOGRAPHY

Measurement of FRC by body plethysmography (BP) is based on an application of Boyle's law.

$$P_1V_1 = P_2V_2$$

or

$$V_1 = \frac{P_2V_2}{P_1}$$

BP does not, as this equation implies, measure absolute values for the new levels $P_2$ and $V_2$. Instead, the amount of *change* in air pressure ($\Delta P$) and volume ($\Delta V$) during breathing is measured and used in the equation. The algebra used to modify Boyle's law into its practical form for BP is demonstrated in Table 4–6.

The BP testing method has an advantage over the gas dilution techniques. Because thoracic volume and pressure changes are measured directly, the total volume of all air contained within the thorax is measured. Unlike gas dilution tests, this includes both air in communication with open airways as well as air trapped within noncommunicating thoracic compartments. For this reason, the volume measured by BP is referred to as the *thoracic gas volume* ($V_{TG}$). Since there is normally no extrapulmonary thoracic gas, in most subjects the $V_{TG}$ reflects the intrapulmonary volume.

During test administration, the subject is required to perform an open-glottis panting maneuver at a rate of approximately one to two breaths per second. The BP shutter is closed suddenly at end-expiration just prior to an inspiration (Figure 4–4). Panting is then continued by the subject for several breaths against the closed shutter.

Air flow is not possible after shutter closure. Therefore, airway pressure changes at the mouth may be assumed to reflect alveolar pressure changes ($\Delta P_A$). The thoracic-pulmonary volume changes ($\Delta V_A$) during panting produce air volume changes within the BP cabinet. Decreases in cabinet volume are an equal inverse response to thoracic volume increases. (As thoracic volumes increase with the panting inspiration, BP cabinet volume decreases.) Changes in the subject's mouth pressure and cabinet air volume are measured by the BP.

Measurement of $V_{TG}$ is generally performed from the FRC level, making FRC the $V_1$ solved for in the equation. Alveolar pressure just prior to inspiration ($P_1$) may be assumed to be equal to atmospheric ($P_{Atm}$). The $P_{Atm}$ used must have the BTPS water vapor pressure (47 mm Hg) subtracted and is generally converted from units of mm Hg to cm $H_2O$.

**TABLE 4–6  Derivation of the Thoracic Gas Volume Equation from Boyle's Law**

$$P_1 \times V_1 = P_2 \times V_2$$

$$P_1 \times V_1 = [P_1 + \Delta P] \times [V_1 \times \Delta V]$$

$$P_1 \times V_1 = [P_1 \times V_1] + [P_1 \times \Delta V] + [\Delta P \times V_1] + [\Delta P \times \Delta V]$$

Subtracting $P_1 \times V_1$ from both sides,

$$0 = [P_1 \times \Delta V] + [\Delta P \times V_1] + [\Delta P \times \Delta V]$$

$V_1$ is isolated for the solution on the left side of the equal sign by subtracting $\Delta P \times V_1$ from both sides.

$$-[\Delta P \times V_1] = [P_1 \times \Delta V] + [\Delta P \times \Delta V]$$

$$-V_1 = \frac{[P_1 \times \Delta V] + [\Delta P \times \Delta V]}{-\Delta P}$$

or

$$-V_1 = \frac{\Delta V \times [P_1 + \Delta P]}{-\Delta P}$$

Since atmospheric pressure is used in the test for $P_1$ and the $\Delta P$ is small by comparison, we can accept $P_1 + \Delta P = P_1$. Therefore, disregarding the minus sign and continuing,

$$V_1 = \frac{\Delta V \times P_1}{\Delta P}$$

or

$$V_1 = \frac{P_1}{\Delta P / \Delta V}$$

With the pressure ($\Delta P_A$) and volume ($\Delta V_A$) changes measured by the plethysmograph during panting, the equation used for determining $V_{TG}$ is

$$V_{TG} = \frac{P_{Atm}}{\Delta P_A / \Delta V_A}$$

An oscilloscope or video display is used to create a graph of the pressure and volume changes during panting. Generally, the results are shown with $\Delta P_A$ on the vertical (Y) axis and $\Delta V_A$ on the horizontal (X) axis. Most displays allow for direct measurement of the angle of the $\Delta P_A / \Delta V_A$ tracing (see Figure 4–4). The value for the angle's **tangent** (slope) provides an average value for $\Delta P_A / \Delta V_A$ over the length of the tracing. The tangent can

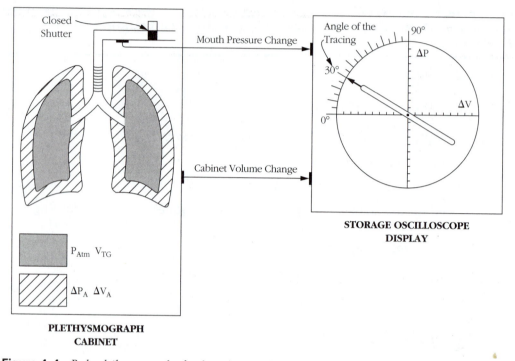

**Figure 4–4** *Body plethysmography for thoracic gas volume determination.*

be indicated directly on the screen display, determined from a chart of angle/tangent conversions, or calculated by computer software. Using this information, the basic equation for determining $V_{TG}$ can then be simplified to

$$V_{TG} = \frac{P_{Atm}}{\text{Tracing Tangent}}$$

A minimum of three acceptable test maneuvers must be performed because the calculation for $V_{TG}$ requires a *mean* value for angle tangent from several test tracings. Table 4–7 provides criteria for $V_{TG}$ test acceptability and selection of data for reporting. If the angle measurement variability is greater than 10%, the values can be used; but the variability should be noted when the results are interpreted. The mean value for the tangents of these angles is used in the equation just given for determining a value for $V_{TG}$.

Three important adjustments are required for the calculation of $V_{TG}$ to reflect the subject's actual FRC volume accurately . The first is a $\Delta P/\Delta V$ calibration factor ($F_{Cal}$) for the cabinet. (The determination of this factor is covered in Chapter 16.) The second is an adjustment for cabinet volume loss that is due to the presence of the subject in the cabinet. This value is based on the cabinet volume when empty ($V_{Cab}$) and the subject's volume. Subject volume is determined by dividing the subject's body weight ($W_{Sub}$) in kilograms

---

**TABLE 4–7 Criteria for $V_{TG}$ Test Acceptability and Selection of Data for Reporting**

---

### Acceptability Criteria

---

A test for $V_{TG}$ may be considered *acceptable* if:

- The panting by the subject is correct in volume and rate. Manufacturer recommendations for use of the plethysmograph equipment can help in evaluating subject panting.

---

### Test Data Reporting Criteria

---

- The data must be taken from three acceptable panting maneuvers.
- The tracing angle for each of the three panting maneuvers should be within 10% of the mean value for all three tracing angles.
- A *mean* tangent value for the three acceptable test tracing angles must be used in the calculation of $V_{TG}$.

---

by the density of the human body (1.07 kg/l). The following equation may be used to calculate the subject volume correction factor ($F_{Sub}$):

$$F_{Sub} = \frac{(V_{Cab} - (W_{Sub}/1.07))}{V_{Cab}}$$

The final adjustment is subtraction of the mouthpiece deadspace volume ($V_{MD}$). The complete equation for determination of $V_{TG}$ is as follows:

$$V_{TG} = \left( \frac{(P_{Atm} - 47 \text{ mm Hg}) \times 1.36 \text{ cm H}_2\text{O/mm Hg}}{\text{Tracing Tangent}} \times F_{Cal} \times F_{Sub} \right) - V_{MD}$$

The value of 1.36 cm $H_2O$/mm Hg is included in the equation to convert the calculation from units of mm Hg to cm $H_2O$.

Because all measurements are made under BTPS conditions, the $V_{TG}$ does not need to be corrected to BTPS. (An example of the use of this equation is presented in the Study Section of this textbook.)

As noted in Chapter 1, there are several methods for measuring changes in plethysmograph cabinet volume. Generally, pressure-type plethysmographs are used. Volume changes measured by these systems are accurate only if cabinet temperature remains stable. The subject should sit within the closed cabinet for a few minutes prior to the actual testing. This will allow the cabinet to reach temperature equilibrium. The subject's exhaled air can also alter cabinet temperature when there are significant changes in minute volume. Use of shallow panting by the subject minimizes this problem.

## COMPARISON OF INDIRECT SPIROMETRY TEST METHODS

Body plethysmography has three advantages over gas dilution methods for FRC determination. The first, as previously described, is the fact that $V_{TG}$ measurement is not affected by the quality of lung ventilation. Gas volume in the lung is measured regardless of whether or not it is trapped behind airway obstructions. The second is that $V_{TG}$ measurements by plethysmography are made more rapidly than in the gas dilution methods—seconds compared with minutes. Finally, tests by plethysmography are readily repeatable. With the gas dilution methods, time is required for gas concentrations in the lung to return to normal prior to additional testing. The primary drawback for body plethysmography is the expense, size, and complexity of the equipment needed. Another drawback is that some subjects may experience anxiety resulting from feelings of confinement.

## COMPARISON OF INDIRECT SPIROMETRY VOLUME DETERMINATIONS

In normal subjects, FRC determinations are the same regardless of which indirect spirometry method is used. It is only in subjects with obstructive airway or bullous disease that differences develop. Use of either of the gas dilution techniques in these subjects may result in significant *underestimation* of the FRC. This is due, as described earlier, to problems with noncommunicating or poorly communicating airways. For some patients with very severe obstructive disease there may be an *overestimation* of FRC with body plethysmography. This is not a frequent problem. It is most likely to occur if the subject is experiencing acute bronchospasm. The panting required during the test appears to accentuate the problem. Even so, body plethysmography is generally considered to provide the most accurate assessment of FRC.

In some laboratories, a subject will have both body plethysmography and a gas dilution test performed. Comparison of the results from both determinations can be clinically useful. It allows for assessment of the problem the subject is having with poorly ventilated airspaces. A greater difference in the test results would indicate a more significant problem with noncommunicating or poorly communicating airways.

## DETERMINATION OF RV AND TLC

Determination of RV and TLC is based on the FRC from indirect spirometry and volumes measured during direct spirometry. There is more than one acceptable method for determining each volume. These methods are presented in Table 4–8.

Some testing systems allow for direct spirometry measurements in conjunction with either gas dilution studies or body plethysmography for FRC determinations (linked spirometry). Less sophisticated systems may require that direct spirometry be performed separate from FRC determination (unlinked spirometry). Linked spirometry permits relatively accurate RV and TLC calculation.

With unlinked spirometry, RV and TLC calculations are based on data from two separate test administrations. Inaccuracies in RV and TLC calculation can result. The problem appears to be due to the subject's FRC shifting to slightly different levels during the

---

**TABLE 4–8  Calculation of RV and TLC After Determination of FRC**

### Residual Volume

| RV = FRC − ERV | or | RV = (FRC + IC) − VC |
|---|---|---|

### Total Lung Capacity

| TLC = FRC + IC | or | TLC = (FRC − ERV) + VC |
|---|---|---|

---

two separate spirometry procedures. This shift may be recognized if the ERV measured and the TLC calculated deviate from predicted normals in opposite directions. For example, a shift exists if the ERV is greater than predicted and the TLC is less. If significant inverse ERV-TLC deviations are noted, repeat testing may be indicated. Despite the possible occurrence of this problem, unlinked spirometry is considered to be an acceptable method for determining RV and TLC.

# NONSPIROMETRIC/RADIOLOGIC ESTIMATION OF LUNG VOLUME

Total lung capacity may be estimated by using measurements made from chest radiographs. Two methods have been developed. In each, the measurements are based on posterior-anterior and lateral chest X rays that are taken at maximum subject inspiration. The *ellipsoid volume method* assumes that the lungs, in a cross section through the chest, are basically elliptical in shape. Measurements are made on the X rays that divide the thorax into a series of five vertical segments. Each segment is treated as a short cylinder. Its volume is determined on the basis of its height, width, and depth dimensions. The addition of these individual segment volumes provides a total thoracic volume. Additional measurements and calculations are made to determine the volume of the heart and space under each of the hemidiaphragms. These volumes are subtracted from the total thoracic volume to determine lung volume.

The *planimetry method* is a second radiographic technique for estimating TLC. It uses **regression equations** to correlate the lung surface areas measured on chest X rays to TLC measurements made by body plethysmography. The surface areas can be determined by use of a device called a **planimeter**. Computerized systems are also available for the calculation of lung surface areas and TLC.

The results of radiographic TLC estimations correlate rather inconsistently with determinations based on indirect spirometry methods. In normal subjects, radiographic and indirect spirometry methods produce comparable results. Subjects with obstructive disorders demonstrate good correlation between the results of radiographic and plethysmographic methods. Gas dilution methods, as stated earlier, tend to underestimate volumes in these subjects. For subjects with significant space-occupying intrathoracic diseases (e.g., pneumonia or pleural effusion) or severe interstitial fibrosis, radiographic determinations may overestimate TLC when the values are compared with measurements made by indirect spirometry in the same subjects.

Radiographic TLC estimation can be useful in large-population **epidemiologic studies** where direct physiologic measurement is impossible. This is especially true with retrospective or serial studies where accuracy is less essential. Subjects with tracheostomies or other unusual problems may also have TLC estimations made by this method. The problems with potential inaccuracies, however, may limit the usefulness of radiographic studies for clinical or diagnostic purposes. Indirect spirometry still provides the best method for routine determination of TLC.

# INTERPRETATION OF PULMONARY VOLUMES AND VENTILATION

As stated in Chapter 2, interpretation of pulmonary function studies is based on comparing a subject's test values with what are *predicted* to be normal values for that subject. Sources for predicted normal values and their use are discussed in Chapter 7. It should be noted that diagnostic interpretation for a subject requires the evaluation of data from many different assessment methods. Pulmonary function studies should be evaluated in conjunction with data from subject history, physical examination, and other types of clinical assessment. The general basis for interpretation of lung volume and ventilation tests results will now be described.

## INTERPRETATION OF PULMONARY VOLUME STUDIES

Normal values for lung volumes are related most directly to height, age, and gender differences between subjects. Volumes increase with greater height, decrease with greater age, and are generally larger for males than for females. Race and weight also play a role in normal values.

The most significant volumes for evaluating the effects of pulmonary disorders are VC, FRC and RV, and TLC. Because IC and ERV both tend to follow the changes exhibited by VC, they are not of significant diagnostic value. It may be noted, however, that some obese subjects demonstrate reductions in ERV out of proportion with reductions of other lung volumes.

A useful tool in evaluating lung volume studies is the *residual volume/total lung capacity ratio* (RV/TLC%). It is calculated by the following equation:

$$RV/TLC\% = \frac{RV}{TLC} \times 100$$

Since the RV/TLC% is reported as a ratio, the calculation may be made regardless of whether both volumes are reported in ATPS or BTPS. In normal, young, healthy adults, the RV/TLC% ranges between 20% and 35%. Abnormalities are indicated when the RV/TLC% becomes greater than 35%. A value greater than 35% indicates *air trapping*

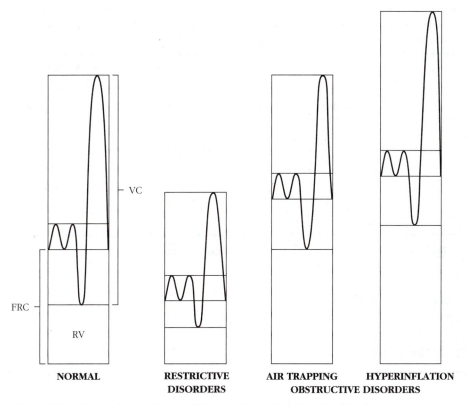

**Figure 4–5** *Alterations in lung volumes with restrictive and obstructive disorders.*

within the lungs. *Hyperinflation* of the lungs is demonstrated when, in addition to the RV/TLC% being greater than normal, the TLC of the subject is also significantly greater than normal. Both of these patterns are demonstrated in Figure 4–5.

It is important to note that lower than predicted values for TLC and VC may be due to poor patient effort during direct spirometry. To detect the possibility of poor patient effort, the technician should evaluate results for internal consistency. The types of alterations or abnormalities shown in different volume subdivisions must be consistent before overall abnormality of the study can be declared. If the alterations present significantly conflicting patterns, the study may need to be repeated. There also should be consistency between the pulmonary function study results and the data gathered from other assessment methods.

Two general patterns of lung volume changes can result from pulmonary disorders. *Restrictive patterns* tend to demonstrate reductions in all lung volumes. *Obstructive patterns*, on the other hand, tend to demonstrate increases in only some volumes. The exception to the general pattern of lung volume increases for obstructive disorders is that either no change or even a decrease in volume for VC may be demonstrated. Table 4–9 indicates the direction of lung-volume change that occurs with each pattern. Figure 4–5 provides graphic

**TABLE 4–9  Patterns of Lung Volume Changes with Restrictive and Obstructive Pulmonary Disorders**

| Volume | Restrictive Pattern | Obstructive Patterns | |
|---|---|---|---|
| | | Air Trapping | Hyperinflation |
| TLC | ↓ | N | ↑ |
| VC | ↓ | ↓ | N |
| FRC | ↓ | ↑ | ↑ |
| RV | ↓ | ↑ | ↑ |
| RV/TLC% | N | ↑ | ↑ |

*N = normal values; ↑ = increased values; ↓ = reduced values.*

representations of these changes. Table 4–10 provides examples of the volumes that may be measured in individuals with obstructive and restrictive patterns of disease.

## Restrictive Patterns

Restrictive lung volume patterns may be the result of a variety of disorders. Space-occupying abnormalities within the thorax (e.g., pleural effusion, pneumonia, tumor), loss of lung volume (e.g., atelectasis, surgical excisions), increased lung elastic recoil (e.g., interstitial fibrosis-sarcoidosis, asbestosis, and complicated silicosis), and deformities of the chest wall (e.g., severe kyphoscoliosis)—all can produce general restrictive patterns. Some abnormalities, such as weakness of the ventilatory muscles, neuromuscular disorders, and CNS depression, can demonstrate a greater reduction in VC than in other lung volumes.

**TABLE 4–10  Comparison of Lung Volumes in Normal, Restrictive, and Obstructive Patterns**

| Volume | Normal | Restrictive Pattern | Obstructive Pattern | |
|---|---|---|---|---|
| | | | Air Trapping | Hyperinflation |
| TLC (ml) | 6000 | 3600 (60% pred.) | 6000 (100% pred.) | 7500 (125% pred.) |
| VC (ml) | 4800 | 2850 (59% pred.) | 3600 (75% pred.) | 4575 (95% pred.) |
| FRC (ml) | 2400 | 1400 (58% pred.) | 3500 (145% pred.) | 4000 (167% pred.) |
| RV (ml) | 1200 | 750 (63% pred.) | 2400 (200% pred.) | 2925 (243% pred.) |
| RV/TLC% | 20% | 20% | 40% | 40% |

Most restrictive disorders will reduce both VC and TLC if the disorder is sufficiently severe. Generally, a reduction in VC will occur before a reduction in TLC is demonstrated in the subject. The RV/TLC% will be normal in subjects with pure restrictive disorders. Significant reductions in lung volumes may increase the work of breathing and limit the ability of the subject to maintain adequate levels of ventilation.

Mild restrictive disorders can be difficult to identify. This is due to the large variability between normal subjects in a reference population. For the early detection of a restrictive disorder, serial test measurements for a subject that demonstrate a growing pattern of restriction have been found to be more useful than the comparison of a single test with normal reference values.

## Obstructive Patterns

Obstructive lung volume patterns are the result of obstructive airway disorders. Diseases such as chronic bronchitis and emphysema are common types of disorders producing this pattern. Inflammatory diseases such as asthma can result in airway obstruction during acute exacerbations but may be fully reversible.

The primary change in an obstructive pattern is an increase in RV. Generally, RV and FRC increase together, although this may not always be the case. Two different obstructive patterns are possible. One is where increases in RV result in a proportional reduction of VC while the TLC remains relatively constant. This is referred to as *air trapping*. In the second pattern, RV increases with little or no change in VC. This causes an increase in TLC in direct proportion to the increase in RV. The term *hyperinflation* is used to describe this pattern. An abnormally increased RV/TLC% will be demonstrated in either situation. In addition to abnormal volumes, subjects with obstructive disorders also demonstrate abnormalities in expiratory flow rates (discussed in Chapter 2).

Significant changes in lung volumes can limit the subject's ability to maintain adequate levels of ventilation. Initial increases in RV may not reduce the ability of the subject to ventilate adequately. As RV increases become more significant and the work of breathing becomes greater, reductions in ventilation can result.

## Mixed Restrictive/Obstructive Patterns

Mixed patterns can occur in some subjects. Examples include:

- Smoking-related COPD superimposed on coal worker's pneumoconiosis.
- Tracheal stenosis occurring in a subject suffering from extreme obesity.

Changes in TLC as a result of mixed patterns are best demonstrated in serial studies. For example, a subject may begin with emphysema and then develop a restrictive process later on. Initially, the subject's TLC would become larger as a result of the emphysema. As the restrictive process develops, a TLC reduction could occur. The TLC may again, over time, approach a normal value. RV/TLC% will be reduced in subjects with mixed disorders.

VC reductions in these subjects can be due to the restrictive process, the obstructive process, or both. Assessment of mixed disorders is difficult when relying solely on lung volume studies. The results of expiratory flow rate tests may be a useful addition for consideration.

**TABLE 4–11  Assignment of Severity for Lung Volume Disorders**

| Volume | Normal | | Abnormal | | |
|---|---|---|---|---|---|
| | | | Mild (%) | Moderate (%) | Severe (%) |
| TLC | 80–120% of predicted* | *Restrictive Disorders* | 70–80 | 60–70 | <60 |
| | | *Obstructive Disorders* | 120–130 | 130–150 | >150 |
| VC | >90% of predicted | *Restrictive Disorders* | 70–90 | 50–70 | <50 |
| | | *Obstructive Disorders* | 70–90 | 50–70 | <50 |
| FRC | 65–135% of predicted† | *Restrictive Disorders* | 55–65 | 45–55 | <45 |
| | | *Obstructive Disorders* | 135–150 | 150–200 | >200 |
| RV | 65–135% of predicted† | *Restrictive Disorders* | 55–65 | 45–55 | <45 |
| | | *Obstructive Disorders* | 35–150 | 150–250 | >250 |

*Note: For VC, <35% of predicted can be used to indicate a very severe impairment.*
*\*Can be expressed as ±20% of predicted.*
*†Can be expressed as ±35% of predicted.*

## Degree of Severity for Lung Volume Changes

Assigning severity labels based on lung volume studies alone is of limited clinical usefulness. This is due to the wide variety of disorders that may be present in subjects. Generally, additional variables such as forced expiratory flow values are also taken into consideration. Approximate guidelines for severity assignment as shown in Table 4–11 can be of some value.

## INTERPRETATION OF VENTILATION STUDIES

Ventilation must be evaluated within the context of *arterial blood gas* (ABG) values. Table 4–12 provides definitions for terms that relate to changes in ventilation. Changes in the level of a subject's ventilation can cause abnormal ABGs. Hypoventilation, for example, will produce hypercapnia and acidosis. It is also possible, however, for ventilation changes to be in response to ABG changes. Abnormally high levels of ventilation may be required to compensate for changes in ABGs that result from a metabolic disorder. Diabetic ketoacidosis will cause a subject to increase ventilation significantly. The resulting hypocapnia may allow the subject to return to a relatively acceptable acid/base status.

A variety of circumstances can lead to changes in a subject's ventilation. Increases in ventilation are caused by disorders or changes from **homeostasis**. Examples include hypoxemia, hypercapnia, acidosis, exercise, anxiety, and an increased pulmonary deadspace volume. Disorders that cause reductions in ventilation include obstructive airway disease, severe restrictive thoracic/pulmonary disorders, neuromuscular disorders, and central nervous system disorders.

Respiratory rate and tidal volume can contribute in different ways to changes in ventilation. Both tidal volume and respiratory rate increase together in situations such as ex-

**TABLE 4–12  Definitions for Ventilation States**

| | |
|---|---|
| *Eupnea* | A normal pattern of tidal breathing. |
| *Tachypnea* | Tidal breathing at a more rapid rate than normal. |
| *Bradypnea* | Tidal breathing at a slower rate than normal. |
| *Hyperpnea* | Tidal breathing with larger volumes than normal; may also indicate a faster rate of breathing. |
| *Hypopnea* | Tidal breathing with smaller volumes than normal; may also indicate a slower rate of breathing. |
| *Hyperventilation* | Ventilation in excess of physiologic need; results in a relative hypocapnia and respiratory alkalosis. |
| *Hypoventilation* | Ventilation insufficient for physiologic need; results in a relative hypercapnia and respiratory acidosis. |

*Note: "Normal" is relative to the height, age, etc., of the subject.*

ercise and diabetic ketoacidosis. In severe thoracic/pulmonary restrictive disorders, the work of breathing (WOB) is less when the subject breathes with smaller tidal volumes. As a result, in order to maintain adequate ventilation, the respiratory rate must be greater than normal. Subjects with flow resistance caused by obstructive disorders experience less WOB at slower respiratory rates. As a result of the slower breathing rate, the tidal volume will be increased to maintain adequate overall ventilation.

It must be noted that *increases in tidal volume and/or respiratory rate can be exhibited by subjects solely as a result of breathing on the pulmonary function apparatus.* This may be due to anxiety over the test. It can also be due, however, to the effects of the nose clips and required mouth breathing.

*Review Questions*

Please use the following review questions to evaluate your learning of information from this chapter. It might be helpful to write out your answers on a sheet of paper. If you are unsure of the answers to these questions, review the chapter to reinforce your learning.

1. What are the volumes and capacities into which the lung can be divided?
2. What are criteria for VC test acceptability and reproducibility and selection of data for reporting?
3. How is measurement for minute ventilation performed?
4. What gas law is used as the basis for the gas dilution techniques for indirect spirometry?
5. What is the basic technique for performing the open-circuit (nitrogen washout) test for FRC determination?
6. What are the criteria for ending a nitrogen washout test?

ısic technique for performing the closed-circuit (helium dilution) test
mination?
riteria for ending a helium dilution test?
is used as the basis for body plethysmography?
_sic technique for performing body plethysmography for $V_{TG}$ determi-
nation?

11. What are the criteria for $V_{TG}$ test acceptability and selection of data for reporting?
12. What are key points in comparing the different test methods used for indirect spirometry?
13. What are key points in comparing the results of the different methods used for indirect spirometry?
14. How are values for RV and TLC determined?
15. How is nonspirometric/radiologic estimation of lung volume performed?
16. How are lung volume measurements used to evaluate the lungs?
17. What are the effects of restrictive, obstructive, and mixed disorders on the lung volumes?
18. How is the severity of lung volume abnormalities described?
19. How are ventilation studies used to evaluate breathing?

# CHAPTER FIVE

# TESTS FOR PULMONARY GAS DISTRIBUTION

## —————— RELATED LEARNING ——————

Prior knowledge of the following related information will facilitate understanding and learning of the material in this chapter. The learner will be aided by being able to

1. Describe the mechanical forces that normally affect the distribution of ventilation within the lung.
2. Describe the operation and use of a nitrogen analyzer, as presented in Chapter 2.
3. Describe the operation and use of spirometers, as presented in Chapter 1.
4. Describe the operation and use of recording systems, as presented in Chapter 1.
5. Describe the administration of tests for FRC determination, as presented in Chapter 4.
6. Describe the use of spirometric methods for evaluation of obstructive pulmonary disorders, as presented in Chapter 2.
7. Describe the normal pattern of blood circulation through the heart, pulmonary circuit, and systemic circuit.
8. Describe the functional disorders related to a condition of pulmonary hypertension.

## —————— LEARNING OBJECTIVES ——————

Upon successful completion of this chapter, the learner should be able to

1. Describe the following methods for measurement of deadspace volume within the lungs, and state the clinical significance of their results:
   a. Fowler method for anatomic deadspace determination
   b. Bohr method for physiologic deadspace determination
2. Describe the following methods for evaluating the distribution of ventilation within the lungs, and state the clinical significance of their results:

    a. general indicators for the uniformity of ventilation that can be used during gas dilution testing for FRC

    b. single-breath nitrogen elimination test, including the determination of closing volume and closing capacity

3. Describe the use of ventilation/perfusion scans, and state the clinical significance of their results.

---

## KEY TERMS

| | |
|---|---|
| albumin | scintiphotographs |
| hypercapnia | scintiscan |
| hyperoxia | technetium |
| iodine | xenox |

The topic of pulmonary gas distribution can be viewed in two different ways. One is the division of the pulmonary volume into regions where gas exchange is and is not possible. This relates to relative proportions of deadspace ventilation and effective alveolar ventilation within the pulmonary system.

A second concern for pulmonary gas distribution is the pattern of how ventilation is distributed within the lung. This relates to the general uniformity of ventilation. It is affected primarily by the mechanical forces that create unequal distribution of ventilation between the upper and lower portions of the lung. Pulmonary gas distribution can be evaluated by use of both pulmonary function and nonpulmonary function testing methods.

---

# DEADSPACE VENTILATION

## DEFINITIONS

The pulmonary volume can be divided into two types of ventilatory regions as they relate to the matching of ventilation with gas exchange perfusion. These are deadspace ventilation regions and effective alveolar ventilation regions. *Deadspace ventilation* occurs in a ventilatory region where gas exchange perfusion is not available. The volume of the conducting airways and possibly some nonperfused alveolar units may be involved in deadspace ventilation. Table 5–1 lists the different types of deadspace ventilation.

The other type of ventilatory region is in alveoli, where gas exchange perfusion is available. Ventilation here is referred to as *effective alveolar ventilation* ($\dot{V}_A$eff). Values for deadspace and effective alveolar ventilation are generally expressed in units of liters per minute (l/min). The values of $V_D$an and $V_D$ are expressed in units of either liters or milliliters.

Test methods are available for determining the volume of a subject's $V_D$an and $V_D$. Each is measured by a separate test procedure.

**TABLE 5–1  Definitions for Different Types of Deadspace**

| | |
|---|---|
| Anatomic Deadspace ($V_Dan$) | The volume of the conducting airways from the mouth/nose down to and including the level of the terminal bronchioles. |
| Alveolar Deadspace ($V_DA$) | The volume of malfunctioning alveoli that are lacking normal gas exchange perfusion. |
| Physiologic Deadspace ($V_D$) | The total volume of deadspace in the pulmonary system; consists of the sum of the anatomic and physiologic deadspace combined; may also be referred to as *functional deadspace.* |
| Ventilation in Excess of Perfusion | Alveolar units where the quantity of ventilation exceeds the quantity of perfusion available; results in a partial deadspace ventilation effect. |

*Note: When the symbol $\dot{V}$ (ventilation) is substituted for V (volume) in the deadspace definitions above, the minute volume of each type of deadspace is being indicated.*

## FOWLER METHOD FOR ANATOMIC DEADSPACE DETERMINATION

The Fowler method for determining deadspace volume measures the volume of a subject's conducting airways. This provides a measure of the subject's anatomic deadspace volume. The volume of expired air from the pulmonary system is measured down to a level where there is a dilution of the freshly inspired gas with gas that was already in the lung prior to inspiration. The procedure is based on the single-breath nitrogen elimination test that will be described in more detail later in this chapter.

### Equipment Required

The key equipment for the Fowler test is a rapid-response gas analyzer for nitrogen ($N_2$) and a spirometer system. Systems for nitrogen washout for FRC determination (Chapter 4) or for the single-breath nitrogen elimination test can be used.

### Test Administration

The Fowler test is based on having the subject inhale and breathe 100% oxygen ($O_2$). It can be performed as a single-breath $O_2$ inspiration test (single-breath $N_2$ elimination) or during the initial breaths of a test requiring prolonged oxygen rebreathing ($N_2$ washout for FRC). With inspiration, the subject's alveoli contain a mixture of $N_2$ and the inspired $O_2$. The presence of $N_2$ results from the preexisting residual volume gas. The conducting airways contain only 100% $O_2$ from the inspired gas. With expiration, the subject's exhaled gas passes through a system set up to analyze the expired $N_2$ concentration ($FEN_2$) and measure the exhaled volume ($V_E$) rapidly.

An illustration of the resulting $FEN_2/V_E$ tracing is shown in Figure 5–1. Initially, as can be seen in the tracing, the exhaled gas is 100% $O_2$ (0.0% $N_2$) from the anatomic deadspace. Then, as alveolar gas begins to be exhaled, the $FEN_2$ rapidly rises (starting at point A). Once the $FEN_2$ tracing reaches a relative plateau (point E), the transition to alveolar gas exhalation is complete.

As can be seen in the tracing, the change from deadspace gas to alveolar gas is not instantaneous. This is because not all areas of the lung empty at the same rate. A theoretical square front (line B-C-D) can be constructed for the curve as shown. The $V_Dan$ is indicated by line B-C-D when it is positioned so that areas A-B-C and C-D-E are equal in size.

A mathematical approach to determining $V_Dan$ from the tracing is possible. This method requires the subject to continue exhaling the breath down to the RV level. An example of a tracing from this maneuver is shown in Figure 5–2. The equation used to calculate $V_Dan$ is based on a modification of the Bohr equation (described later) and is demonstrated in Table 5–2. Application of both of these methods is simplified by use of a

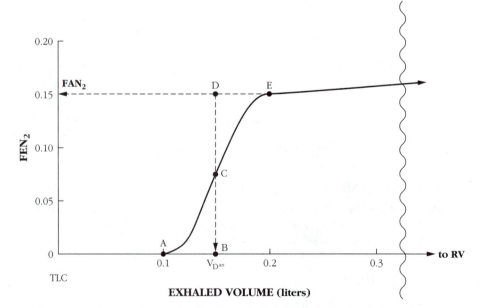

**Figure 5–1** *$FEN_2$/volume tracing for the Fowler method of anatomic deadspace determination.*

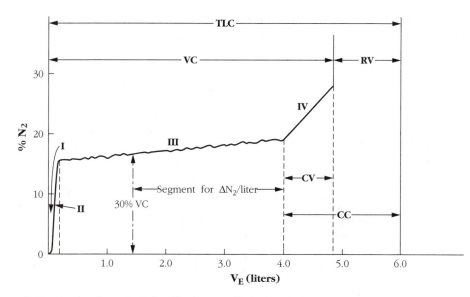

**Figure 5–2** *Tracing for a single-breath nitrogen elimination test.*

planimeter or computer system for determining the area of certain portions of the test tracings.

A similar test can be performed using a carbon dioxide ($CO_2$) meter in the spirometer. The test is based on the same principle just described. It differs, however, in that it allows room air—instead of 100% $O_2$—to be inhaled for the test. The tracing and calculations are based on $FECO_2$ values measured during exhalation.

---

**TABLE 5–2  Mathematical Approach to the Fowler Method of $V_D$an Determination**

---

$$V_D an = \left[ \frac{FAN_2 - F\bar{E}N_2}{FAN_2} \right] V_E$$

where

$V_E$ = volume exhaled by subject.

$FAN_2$ = alveolar $FN_2$ that is indicated by start of plateau level for $FEN_2$. (See start of Phase IV on Figure 5–2.)

$F\bar{E}N_2$ = mean value for exhaled $FN_2$. This is calculated by dividing area under $FEN_2$ curve by $V_E$ measured during VC maneuver.

---

## BOHR METHOD FOR PHYSIOLOGIC DEADSPACE DETERMINATION

The Bohr equation is expressed as

$$\frac{V_D}{V_T} = \frac{(FACO_2 - F\bar{E}CO_2)}{FACO_2}$$

The usefulness of this equation is based on the assumption that the $CO_2$ within expired gas comes only from alveoli that have effective gas exchange perfusion. Physiologic deadspace, on the other hand, contributes no $CO_2$ to the expired gas. A derivation of the Bohr equation, as arranged to determine $V_D/V_T$, is provided in Table 5–3.

---

**TABLE 5–3   Derivation of the Bohr Equation for Physiologic Deadspace**

---

The volume of $CO_2$ in exhaled air can be calculated by relating lung volumes to $CO_2$ concentrations (either within the lung or within exhaled air). Therefore,

$$VECO_2 = (V_D \times FDCO_2) + (V_A \times FACO_2)$$

or

$$VECO_2 = V_T \times F\bar{E}CO_2$$

Given these relationships, the following statement can be made:

$$(V_D \times FDCO_2) + (V_A \times FACO_2) = V_T \times F\bar{E}CO_2$$

The value for $FDCO_2$ is identical to the $FICO_2$. Because the $FICO_2$ is normally .0003, its value may be assumed to be 0.0. As a result, the following basic proportional relationship exists between pulmonary volumes and related fractions of $CO_2$.

$$V_A \times FACO_2 = V_T \times F\bar{E}CO_2$$

Because $V_A = V_T - V_D$, we can make the following substitution:

$$(V_T - V_D) \times FACO_2 = V_T \times F\bar{E}CO_2$$

or

$$(V_T \times FACO_2) - (V_D \times FACO_2) = V_T \times F\bar{E}CO_2$$

We rearrange to simplify for $V_T$ as follows:

$$-(V_D \times FACO_2) = (V_T \times F\bar{E}CO_2) - (V_T \times FACO_2)$$

or

$$-(V_D \times FACO_2) = V_T (F\bar{E}CO_2 - FACO_2)$$

After multiplying both sides of the equation by $-1$,

$$V_D \times FACO_2 = V_T(FACO_2 - F\bar{E}CO_2)$$

**TABLE 5–3** (*Continued*)

We finally solve for $V_D/V_T$:

$$\frac{V_D}{V_T} = \frac{(FACO_2 - F\bar{E}CO_2)}{FACO_2}$$

where

$FACO_2$ = fraction of $CO_2$ contributed by effectively perfused alveoli.

$FDCO_2$ = fraction of $CO_2$ in deadspace air.

$F\bar{E}CO_2$ = fraction of $CO_2$ in mixed exhaled air that was collected from tidal breathing.

$FICO_2$ = fraction of $CO_2$ in inspired air.

$V_A$ = volume of effectively perfused alveoli.

$V_{ECO_2}$ = volume of $CO_2$ in exhaled air.

$V_D$ = volume of physiologic deadspace.

$V_T$ = volume of tidal breathing.

Adjustments can be made to make this equation more clinically applicable. Because the fraction of a gas in a sample is proportional to its partial pressure, $PCO_2$ values can be substituted for $FCO_2$ values. Additionally, $PACO_2$ can be determined by more than one method. The value for arterial $PCO_2$ ($PaCO_2$) is commonly accepted as being approximately equal to the $PACO_2$. Alternatively, $PCO_2$ measurements made on exhaled gas that is sampled toward the end of expiration can be used to provide a value for $PACO_2$. This type of sampling provides what is referred to as an *end-tidal* $PCO_2$ value ($PetCO_2$). The value for $P\bar{E}CO_2$ is meant to represent the subject's average exhaled $PCO_2$. It is based on the analysis of a gas sample taken from a large volume of the subject's exhaled air. The exhaled air is collected during the test procedure. The clinical equation used for determining $V_D/V_T$ is

$$V_D/V_T = \frac{PACO_2 - P\bar{E}CO_2}{PACO_2}$$

Values for either the subject's $PaCO_2$ or $PetCO_2$ can be used as a substitute for $PACO_2$. The results of the calculation are expressed as a decimal fraction—for example, $V_D/V_T =$ .35.

A value for the subject's $V_D$ can be determined in the following manner:

$$V_D = (V_D/V_T) \times V_T$$

A sample calculation for deadspace determination by the Bohr method is provided in the Study Section of this textbook.

## Equipment Required

The equipment needed to perform the Bohr test includes a spirometer for measuring exhaled volumes, a **Douglas bag** for collecting an exhaled gas sample, a $CO_2$ analyzer, and an end-tidal $PCO_2$ analyzing system or equipment for arterial blood sampling and analysis. The breathing circuit must include a valve system to allow the subject to inhale room air and exhale into the spirometer/Douglas bag. Nose clips are required to ensure complete exhaled gas collection.

## Test Administration

Exhaled gas collection can begin once the subject is connected to the breathing circuit and is performing regular tidal breathing. Exhaled gas collection should continue until the Douglas bag nearly reaches its capacity. Collection times of 5–10 minutes are typical. Larger-volume collections increase the accuracy of the test. The subject's end-tidal $PCO_2$ values must be recorded and averaged, or an arterial blood sample must be drawn and analyzed to provide for a $PACO_2$ determination. To make the test most accurate, the arterial blood sampling should be performed during the time of exhaled gas collection. The subject's average $V_T$ during gas collection must be determined. Once the data has been gathered, $V_D/V_T$ and $V_D$ can be calculated.

## INTERPRETATION OF TEST RESULTS

The normal value for $V_D$an (ml) approximates a subject's ideal body weight in pounds. Thus, a subject whose ideal body weight is estimated at 150 lb should have a $V_D$an of approximately 150 ml. Values for $V_D$an increase directly with height and (slightly) age. Taller and, to some degree, older subjects will demonstrate greater values for $V_D$an. Males have slightly larger values than females.

For $V_D/V_T$, normal values range between .20 and .40 (.25 and .35 in some references). In normal subjects, the values for $V_D$an and $V_D$ should be approximately equal. This is because alveolar deadspace does not normally exist to a significant degree. The only deadspace volume making up the $V_D$ in the lungs would be the volume of the conducting airways ($V_D$an).

It is only in pathologic states that alveolar deadspace begins to develop measurably and that $V_D$ increases to become greater than the $V_D$an. Table 5–4 lists factors that can cause alterations in pulmonary deadspace volumes.

Comparing a subjects's estimated $V_D$an value with a measured value for $V_D$ can provide a basis for evaluating lung ventilation/perfusion relationships. If the subject's $V_D$ becomes measurably greater than $V_D$an, it indicates the development of alveolar deadspace. Alveolar deadspace signifies the presence of alveolar ventilation/perfusion abnormalities within the lung.

$\dot{V}_A$eff can be calculated by the following equation:

$$\dot{V}_A\text{eff} = f \times (V_T - V_D)$$

Because of the possible wide variations for f, $V_T$, and $V_D$ that may be exhibited by subjects, normal values for $\dot{V}_A$eff may range from 3 l/min to 8 l/min. Relative increases in

**TABLE 5–4  Factors That Cause Alterations in Deadspace Volume**

### Anatomic Deadspace

#### Increases in $V_D$an

- Disorders that cause destruction or dilation of the airway walls (*bronchiecta-sis*).
- Breathing at a greater FRC level or with larger inspiratory volumes (*air trapping/hyperinflation*).
- Bronchodilator agents.

#### Decreases in $V_D$an

- Disorders that cause constriction (*asthma*) or obstruction (*carcinoma*) of the airways.
- Bronchoconstrictor agents.

### Alveolar Deadspace (Increases only)

#### Loss of Pulmonary Perfusion

- *Pulmonary embolism.*

#### Reduced Pulmonary Perfusion

- *Decreased cardiac output/hypotension.*
- *Acute pulmonary hypertension.*

### Ventilation in Excess of Perfusion (Increases only)

#### Alveolar septal destruction

*Note: Though not a disorder itself, positive pressure ventilation also causes ventilation in excess of perfusion.*

$\dot{V}_A$eff can result in **hyperoxia** and **hypocapnia**. Decreases in $\dot{V}_A$eff can cause **hypoxemia** and **hypercapnia**.

It should be remembered that the relative impact of deadspace ventilation on gas exchange can change depending on the subject's pattern of ventilation. For example,

- If a rapid, shallow breathing pattern is adopted by the subject, there will be relatively more deadspace ventilation and less effective alveolar ventilation.
- If a slower, deeper breathing pattern is adopted by the subject, there will be relatively less deadspace ventilation and more effective alveolar ventilation.

# DISTRIBUTION OF VENTILATION

The lungs, unlike simple balloons, are incredibly complex organs of gas exchange. Normal ventilation is not evenly distributed throughout the 300 million alveoli in the adult lung. At rest, the alveoli in the upper lung regions are larger than alveoli in the lower regions. Because of their initial smaller size, alveoli in the lung bases receive more ventilation than those in the apices. This is the result of intrathoracic pressure relationships. The alveoli in peripheral, outer lung tissue receive more ventilation than alveoli deeper within the lung. This is the result of intrapulmonary tissue force relationships. In normal ventilation, the greater part of inspiratory/expiratory volume exchange occurs in the lung bases. The upper lung regions are responsible for holding a larger portion of the FRC volume.

Pulmonary disorders can create pathologic problems in the distribution of ventilation (Table 5–5). It must be noted that these disorders generally do not create consistent changes throughout the lungs. The abnormalities that result usually demonstrate a significantly uneven pattern of ventilatory distribution.

**TABLE 5–5   Disorders That Affect the Distribution of Ventilation**

**Disorders Affecting Lung Compliance**

*Increased Compliance*

- *Emphysema.*

*Reduced Compliance*

- *Fluid or exudate collecting in the alveoli or interstitial spaces.*
- *Atelectasis.*
- *Tumors.*
- *Fibrotic pulmonary disorders.*

**Disorders Increasing Airway Resistance**

*Partial Obstruction*

- *Asthma.*
- *Bronchitis.*
- *Peribronchiolar or intrabronchial tumors.*

*Check Valve Expiratory Obstruction*

- *Emphysema.*

## TESTS FOR UNIFORMITY OF VENTILATION

General indicators for the uniformity of ventilation are based on previously described tests for FRC determination (Chapter 4). These tests involved either the washout ($N_2$) or equilibrium (He) of gases in the lung. The particular test for uniformity of ventilation selected by a laboratory will depend on the method already established for FRC determination.

When disorders affecting the distribution of ventilation are present, the processes of gas equilibrium or washout will be affected. These processes will proceed more slowly and will require a greater number of breaths or a greater level of ventilation for equilibrium to be achieved.

Establishing indicators for the rate of equilibrium or washout allows the uniformity of ventilation to be evaluated. A number of methods have been devised for doing this. Table 5–6 lists some of these methods. It is beyond the scope of this text to expand on each method. The one most accepted clinically is the index based on the volume of ventilation required to achieve end-tidal $N_2$ concentrations of 2%.

### Interpretation of Test Results

There can be a wide variability in the results of these indicators for uniformity, even within an individual subject. Regardless, the indicators have reasonable sensitivity to significant disorders in the distribution of ventilation.

---

**TABLE 5–6  Methods for Assessing the Uniformity of Distribution**

---

#### Based on Helium Dilution Method for FRC Determination

---

1. Noting the amount of time required for the subject to achieve complete or 90% equilibrium.*
2. Calculating an index upon dividing the theoretical number of breaths to achieve equilibrium (also calculated) by the number of breaths actually required by the subject to achieve 90% equilibrium (normal = .45–.80).
3. Calculating an index based upon the measured ventilation ($\dot{V}_E$) required by a subject to achieve 90% equilibrium divided by the subject's FRC volume (normal = 7.0 + 1.7).

---

#### Based on the Nitrogen Washout Method for FRC Determination

---

1. Measuring the percent increase in $N_2$ during a forced expiration after seven minutes of breathing $O_2$ (normal = <2.5% increase).*
2. Calculating an index based upon the measured ventilation ($\dot{V}_E$) required by a subject to achieve end-tidal $N_2$ concentrations of 2% divided by the subject's FRC volume (normal = 5–9).

---

*Indicates that the results of these tests are affected negatively by such factors as the subject's respiratory rate, $V_T$, and FRC volume. These effects can create inconsistencies in the test results.

## SINGLE-BREATH NITROGEN ELIMINATION TEST

The *single-breath nitrogen elimination* test (SBN$_2$), sometimes referred to as the *single-breath oxygen* test (SBO$_2$), involves having the subject inhale a breath of 100% oxygen. The breath must be an inspiratory VC maneuver starting from the RV level. Based on the normal pattern of ventilation, more of the inspired O$_2$ enters alveoli in the dependent lung regions (bases) than it does the upper regions (apices).

Once the 100% oxygen is inhaled, the subject then exhales slowly back to the RV level. During exhalation, the volume exhaled (V$_E$) and percent N$_2$ (% N$_2$) of the exhaled gas are both continuously monitored. The resulting tracing is demonstrated in Figure 5–3. This tracing can be divided into four phases of % N$_2$ changes. *Phase I* is the initial 0.0% N$_2$ concentration measured during the emptying of the V$_D$an. No N$_2$ is measured because only 100% O$_2$ was present in the conducting airways at the end of inspiration. *Phase II* is the rapid increase in % N$_2$ that indicates the transition from V$_D$an to alveolar gas. This is determined as described earlier in the chapter for V$_D$an determination.

*Phase III* is the relative % N$_2$ plateau that results from the emptying of mixed gas from the alveoli during expiration. The mixture is a combination of the inhaled O$_2$ and the N$_2$ containing FRC gas that was present at the start of the inhalation. Most of the gas leaving the lungs during this phase is from alveoli in the lower lung regions. The plateau is not usually flat. It generally demonstrates a slight increase in % N$_2$ during expiration. If the subject's expiratory flow rate is too slow, notable oscillations may be demonstrated in the tracing. These oscillations are thought to be the result of fluctuations in alveolar N$_2$ concentrations that are caused by the pulsations of pulmonary capillary blood flow.

*Phase IV* occurs toward the end of the expiration in most subjects. It is a relatively rapid increase in % N$_2$ from the Phase III plateau that continues with exhalation to the RV level.

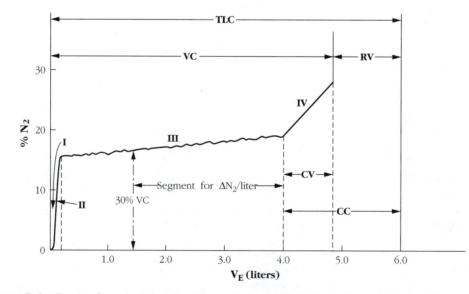

**Figure 5–3**  *Tracing for a single-breath nitrogen elimination test (this is Figure 5–2 repeated).*

Phase IV indicates the point where airways in the lung bases are contributing less of the exhaled volume. This lesser contribution is probably the result of forces, such as dynamic compression, that cause closure of the airways. Consequently, a greater proportion of alveolar gas volume from the upper lung regions begins to be exhaled. Because less of the originally inhaled $O_2$ goes to this region, there is a rapid increase in % $N_2$ until RV is reached.

## Equipment Required

The primary pieces of equipment required for the SBN$_2$ test are a gas analyzer for measuring the % $N_2$ of the exhaled gas, a spirometer system for measuring exhaled volume, and a system for recording and producing tracings for the % $N_2$ and $V_E$ changes. It is helpful to have a feedback system included to indicate inspiratory and expiratory flow rates to the subject. Modern pulmonary function testing systems include all of the components required to perform this procedure. Additionally, computer technology allows rapid determination of a number of parameters, including $V_D$an, from the test results.

## Test Administration

With nose clips on, and while breathing through the system circuit, the subject should take two deep breaths and then exhale down to the RV level. Once this has occurred, the breathing circuit must be changed over to provide 100% $O_2$ for the inspiratory gas. The subject should inhale to the TLC level with a flow rate of approximately 0.3–0.5 (ideally 0.4) l/sec. The flow-rate feedback system can help the subject maintain this flow rate. Once TLC is reached, the subject should, without a pause, begin exhaling at approximately the same flow rate. Once RV is reached, the subject may resume normal air breathing. The test should be repeated twice more, with a few minutes' rest between procedures. Table 5–7 provides criteria for SBN$_2$ test acceptability and selection of data for reporting.

## Interpretation of Test Results

A number of pulmonary function parameters can be determined from an SBN$_2$ elimination test. These include the VC, $V_D$an, uniformity of ventilatory gas distribution, effects of pulmonary mechanics on small airway closure, TLC, and RV. Each of these will be discussed in turn.

The VC can be read as the total of the volume exhaled by the subject. As described earlier in the chapter, $V_D$an can be determined from the maneuver by use of the Fowler method. The % $N_2$ change in Phase II allows this to be done. Computer integration with modern testing systems can provide automated measurement of a square front for Phase II. It can also be used to determine the area under the entire curve for $V_D$an measurement by that technique.

The uniformity of ventilation in the lung can be evaluated based on measurements made from the % $N_2$ changes during Phase III of the tracing. The *change* (increase) *in %* $N_2$ *between the 750 ml point and 1250 ml point of the exhaled volume* ($\Delta$ %$N_2$750–1250) provides one measure (Figure 5–4). If there is too much unevenness in this region of the tracing, a best-fit line must be drawn along Phase III in order to evaluate the changes in %

---

**TABLE 5–7  Criteria for SBN$_2$ Test Acceptability and Selection of Data for Reporting**

---

### Acceptability Criteria

A test for SBN$_2$ can be considered *acceptable* if:

- The mean expiratory flow rate, especially the first 500 ml of $V_E$, is $\leq$0.5 l/sec.
- Except for the first 500 ml, transient expiratory flow rate increases (lasting for $\geq$300 ml of $V_E$) must not exceed 0.7 l/sec.
- The inspiratory and expiratory VC volumes must not differ by more than 5%.
- The VC volumes between procedures must not differ by more than 10%.
- A notable steplike change in %N$_2$ with continued cardiac oscillations must not be exhibited in the tracing. This steplike change can cause misjudgment of the start of phase IV.

---

### Test Data Reporting Criteria

- The *mean* value for the results of three acceptable tests is reported as the test result.
- The averaged results of only two acceptable procedures can be reported if that is all that is available.
- If only one acceptable procedure is accomplished, no test results should be reported.
- The tracing angle for each of the three panting maneuvers should be within 10% of the mean value for all three tracing angles.
- A *mean* tangent value for the three acceptable test tracing angles must be used in the calculation of $V_{TG}$.

---

N$_2$. Increases of no more than 1.5% are normal for young, healthy adults. This value may increase to as much as 3.0% in older normal subjects. Greater than normal values for $\Delta$%N$_2$750–1250 indicate a nonuniformity of ventilation within the lung. Values of 6.0% to as great as 10% can be demonstrated by some subjects with severe obstructive disorders.

The *change in % N$_2$ per liter of exhaled volume* ($\Delta$%N$_2$/liter) is a second indicator of the uniformity of ventilation. It is measured on the segment of the tracing between the 30% VC point to where Phase IV begins (see Figure 5–3). Normal values have been reported to range from 0.5% to nearly 1.0% per liter of exhaled volume. Values greater than normal, as with the $\Delta$%N$_2$750–1250, indicate a nonuniformity of ventilation.

The *closing volume* (CV) and *closing capacity* (CC) are based on the point at which the % N$_2$ increase of Phase IV occurs (see Figure 5–3). CV is the volume exhaled from the start of Phase IV to the end of expiration at the RV level. CC consists of the CV plus the RV. Generally, CV is expressed as a percentage of VC (CV/%VC), and CC is expressed as a percentage of TLC (CC/% TLC). The VC maneuver performed by the subject for CV and CC determination must be within 5% of the VC measured by other tests. If it is not, the calculated results for CV/%VC and CC/%TLC may be in error.

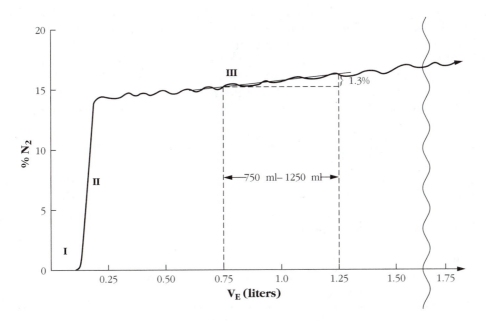

**Figure 5–4** *Changes in percent N$_2$ between 750 ml and 1250 ml.*

Normal values for CV and CC are slightly greater for females than for males and increase with advancing age. Table 5–8 provides normal values for CV and CC. As stated earlier, the start of Phase IV identifies the point at which airways in the lung bases are exposed to forces that cause their closure. Small airway disorders cause airway closure to occur earlier in expiration and with a greater volume remaining in the lung.

Subjects with COPD or disorders that result in edematous airways will demonstrate greater than normal values for CV/%VC and CC/%TLC. These parameters can be used to identify the presence of small airway disorders even before they are detectable by the use of spirometric methods. They may provide an excellent means for the early identification of COPD in subjects. There is evidence that CC/%TLC may be a more sensitive indicator of small airway disorders than the CV/%VC.

With restrictive processes, because of the reductions in lung volume overall, airway closure may occur earlier in the VC maneuver. As a result, Phase IV and the CV can start at a volume greater than the FRC level. This produces a significant risk for atelectasis and

**TABLE 5–8   Normal Values for Closing Volume and Closing Capacity**

|  | Male | Female |
|---|---|---|
| CV/%VC | 7.7% | 8.7% |
| CC/%TLC | 24.8% | 25.1% |

*Note: Subject age = 20 yrs.*

hypoxemia in the subject. For these subjects, when they are under the influence of anesthetic or narcotic agents, the risk is even greater.

TLC can be calculated based on the area under the % $N_2$ curve on the $SBO_2$ tracing. This area can be determined by planimetry or by electronic integration of the % $N_2$ signal from the gas analyzer. Table 5–9 demonstrates the calculation of TLC from the $SBO_2$ tracing. RV is determined by subtracting the VC measured during the procedure from the TLC calculated from the tracing.

## VENTILATION/PERFUSION LUNG SCANS

Techniques using radioactive substances have been developed to evaluate the distribution of both ventilation and perfusion in the lungs. Although they are not part of the domain of a pulmonary function laboratory, these procedures play an important role in the evaluation of pulmonary disorders.

---

**TABLE 5–9   Determination of TLC from $SBO_2$ Test**

---

Calculation of the mean fraction of exhaled $N_2$ ($FEN_2$):

$$FEN_2 = \frac{(A/V_E)(\% \ N_2 cal)}{100}$$

where

A = area under % $N_2$ curve ($cm^2$).

$V_E$ = exhaled volume (cm; based on length of $V_E$ from the tracing).

% $N_2 cal$ = calibration factor relating distance (cm) on the vertical axis to the % $N_2$.

Calculation of the $V_D$ admixture correction for the mean fraction of exhaled $N_2$ ($FV_D N_2$):

$$FV_D N_2 = \frac{(FEN_2)(V_E)}{V_E - V_D}$$

Calculation of TLC (liters):

$$TLC \ (liters) = \frac{(V_I)(FAN_2) - (V_D)(FV_D N_2)}{FAN_2 - FV_D N_2}$$

where

$V_I$ = inhaled volume.

$FAN_2$ = alveolar $N_2$ fraction; assumed to be equal to 0.80.

---

## Ventilation Scans

Ventilation scans involve having the subject breathe the radioactive gas **xenon** 133 ($Xe^{133}$). A **scintiscan** is made of the lungs during the breathing of the gas. During the scan, **scintiphotographs** are made to record the process and pattern of the distribution of the $Xe^{133}$ in the lungs. These scans allow a visual evaluation of distribution of ventilation in the lungs. The pattern of distribution can be quantified by dividing the lung into zones and recording the $Xe^{133}$ accumulation in each zone.

Ventilation scans are useful in a number of clinical circumstances. With bronchiectasis and bullous lung disorders, the scans can more precisely quantitate the severity and extent of the disorder. The presence of such abnormalities as a foreign body, cancer, or other airway masses may be localized. This information can be beneficial prior to the use of other, more invasive studies, such as bronchograms or bronchoscopy.

## Perfusion Scans

Perfusion scans involve the intravenous injection of a radioactively tagged substance. **Iodine** 131 ($I^{131}$) and **technetium** 99 ($TC^{99}$) are examples of isotopes that can be used to radioactively tag the carrier substance. A commonly used carrier is human **albumin**. It is processed into microspheres, or particles that are large enough to be caught and held in the pulmonary capillary circulation.

When the carrier substance is injected into the venous circulation, it passes through the right heart and enters the pulmonary circulation. The carrier substance particles lodge in the capillary beds. The pattern of how the carrier particles have lodged within the capillary bed matches the pattern of pulmonary perfusion within the lungs. Scintiphotographs are made once the carrier has reached the pulmonary circulation. Anterior, posterior, and left and right lateral views are photographed.

With normal doses of the carrier substance, only about 0.1 percent of the pulmonary circulation is blocked. Generally, no functional abnormality is detectable as a result of these particles being trapped within the lungs. After a time, the carrier particles break up and pass through the pulmonary circulation. They are then removed from the blood and are processed for elimination by the liver and spleen.

Perfusion scans are very useful for detecting and locating the site(s) of obstruction within the pulmonary circulation. Such obstruction can be the result of an embolism or a tumor. The reduction or cessation of pulmonary circulation that may result from an intrapulmonary disease process can also be detected.

Perfusion scans may be contraindicated for subjects with severe pulmonary hypertension or anatomic right-to-left vascular shunts. In pulmonary hypertension, the subject may already have a significant reduction in the cross-sectional area of the pulmonary capillary bed. The additional loss of pulmonary perfusion from the test procedure can create a functional disorder in pulmonary gas exchange.

An anatomic right-to-left shunt can allow the carrier particles to pass unchanged directly into the systemic circulation. The particles may then become lodged in the capillary beds of the brain, heart, kidneys, or other organs. The resulting loss of perfusion to these important organ systems could be life-threatening.

## Combined Ventilation and Perfusion Scan Results

Combining the results of ventilation and perfusion scans provides useful clinical information. A region of the lungs that demonstrates a perfusion defect but has normal ventilation is strongly indicative of pulmonary embolism. Subjects with COPD often show matching ventilation and perfusion defects throughout the lung fields.

## *Review Questions*

Please use the following review questions to evaluate your learning of information from this chapter. It might be helpful to write out your answers on a sheet of paper. If you are unsure of the answers to these questions, review the chapter to reinforce your learning.

1. What is the basic technique for performing the Fowler method for anatomic dead-space determination?
2. What is the basic technique for performing the Bohr method for physiologic dead-space determination?
3. Relating to the clinical use of deadspace measurement:
   a. How do deadspace measurements relate to clinical evaluation of subjects?
   b. What are factors that can cause alterations in deadspace volume?
4. How can general indicators used during gas dilution tests provide information on the distribution of ventilation?
5. Relating to the single-breath nitrogen elimination test,
   a. How is the single-breath nitrogen elimination test performed?
   b. What are the four phases defined on the graph during the test, and what is their significance?
   c. What are the criteria for acceptability and selection of data for reporting for single-breath nitrogen elimination tests?
   d. What is the clinical significance of the following measurements made during a single-breath nitrogen elimination test:

   - Change in $\%N_2$ between the 750 ml point and 1250 ml point of exhaled volume
   - Change in $\%N_2$ per liter of exhaled volume, closing volume, closing capacity

   e. How do obstructive and restrictive disorders affect the preceding measurements?
6. Relating to ventilation scans and perfusion scans,
   a. How are ventilation scans performed?
   b. How are perfusion scans performed?
   c. How can these scans provide clinically useful information?

# CHAPTER SIX

# TESTS FOR PULMONARY GAS DIFFUSION

## RELATED LEARNING

Prior knowledge of the following related information will facilitate understanding and learning of the material in this chapter. The learner will be aided by being able to

1. Explain the basic concepts of diffusion.
2. Describe the anatomic pathway for diffusion of oxygen from alveolar gas to attach to hemoglobin in the pulmonary capillary blood.
3. Describe the operation of CO, He, $N_2$ gas analyzer systems, as presented in Chapter 3.
4. State the alveolar air equation as used for determining $PAO_2$ values.
5. Explain the significance of the respiratory exchange ratio.

## LEARNING OBJECTIVES

Upon successful completion of this chapter, the learner should be able to

1. Describe the following techniques for measuring diffusion within the lungs:
   a. fractional carbon monoxide (CO) uptake
   b. single-breath method for measuring CO diffusing capacity
   c. steady-state methods for measuring CO diffusing capacity:

   • deadspace-compensated techniques:
   • estimated-deadspace technique
   • assumed-deadspace technique
   • alveolar gas sampling technique

   d. rebreathing methods for measuring CO diffusing capacity:

   • reservoir-sampling technique
   • washout-sampling technique

2. Describe the administration of a single-breath CO diffusing capacity test.
3. Interpret the results of diffusing capacity testing.

---
## KEY TERMS
---

end-tidal sampling          $P_{H_2O}$                              STPD

Diffusion is the process by which oxygen and carbon dioxide transfer along the intra-pulmonary gas exchange pathway that crosses the alveolocapillary (A-c) membrane. This diffusion pathway consists of alveolar air, the A-c membrane, the pulmonary capillary plasma, erythrocytes, and hemoglobin. Movement along this pathway across the A-c membrane can be in either direction depending on which end has the higher gas concentration. Oxygen has a slower rate of diffusion along the pathway than does carbon dioxide. This is because of oxygen's lesser solubility in the body fluids. As a result, oxygen transfer within the lungs will be affected much more than carbon dioxide's when diffusion abnormalities are present in a subject. Diffusion defects can produce clinically significant problems with arterial blood oxygen levels.

## TEST DESCRIPTION

Tests for pulmonary gas diffusion ($D_L$) measure the lungs' ability to permit transfer of an alveolar gas along the A-c pathway into blood, where it can combine with hemoglobin molecules. The force driving this transfer is the difference (*gradient*) between the gas's partial pressure in the alveolus (PAgas) and its partial pressure in the capillary blood (Pc-gas).

*Diffusing capacity* ($D_L$gas or $D_{gas}$) relates to the quantity of a specific gas that can diffuse along the A-c pathway in response to a given pressure gradient. If pathway conditions remain unchanged, a greater A-c pressure difference will result in a greater quantity of the gas being transferred.

For a gas of known solubility, $D_L$gas is defined by two factors:

- The volume of gas transferred between the alveoli and the pulmonary capillary blood per unit of time ($V_{gas}$; ml/min).
- The pressure gradient (PAgas − Pcgas; mm Hg) available along the diffusion pathway to drive the transfer.

The following equation demonstrates the relationship between these factors:

$$D_L gas = \frac{V_{gas}(\textbf{STPD})}{PAgas - Pcgas}$$

Values used for PAgas and Pcgas must represent the mean value for gas partial pressure in each physiologic compartment.

The gas transfer factors relating to diffusing capacity are not affected by the process of diffusion alone. Ventilation/perfusion relationships can also limit gas transfer in the lungs. Additionally, the measurement process used to determine $D_L$gas does not truly indicate the lungs' capacity for diffusion. Because these multiple factors affect gas transfer in the lungs, it has been suggested that *gas transfer factor* ($T_{gas}$) would be a more accurate term than $D_L$gas. Unfortunately the term $D_L$gas is still much more commonly applied.

The gas used to measure $D_L$gas must be capable of two physiologic actions:

- The gas must be capable of diffusing along the A-c pathway.
- The gas must be capable of being transported by hemoglobin.

For this reason, only two gases—oxygen and carbon monoxide—can be considered. Use of oxygen for diffusing capacity determination would be of direct clinical significance. There is, however, a serious limitation to measurement of oxygen diffusing capacity ($D_LO_2$). $PcO_2$ values are not constant. Instead, they increase in a nonlinear manner as blood flows past the alveolus. Although mean $PcO_2$ values can be determined, the process is complex and is sometimes inaccurate. This can seriously affect the accuracy of $D_LO_2$ measurement.

Carbon monoxide (CO) is ideal for $D_L$gas determination. It is subject to the same diffusion-pathway considerations as oxygen. Additionally, hemoglobin has a significant affinity for combining with CO (210 times greater affinity than for oxygen). Consequently, little or no CO remains dissolved in the plasma during the transfer process. The result is a mean PcCO value of zero (0) mm Hg. For this reason, *the PACO-PcCO difference (gradient) can generally be assumed to be equal to the value for PACO.*

The measurement of *carbon monoxide diffusing capacity* ($D_LCO$) is based on the number of milliliters per minute of CO transferred ($\dot{V}_{CO}$) for a given PACO value. The following equation expresses this relationship:

$$D_LCO = \frac{\dot{V}_{CO}(STPD)}{PACO}$$

The unit of measure for $D_LCO$ is milliliters of CO/minute/mm Hg STPD.

# TECHNIQUES FOR MEASUREMENT

There are different methods for using CO to assess diffusion in the lungs. They include measurement of fractional uptake of CO and the single-breath, steady-state, and rebreathing methods for measuring diffusing capacity. Each of these techniques will be described. Despite their apparent complexity, these techniques are all based on the basic principles just described.

## FRACTIONAL CO UPTAKE

*Fractional CO uptake* (FuCO) provides an index to indicate possible diffusion disorders in the lung. It is determined by having the subject breathe in a gas containing a small fraction (.001 or, in percent, 0.1%) of CO (FICO). The subject's exhaled air is collected in a spirometer or baglike reservoir. After a few minutes of having the subject breathe in this manner, a sample is taken from the exhaled air reservoir. The fraction of exhaled CO (FECO) in the sample can be measured with a gas analyzer. The following equation is used to determine FuCO and to express it as a percent.

$$FuCO = \frac{FICO - FECO}{FECO} \times 100$$

FuCO is affected by the level of the subject's ventilation. A less than normal subject minute volume during the measurement period can result in an erroneously small FuCO value. This is true even if there is no actual change in the subject's diffusing capacity.

A value for $D_LCO$ cannot be assessed because no attempt is made to determine the subject's PACO during the procedure. FuCO does provide, however, a simple screening tool. Given a relatively unchanged minute ventilation, if the FuCO results are normal, it is unlikely that the subject has a serious diffusion impairment or ventilation/perfusion abnormality. A reduced FuCO may indicate diffusion impairment.

## CARBON MONOXIDE DIFFUSING CAPACITY

As stated earlier, values for $\dot{V}_{CO}$ and the PACO must be available in order for $D_LCO$ to be determined. The methods used for acquiring these values and measuring $D_LCO$ fall into three basic categories of procedures: single-breath method ($D_LCO$-SB), steady-state method ($D_LCO$-SS), and rebreathing method ($D_LCO$-RB).

All three methods determine $\dot{V}_{CO}$ by some process that uses the difference between the inspired and expired fractions of CO (FICO and FECO, respectively). When these values are related to the lung volumes ($V_L$) used in their measurement, a value for $\dot{V}_{CO}$ can be calculated. Stated more simply,

$$FxCO \times V_L = V_{xCO} \quad \text{(where either I or E can be substituted for x)}$$

The difference between the $V_{ICO}$ and $V_{ECO}$ establishes a value for $\dot{V}_{CO}$.

There are significant differences between the three test methods. These differences fall primarily into the following areas:

- The type of breathing maneuver that the subject is required to perform during the procedure.
- Whether the values used for determining PACO are based on direct measurements, estimations, or assumptions.
- The number of different measurements and complexity of equipment required for performance of the procedure.
- The degree to which the test results are affected by ventilation/perfusion abnormalities.

The specifics of each measurement method will be described.

## Single-Breath (Modified Krogh) Method

The $D_LCO$-SB method uses a reasonably straightforward procedure for gathering the data needed to determine the partial pressure of alveolar CO (PACO). However, the subject must perform an unusual and possibly difficult breathing maneuver.

The procedure requires the subject to exhale down to the RV level. Then, breathing in a special gas mixture, she or he must perform a maximal inspiration to TLC and hold in the breath for a period of time ($T_{Hold}$). The subject must then exhale back down to the RV level. A valve system is used to control the source of inspired gas and the location to which the exhaled gas is directed.

Subject breathing must progress in a very controlled manner. A single, *rapid* inspiratory VC maneuver from RV is required. Inspiration must be held at the TLC level for approximately 10 seconds (9–11 seconds). The subject has to then exhale *rapidly* back down to the RV level. This is necessary to keep the CO diffusion time period controlled and limited. Prolonged expiration may artificially extend the CO diffusion time and produce an overestimation of $D_LCO$. In some circumstances, prolonged expiration may occur and be beyond the technologist's control. Subjects with obstructive airway disorders may uncontrollably create this problem.

The inspired gas mixture used for the procedure includes 0.3% CO, helium (He) (commonly 10%, although another inert gas, such as neon, may be used), and room air as the remaining balance of gas. This mixture provides values for the fractions of inspired CO (FICO) and He (FIHe).

During the subject's expiration, an alveolar gas sample is taken from the exhaled air. Alveolar gas sampling is performed after the first approximately 1000 ml are exhaled. This ensures that deadspace gas is not accidentally sampled. The sample is analyzed for a fractional value of exhaled He (FEHe) and a final fractional value for alveolar CO ($FACO_F$). The subject's VC volume ($V_{VC}$) must be measured and recorded during the procedure. In addition, barometric pressure ($P_{Atm}$) and water vapor pressure at BTPS ($P_{H2O}$) are required.

The equations used for $D_LCO$-SB determination are demonstrated in Table 6–1. The data collected during the test are applied in the following ways:

- FICO, FIHe, and FEHe are used together for calculation of an initial concentration of alveolar CO ($FACO_I$).
- FIHe and FEHe are used for calculation of the alveolar volume ($V_A$). (This is the term generally used to describe the end-inspiratory TLC lung volume level.) The method is similar to the helium dilution technique for measuring FRC.

Determination of $\dot{V}_{CO}$ is accomplished by the method described earlier. Unfortunately, this is not apparent in the final equation of Table 6–1. The relationships between $FACO_I$, $FACO_F$, and $V_A$ do relate to the inspiratory and expiratory values for $V_{CO}$, however, and work to provide a value for $\dot{V}_{CO}$ in the equation.

Determination of a value for mean PACO is performed using the simple data measurements described earlier. Mean PACO is based, however, on a complex set of physiologic variables. The relationship between $FACO_I$ and $P_{Atm} - P_{H_2O}$ establishes an initial

---

### TABLE 6–1  Determination of $D_LCO$ from a $D_LCO$-SB Procedure

---

Calculation of the initial fraction of CO in alveolar air at the start of $T_{Hold}$(FACO$_I$):

$$FACO_I = FICO \times \frac{FEHe}{FIHe}$$

Calculation of the alveolar volume $(V_A)$STPD:

$$V_A(STPD) = \frac{V_{VC}(STPD)}{FEHe/FIHe}$$

where

$$V_{VC}(STPD) = V_{VC}(ATPS) \times STPD \text{ factor}$$

Calculation of $D_{LCO}$SB, where $P_{H_2O}$ is equal to the vapor pressure of water in the alveoli at BTPS (47 mm Hg):

$$D_LCO\text{-}SB = \frac{V_A(STPD) \times 60}{(P_{Atm} - P_{H_2O})(T_{Hold})} \times Ln \frac{FACO_I}{FACO_F}$$

---

*Note: The number 60 is used to correct the calculation from seconds to minutes.*

value for PACO at the start of $T_{Hold}$. The complication is that PACO (and therefore FACO) is not constant during $T_{Hold}$ because of the diffusion of CO out of the alveoli. The value for FACO decreases exponentially (e) until the FACO$_F$ is reached just before expiration. This process is described in the following equation:

$$FACO_F = FACO_I \times e^{KT_{Hold}} \qquad \text{(Equation A)}$$

The value for K is determined by

$$K = \frac{D_LCO \times (P_{Atm} - P_{H_2O})}{V_A \times 60} \qquad \text{(Equation B)}$$

By taking the natural logarithm (Ln) of Equation A and by substituting and rearranging the values from Equation B, we can develop the final equation for determining $D_LCO$-SB (see Table 6–1). The actual process for derivation of the equation is beyond the scope of this text.

The time period for $T_{Hold}$ during the procedure must be precisely measured. Several different methods are used. *Each is based on times when diffusion is assumed to start (S) and end (E).* Figure 6–1 provides a tracing of the $D_LCO$-SB breathing maneuver and illustrates the different methods for $T_{Hold}$ determination.

- *Method A* measures $T_{hold}$ from the start of inspiration ($A_S$) to the start of alveolar sampling ($A_E$).
- *Method B* measures $T_{hold}$ between the point where the first one third of inspiration is completed ($B_S$) and the halfway point of the alveolar gas sampling ($B_E$).

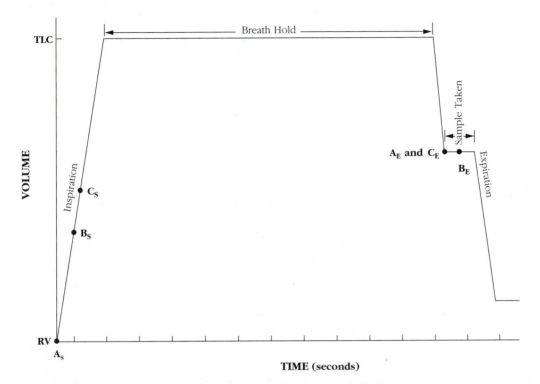

**Figure 6–1** *$D_LCO$-SB spirometer tracing demonstrating the methods for determining $T_{Hold}$.*

- *Method C* measures $T_{hold}$ between the halfway point of inspiration ($C_S$) and the beginning of alveolar sampling ($C_E$).

As inspiration and expiration are performed more rapidly by the subject, differences in the results between these three methods are minimized. Method B is the one currently recommended for use. The timing method selected by a laboratory should, if at all possible, match the one used by the source(s) of the predicted normal values.

The single-breath method is the one most widely used for determining $D_LCO$. Table 6–2 lists its advantages and disadvantages.

## Steady-State Methods

The $D_LCO$-SS methods allow for measurements to be made with the subject performing relatively normal tidal breathing. A gas mixture containing 0.1% CO, with the remaining balance air, is inhaled by the subject with each breath. The lower concentration of CO used with these procedures minimizes development of a significant PcCO level. If increased PcCO levels were to develop, the effect on the diffusion gradient would limit the benefits of using CO to perform the test.

During the last two minutes of breathing ($T_{Col}$), the subject's exhaled air is collected in a Douglas bag. A sample volume ($V_{Sam}$) is taken from the exhaled air. Values for $F\bar{E}CO$,

---

### TABLE 6–2  Overview of $D_L$CO-SB Method

---

#### Advantages

---

- Does not require the use of invasive measuring procedures.
- Analysis of only two gases is required.
- Test is easily and rapidly performed and can be repeated within a reasonably short period of time.

---

#### Disadvantages

---

- Nature of the breathing maneuver. The subject may have difficulty achieving a full inspiration, full expiration, sufficiently deep breath, or a 10-second breath hold.
- Not practical for use during exercise testing.
- Less than maximal inspired VC volumes affect measurement accuracy.
- Maldistribution of ventilation can affect the test results. Because a large inspired volume is used, however, the effects of ventilation/perfusion mismatches are minimized.

---

$\overline{\text{FE}}\text{CO}_2$, and $\text{FEN}_2$ are measured from the sample. The volume of $V_{Sam}$ and the remaining volume of collected air ($V_{Col}$) are measured. As will be described later, all of these measurements are used to determine values for $\dot{V}_{CO}$ and PACO. $D_L$CO-SS is then calculated by the simple equation,

$$D_L\text{CO-SS} = \frac{\dot{V}_{CO}(\text{STPD})}{\text{PACO}}$$

Determination of a value for $\dot{V}_{CO}$ is based on the principle described earlier. The required equations are provided in Table 6–3. With this calculation, the following adjustment factor is used in the third equation:

$$\left(\text{FICO} \times \frac{\text{FEN}_2}{\text{FIN}_2}\right)$$

It serves to compensate for the expired/inspired air volume difference that results from the respiratory exchange ratio. Calculation of $\text{FEN}_2$ and $\text{FIN}_2$ is based on the respiratory exchange difference of oxygen and carbon dioxide with breathing.

PACO is more difficult by steady-state testing than by single-breath testing. PCO analysis of a sample taken from collected, steady-state exhaled air cannot be used directly as a value for the subject's PACO. The alveolar gas in the sample is contaminated with gas from the subject's physiologic deadspace volume ($V_D$). Presence of $V_D$ gas lowers the exhaled PCO value in comparison to the actual value for PACO. The $D_L$CO-SB method avoids the problem of $V_D$ gas contamination because **end-tidal alveolar sampling** from a single large breath is used.

**TABLE 6–3   Calculation of $\dot{V}_{CO}$ for $D_LCO$-SS Determination**

$$\dot{V}_E(ATPS) = \frac{V_{Col} + V_{Sam}}{T_{Col}}$$

$$\dot{V}_E(STPD) = \dot{V}_E(ATPS) \times STPD\ factor$$

$$\dot{V}_{CO} = \dot{V}_E(STPD) \times \left[\left(FICO \times \frac{FEN_2}{FIN_2}\right) - FECO\right]$$

where $FIN_2$ and $FEN_2$ are determined by

$$FEN_2 = 1 - (FEO_2 + FECO_2)$$

$$FIN_2 = 1 - (FIO_2 + FICO_2)$$

Two possibilities exist for overcoming the difficulty of PACO determination with steady-state testing:

- *Compensate for the deadspace effects* on the PACO when determination is based on a sample of collected, exhaled air.
- *Sample "alveolar" gas* and measure the PACO directly.

Techniques that use these two principles are described here.

*Deadspace-Compensated Techniques.*   Two deadspace-compensated procedures are used. The *estimated-deadspace technique* incorporates calculation of a value for $V_D$ into the determination of PACO. The Bohr method for $V_D$ calculation, described in Chapter 5 and demonstrated in Table 5–3, is used. The application of this, as it relates to PACO determination, is demonstrated in Table 6–4.

The second deadspace-compensated procedure is the *assumed-deadspace technique*. With this procedure, an assumed value of $V_D$ is used in determining PACO. The assumed $V_D$ is based on the following relationship.

$V_D = 1$ ml/lb of the subject's lean body weight

A value for lean body weight can generally be obtained from charts that relate weight to the subject's height. Given an assumed value for $V_D$, the calculation of PACO is provided in Table 6–5.

Misestimation of $V_D$ can lead to errors in $D_LCO$ determination by this method. The technique is very useful for $D_LCO$ measurement during exercise, however. The large tidal volumes that occur during exercise, in relation to the unchanging deadspace volume, make any misestimation of $V_D$ a less significant concern.

*Alveolar Gas Sampling Technique.*   The alveolar gas sampling technique eliminates the problem of $V_D$ and PACO that is associated with the other steady-state methods. The

---

**TABLE 6–4  Calculation of PACO by Estimated-Deadspace Technique**

---

An estimated value for $FACO_2$ can be determined by using the $PaCO_2$ from an arterial blood gas sample in the following equation:

$$FACO_2 = \frac{PaCO_2}{P_{Atm} - P_{H_2O}}$$

Assuming that the $V_D/V_T$ calculation based on CO values is the same as for $CO_2$ values,

$$\frac{V_D}{V_T} = \frac{FACO_2 - F\bar{E}CO_2}{FACO_2} = \frac{FACO - F\bar{E}CO}{FACO - FICO}$$

Solving the above equation for FACO:

$$FACO = \left(FICO - \frac{FACO_2}{F\bar{E}CO_2}\right)(FICO - F\bar{E}CO)$$

Since

$$PACO = (P_{Atm} - P_{H_2O}) \times FACO$$

a value for PACO can be calculated by

$$PACO = (P_{Atm} - P_{H_2O}) \times \left[\left(FICO - \frac{FACO_2}{F\bar{E}CO}_2\right)(FICO - F\bar{E}CO)\right]$$

---

*Note: The $FICO_2$, as described in Table 5–3, is not needed in the $CO_2$ calculation of $V_D/V_T$ because it has a relative value of 0.0 mm Hg. In the CO calculation, FICO has a value and must be included in the equation.*

---

**TABLE 6–5  Calculation of PACO by Assumed-Deadspace Technique**

---

The effects of an assumed $V_D$ on FACO can be taken into account by the following proportional relationship:

$$FACO = \frac{(V_T \times F\bar{E}CO) - (V_D \times FICO)}{V_T - V_D}$$

PACO can then be calculated from FACO the same way it is in the estimated-deadspace technique.

$$PACO = (P_{Atm} - P_{H_2O}) \times FACO$$

technique uses direct sampling of the subject's end-tidal exhaled air during the last two minutes of the steady-state procedure. With breath-by-breath analysis, a mean partial pressure of CO in end-tidal exhaled air ($P\overline{e}tCO$) can be determined. The $P\overline{e}tCO$ is then assumed to be equivalent to the subject's PACO and is used directly to calculate $D_LCO$-SS. $\dot{V}_{CO}$ is still determined by the method described earlier.

The difficulty with this technique is that it is not always correct to assume that the value for $P\overline{e}tCO$ is equal to the PACO. Small or uneven tidal breathing volumes can make proper sampling difficult and can create differences in these values. Additionally, $P\overline{e}tCO$ values may differ significantly from PACO values during exercise.

*Summary for the $D_LCO$-SS Methods.*    Table 6–6 lists the advantages and disadvantages of the $D_LCO$-SS methods. The different steady-state techniques, if performed on a single subject, will generally produce the same approximate value for $D_LCO$. Overall, however, values for $D_LCO$-SS are smaller than $D_LCO$-SB values. The differences are even greater in subjects with disorders that affect the distribution of ventilation. The $D_LCO$-SB breathing maneuver probably allows the lungs to overcome mechanical differences in the distribution of ventilation. As a result, the test is less affected by ventilation disorders that affect ventilation/perfusion relationships. The adverse effects of ventilation disorders on steady-state procedures are a major reason they are not often used.

Another problem with the steady-state methods is the assumption that PcCO has a value of 0.0 mm Hg. Because of prolonged breathing on the test gas, a significant quantity of carboxyhemoglobin (COHb) may develop in the capillary blood. This can produce a PcCO back pressure that will affect the alveolocapillary CO diffusion gradient and the rate of diffusion. It is possible to estimate the gradient under these conditions, but the process increases the complexity of performing the $D_LCO$-SS methods.

## Rebreathing Methods

The $D_LCO$-RB methods, like the $D_LCO$-SS methods, allow for measurements to be made during tidal breathing by the subject. There are two rebreathing method techniques: the reservoir-sampling technique and the washout-sampling technique.

Both techniques involve having the subject rebreathe a gas mixture from a bag or balloonlike reservoir. The gas mixture used contains 0.3% CO and 10% He with the remaining balance of gas being air. The volume of the reservoir is approximately equal to the volume of the subject's $FEV_1$.

The subject first exhales down to the RV level and then begins rebreathing from the reservoir at this level. During rebreathing, the subject should maintain a breathing rate as close to 30 breaths per minute as possible. The reservoir must be emptied completely with each inspiration. From this point on, the two rebreathing techniques differ.

*Reservoir-Sampling Technique.*    In reservoir sampling, the subject rebreathes the gas mixture for a timed period ($T_{RB}$) of approximately 30–45 seconds. A sample of rebreathed gas is then taken from the reservoir, and the concentrations of CO, He, and $O_2$ are mea-

TABLE 6–6   **Overview of the D$_L$CO-SS Methods**

### All D$_L$CO-SS Methods

#### *Advantage*

- Allow a more natural breathing maneuver and allow for measurements to be made under a greater variety of clinical conditions (exercise, sleep, anesthesia).

#### *Disadvantages*

- Generally more complex and difficult to perform because of the difficulty in determining PACO.
- Allow the possibility for COHb buildup, which can be the source of PcCO back pressure.
- More affected by ventilation/perfusion abnormalities because of the smaller lung volumes used. This can produce more error than a properly performed D$_L$CO-SS test.

### Deadspace-Compensated Technique

#### *Advantage*

- Avoids errors that can occur with end-tidal PACO measurement.

#### *Disadvantage*

- Misestimation of V$_D$ can result in inaccurate PACO and therefore inaccurate D$_L$CO-SS calculation. This is less of a problem with testing during exercise where larger tidal volumes make V$_D$ a smaller portion of the V$_T$. As a result, V$_D$ misestimation produces less error.

### Estimated-Deadspace (Filey) Technique

#### *Advantage*

- Provides a more accurate value for V$_D$ than does the assumed V$_D$ technique.

#### *Disadvantage*

- Requires an arterial blood gas sample.

### Assumed-Deadspace Technique

#### *Advantage*

- Avoids the need for arterial blood sampling.

## TABLE 6–6 (Continued)

### Disadvantage

- Poses greater risk of $V_D$ misestimation (although this does not prevent the procedure from being useful for testing during exercise).

### Alveolar Gas Sampling Technique

### Advantage

- Avoids errors associated with $V_D$ misestimation.

### Disadvantage

- Possible error in assuming that PetCO is equivalent to the mean PACO value. This is most likely when $V_T$s are small or uneven or when sampling is done during exercise.

sured. Given this data, the process for determining $D_LCO$-RB is similar to that used with the $D_LCO$-SB method (see Table 6–1). It is demonstrated in the following equation:

$$D_LCO\text{-}RB = \frac{V_{SR}(STPD) \times 60}{(P_{Atm} - P_{H_2O})(T_{RB})} \times Ln\ \frac{FACO_I}{FACO_F}$$

where $V_{SR}$ = the volume of the subject and reservoir combined.

The value for $V_{SR}$ is found by taking the initial reservoir volume ($V_R$), after converting it to STPD, and performing the following calculation:

$$V_{SR} = V_R \times \frac{FIHe}{FEHe}$$

*Washout-Sampling Technique.* In washout sampling, rebreathing continues until a gas concentration equilibrium is reached between the reservoir and the subject's lungs. The subject is then switched to inhaling air. Exhalation washes the gas mixture from the subject's lungs and allows for the concentrations of CO and He to be analyzed. Rapid-response analyzer systems are used, and the results are recorded.

Determination of $D_LCO$-RB by this technique is based on the following principle: During the washout period, CO is lost from the lungs both through ventilation and through diffusion into the blood stream. Helium is lost only through ventilation. As a result, *the analyzed concentrations of CO in the exhaled air will reduce at a faster rate than will the concentrations of He.* Determination of diffusion is based on this difference in washout rates.

Again, a series of equations similar to those in Table 6–1 are used to calculate $D_LCO$-RB by this technique. One difference, however, is that a logarithmic expression relating to the ratio of the initial and final fractions of He is added to the last equation in Table 6–1.

---

**TABLE 6–7  Overview of the $D_LCO$-RB Methods**

---

### *Advantage*

---

• $D_LCO$ method least affected by ventilation/perfusion abnormalities or by changes in the subject's lung volume at the time of measurement.

---

### *Disadvantages*

---

• Complexity of the instrumentation and equations required.
• Results can be affected by PcCO buildup during the procedure unless it is compensated for by complex calculations.
• The results of repeat testing may not always be reproducible because of the need for subject cooperation with breathing and the possibility of PcCO back pressure.

---

The washout-sampling technique is the $D_LCO$ method least affected by ventilation/perfusion abnormalities or by changes in the subject's lung volume at the time of testing. Unfortunately, because of the significant complexity of instrumentation and the calculations required, this technique is generally limited to research applications.

*Summary for the $D_LCO$-RB Methods.*  The advantages and disadvantages for $D_LCO$-RB determination are listed in Table 6–7. These techniques are not generally useful for performing routine $D_LCO$ determination. It must be noted, however, that the $D_LCO$-RB techniques are the ones least affected by ventilation/perfusion abnormalities.

## Comparison of the $D_LCO$ Methods

Table 6–8 provides a summary comparison of the $D_LCO$ methods. As stated earlier, the single-breath method is the one most often used for routine $D_LCO$ determination. In general, the steady-state methods are not used because of their greater risk of error when ventilation-based ventilation/perfusion abnormalities are present in the subject.

## ESTIMATION OF MEMBRANE DIFFUSING CAPACITY AND PULMONARY CAPILLARY BLOOD VOLUME

CO diffusion is a process of gas conductance along the pulmonary diffusion pathway. As a result of abnormalities, changes in the pathway's characteristics can increase resistance to CO conductance. This resistance can cause a reduction in the measured $D_LCO$.

Both physical and chemical pathway characteristics affect conductance and $D_LCO$ (Table 6–9). The two physical characteristics of the alveolocapillary membrane, together, influence what is referred to as the *membrane diffusing capacity* ($D_M$). Individually, the physical and chemical characteristics of the diffusion pathway are approximately equal in the

## TABLE 6–8 Overview of the $D_L$CO Methods

### Single-Breath Methods

- Simplest of the methods in terms of instrumentation and calculations, but it requires the subject to perform a potentially difficult breathing maneuver.
- It is moderately affected by ventilation/perfusion abnormalities.
- Changes in lung volume at the time of measurement can significantly affect test results.

### Steady-State Methods

- More natural subject breathing is permitted, but the test procedures are moderately complex.
- Most likely to be affected by ventilation/perfusion abnormalities.

### Rebreathing Methods

- Least affected by ventilation/perfusion abnormalities.
- The required test procedures and instrumentation are the most complex of all the methods.

amount of resistance they produce. The pathophysiologic factors affecting $D_M$, $\theta_{CO}$, and $V_c$ are listed in Table 6–10.

It is possible to relate CO conductance and $D_L$CO to the potential sources of physical and chemical resistance that can affect them. Because resistance is expressed as the reciprocal of conductance, the summing of the resistances to CO diffusion can be demonstrated in the following way:

$$\frac{1}{D_L CO} = \frac{1}{D_M} + \frac{1}{\theta_{co} V_c}$$

## TABLE 6–9 Characteristics of Pulmonary Diffusion Pathway Affecting $D_L$CO

### Physical Characteristics of the Alveolocapillary Membrane (Determinants of $D_M$)

- Surface area of the alveolar-capillary interface.
- Thickness of the alveolocapillary membrane pathway.

### Chemical Characteristics of the Blood

- Reaction rate of CO with hemoglobin in the blood ($\theta_{CO}$ – ml of CO/min/mm Hg/ml of blood).
- Capillary red blood cell volume ($V_C$ – ml of blood).

## TABLE 6–10  Factors Affecting $D_M$, $\theta_{CO}$, and $V_c$

### $D_M$

#### Surface Area of the Alveolocapillary Membrane

- Changes in actual surface area because of loss of pulmonary parenchymal tissue.
- Changes in effective surface because of ventilation abnormalities that produce ventilation/perfusion inequalities.

#### Thickness of the Alveolocapillary Membrane Pathway

- Alveolar filling and edema.
- Interstitial edema.
- Alveolocapillary parenchymal thickening.

### $\theta_{CO}$

- Changes in $P\bar{c}O_2$.
- Changes in quantity of functional red blood cells/hemoglobin.

### $V_c$

- Changes in number and volume of perfused pulmonary capillaries. These changes may be due to changes in cardiac output/pulmonary artery pressure or in body position that redistribute the pattern of pulmonary perfusion.

This equation provides a basis for clinical evaluation of the $D_M$ and $V_C$ sources of resistance to CO diffusion. The key is the reaction rate of CO with hemoglobin, $\theta_{CO}$. The value for $\theta_{CO}$, given a known $PcO_2$, has been established through experimental testing. It is indirectly related to the amount of oxygen attached to hemoglobin. As blood $PO_2$ increases and more oxygen is attached to hemoglobin, less CO can be taken up and transported by hemoglobin.

With this background, the determination of $D_L CO$ pathway resistance is based on performing the $D_L CO$-SB procedure at different levels of inspired oxygen. A different value for $PAO_2$ results at each $FIO_2$ that is used. This value is easily determined by application of the alveolar air equation. The value for $PcO_2$ at each $FIO_2$ can be assumed to be equal to the $PAO_2$. As stated earlier, for each $PcO_2$ value, there is a corresponding known value for $\theta_{CO}$.

If the value for $1/D_L CO$-SB is plotted against the value for $1/\theta_{CO}$ at which it is measured, both $1/D_M$ and $1/V_c$ can be determined (Figure 6–2). A line is drawn along the points that are plotted. The value for $1/D_M$ is established by extending the line to the Y axis. This line represents the resistance to gas diffusion that is due only to membrane char-

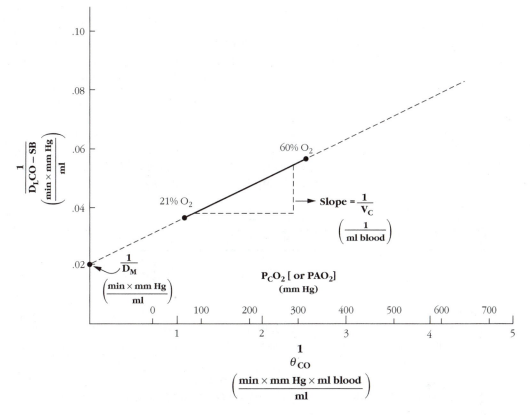

**Figure 6–2** *Determination of $D_M$ and $V_c$.*

acteristics. A value for $1/V_c$ can be determined by calculating the slope of the line. The slope represents the diffusion resistance that results from the capillary red blood cell volume.

## EQUIPMENT REQUIRED

Because the $D_LCO$-SB method is the one most frequently used, the equipment requirements for that method will be discussed here. This equipment includes

- An inspired gas source. A sealed spirometer or bag-in-box arrangement prefilled with the test gas could be used. A demand breathing system connected directly to a tank containing the test gas is also possible. The test gas, at sea level, should consist of 0.3% CO, 10% He, 21% $O_2$, and the remainder $N_2$. At altitudes greater than sea level, the $O_2$ percent should be increased to produce a $PIO_2$ of 150 mm Hg. If this is not possible, the test results may be adjusted for the increased altitude in the following manner:

$$D_LCO \text{ Adjusted} = D_LCO \text{ Measured} \times [1.0 + 0.0035(P_{Atm} - P_{H_2O})]$$

- A five-way breathing valve to direct the subject's inspiratory and expiratory air flows as required for inspiration, volume measurement, and gas sampling.
- An end-tidal gas sampling/analysis system for CO and He.
- A spirometer/recording system. This system must be linked to measure and record both the volume of inspired test gas and the subject's exhaled air volume.

Figure 6–3 illustrates a possible $D_L$CO-SB breathing circuit. A bag-in-box inspired gas source is used. It is linked to the spirometer system in order to allow measurement of the inspired gas volume.

Modern laboratory systems for performing $D_L$CO procedures are highly automated. Such functions as position changes of the five-way valve, end-tidal sampling, and electronic monitoring of $T_{Hold}$ are performed automatically by the system.

## TEST ADMINISTRATION

In order for a $D_L$CO-SB test to be performed successfully, certain pre-test conditions must be met:

- The subject should refrain from smoking for at least 24 hours before the test. This is because a heavy smoker can have a COHb level of as much as 10%–12%. Such elevated COHb levels negate the assumption that the PcCO is zero during the test and thus affect test results. The time of the subject's last cigarette should be recorded.
- The subject should refrain from consuming alcohol for at least four hours before the test. This is because alcohol consumption has been found to reduce $D_L$CO measurements.

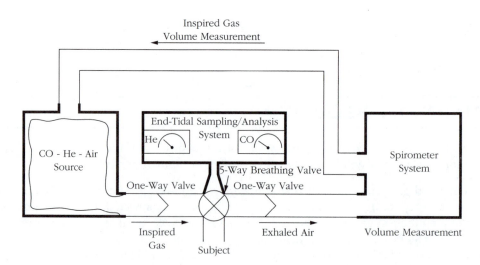

**Figure 6–3**  $D_L$CO-SB breathing circuit.

- The subject should refrain from eating for at least two hours before the test. This is because digestion of heavy meals can alter pulmonary capillary blood volume and thus affect test results.
- The subject should refrain from any strenuous exercise before the test because of its effects on pulmonary capillary blood volume.
- An oxygen-enriched gas mixture should not be breathed by the subject immediately prior to administration of the test. A time of at least 20 minutes is recommended between the administration of nitrogen washout and/or shunt studies and the administration of a $D_LCO$ test.
- The subject should sit and rest for at least five minutes before the test. This is, again, to minimize the effects of exercise on pulmonary capillary blood flow.
- Supplemental oxygen should be discontinued at least five minutes before the test. If the lack of supplemental oxygen is not tolerated by the subject for that long, test results will have to be interpreted with caution.

A rest of at least four minutes is recommended between repeats of the procedure. This is to allow residual CO to be washed from the lungs prior to the next test. The test should be performed with the subject in a sitting position and wearing nose clips. The subject should remain sitting throughout the test sequence.

Also, both inspiration from RV to TLC and exhalation back down to RV should be as rapid as possible. During the breath-hold, the subject should be instructed to simply relax against a closed glottis or, if the system allows, closed breathing valve.

The exhaled washout volume prior to alveolar sampling should be 750 ml–1000 ml. In subjects having a VC of less than 2.0 liters, the washout volume may be reduced to 500 ml. Generally, the volume of the alveolar sample taken after washout should be between 500 ml and 1000 ml, and the sample should be collected in less than four seconds.

The criteria for $D_LCO$-SB test acceptability and reproducibility and selection of data for reporting are stated in Table 6–11.

As mentioned earlier, a break of at least four minutes should take place before a $D_LCO$ test is repeated. This is to allow residual CO to be washed from the lungs before the next test. During this break, the subject should remain seated. Patients with COPD can be instructed to take several deep breaths during the break to rid themselves more effectively of the CO.

The He dilution process used to determine $V_A$ during the $D_LCO$ test can present a problem for patients with moderate to severe obstructive disorders. This is the same problem experienced with the He dilution test for FRC; the subject's poor-quality ventilation can cause a misestimation of the true volume. In this case, the subject's $V_A$ may be estimated as being lower than its actual value. Consequently, a less than actual determination of $D_LCO$ will result. To avoid the problem, some technologists use a previously measured value for RV, added to the VC measured during the $D_LCO$ procedure, as a value for $V_A$. If this is done, the results of both the original and modified methods should be reported and clearly identified.

---

**TABLE 6–11 Criteria for D$_L$CO-SB Test Acceptability, Reproducibility, and Selection of Data for Reporting**

---

### Acceptability Criteria

---

A test for D$_L$CO may be considered *acceptable* if:

- The initial inspiration from RV to TLC must have a volume that is ≥90% of the patient's previously measured VC volume. The inspiration must be performed within four seconds.
- A stable end-inspiratory breath-hold at TLC must be performed for nine to eleven seconds. There should be no evidence of system leaks or a Valsalva or Müller maneuver performed by the subject.
- The expiration back down to RV after the breath-hold must be performed within four seconds.
- Adequate clearance of deadspace volume must occur before alveolar sampling for CO and He is performed.

---

### Reproducibility Criteria

---

At least two acceptable tests for D$_L$CO must be performed, with *reproducibility* being demonstrated if:

- The D$_L$CO measurements from the tests are within 10% or 3 ml CO (STPD)/min/mm Hg of the average D$_L$CO value from the tests.

---

### Data Reporting Criteria

---

Based on acceptable test results:

- The *mean* value from two reproducible D$_L$CO tests should be reported.
- If the patient's best effort at performing the tests is suboptimal, then the average results of the two better performed tests should be reported with a notation on concerns for the quality of the tests.

---

# INTERPRETATION OF TEST RESULTS

Predicted normal D$_L$CO values are directly related to the subject's height or *body surface area* (BSA), and blood hemoglobin level. Greater height (BSA) and levels of hemoglobin will result in a greater D$_L$CO. For each gram of change in the subject's hemoglobin level, the D$_L$CO value will change by approximately 7%. This adjustment factor is included in some regression equations used to generate predicted normal values for D$_L$CO.

Prediction equations that do not include this factor require that the subject's measured value be adjusted before a comparison can be made to predicted values. The following equations are used:

$$\text{Hb Correction Factor} = \frac{1}{0.07 \times \text{gm Hb}}$$

Adjusted $D_L CO$ = Measured $D_L CO \times$ Hb Correction Factor

The adjusted $D_L CO$ can then be compared to the predicted values. With this adjustment, Hb values greater than 14.4 grams will produce an adjusted $D_L CO$ that is less than the original measured value. With an Hb less than 14.4 grams, the adjusted $D_L CO$ will be greater.

Normal $D_L CO$ values are indirectly related to age. Older subjects will have smaller $D_L CO$ values. Male subjects will generally have greater $D_L CO$ values than female subjects. Normal values for children are affected by fewer variables. Values for children are affected by height but not by either age or gender.

A value for $D_L O_2$ can be derived from the measurement of $D_L CO$ by use of the following equation:

$$D_L O_2 = D_L CO \times 1.23$$

A typical normal resting value for $D_L CO$-SB is approximately 25 ml CO/min/mm Hg. $D_L CO$ measured in the same subject by a steady-state technique will generally have a value that is less by about 30%. It has been found that $D_L CO$ values, beginning about mid-morning, decrease 1.2–2.2% per hour throughout the course of the day. This fact can affect reproducibility if repeat tests for the same subject are performed at different times of the day.

$D_L CO$ can increase or decrease in response to changes in a subject's condition. If a $D_L CO$ value is measured to be within ±20% of predicted, it can be considered normal. This guideline is not a particularly sensitive one, however. A more subtle discrimination of normal from abnormal is provided by use of 95% confidence limits for the predicted values. This concept is covered in detail in Chapter 7.

Table 6–12 lists the conditions that can cause changes in $D_L CO$. Increased $D_L CO$ values due to increases in $V_c$ can occur as a result of several different mechanisms. In left-to-right cardiovascular shunt abnormalities and in indigenous (native) populations living at high altitudes, the increased $V_c$ is due to mild pulmonary hypertension. Increased pulmonary blood flow and/or pressure is responsible for the increased $V_c$ and greater $D_L CO$ values seen during exercise. This mechanism also occurs in subjects with left heart failure. Movement of a subject from an upright to a supine body position causes the redistribution of intrapulmonary blood flow. *With each of these mechanisms, there is an increase in the amount of blood flow to the apical pulmonary capillaries that normally have little perfusion.* It is this factor that is primarily responsible for increases in $V_c$ and $D_L CO$.

Decreases in $D_L CO$ are produced by a wide variety of pathologic changes. These changes can occur in combination with an increase in lung volume. Emphysema is an ex-

---

### TABLE 6–12 Conditions That Produce Changes in D$_L$CO

---

#### Increased D$_L$CO

---

Left-to-right cardiovascular shunt abnormalities (1)
Indigeuous peoples living at high altitude (1)
Exercise (1)
Left heart failure (1)
Supine body position (1)
Early polycythemia (2)

---

#### Decreased D$_L$CO

---

Emphysema (3)
Pulmonary resection (4)
Asbestosis (4)
Chronic hypersensitivity pneumonitis (4)
Lymphangitic spread of carcinoma (4)
Hamman-Rich disease (chronic interstitial pneumonitis) (4)
Histiocytosis (4)
Oxygen toxicity (4)
Radiation-induced fibrosis (4)
Sarcoidosis (4)
Scleroderma lung disease (4)
Systemic lupus erythematosus (4)
Pulmonary alveolar proteinosis (4)
Anemia (5)
Pulmonary emboli (6)
Early collagen-vascular disorders (6)
Early miliary tuberculosis (6)
Early sarcoidosis (6)

---

1 = increased pulmonary capillary blood volume with relatively unchanged lung volumes (increased $V_c$/normal $V_A$).

2 = increased number of red blood cells with relatively unchanged lung volumes (increased $\theta_{CO}$/normal $V_A$).

3 = loss of functional alveolocapillary tissue with an increase in lung volume (decreased $D_M$/increased $V_A$).

4 = loss of functional alveolocapillary tissue with a decrease in lung volume (decreased $D_M$/decreased $V_A$).

5 = reduced number of red blood cells with relatively unchanged lung volumes (decreased $\theta_{CO}$/normal $V_A$).

6 = loss of pulmonary capillary bed with relatively unchanged lung volumes (decreased $V_c$/normal $V_A$).

TABLE 6–13   **Assignment of Severity for Diffusion Disorders**

| | |
|---|---|
| Normal | 80%–120% of predicted |
| Mild | 60%–79% of predicted |
| Moderate | 40%–59% of predicted |
| Severe | 20%–39% of predicted |
| Very severe | <20% of predicted |

ample. More often, however, the reduction in $D_LCO$ is in conjunction with a loss of functional lung volume.

Assignment of severity for abnormal $D_LCO$ values is somewhat arbitrary. General guidelines are given in Table 6–13. The specific diffusion disorders present in a subject can greatly affect the usefulness of this rating system, however. $D_LCO$ value of less than 40% demonstrates a severe impairment when a diffuse interstitial pulmonary disorder is present.

$D_LCO$ measurements are not useful for evaluating the severity of COPD. Expiratory flow-rate measurement with an FVC test is far more sensitive for quantitating the severity of COPD. On the other hand, measurement of $D_LCO$ aids the differentiation of the sources of chronic airway obstruction. For a given severity of airway obstruction, $D_LCO$ will be relatively close to normal if the primary disorder is chronic bronchitis. If emphysema is the primary disorder, though, $D_LCO$ values will be less than normal.

An abnormal $D_LCO$-SB value alone may not present a complete picture of the pulmonary changes that have taken place in a subject. Evaluation can be aided by taking into account the lung volume at which the $D_LCO$-SB value was measured. An accepted method for doing this is demonstrated in the following equation:

$$D_L/V_A = \frac{D_LCO\text{-SB}}{V_A}$$

$D_L/V_A$ allows for easier differentiation of the change or pathophysiology involved. This is especially true for abnormally reduced $D_LCO$-SB values. The conditions that affect $D_L/V_A$ can be differentiated into ones that

1. Increase $D_L$ but leave $V_A$ relatively unchanged. *The $D_L/V_A$ in this case is increased.*
2. Decrease $D_L$ in conjunction with a decrease in $V_A$. *This results in either a normal, slightly increased, or slightly decreased $D_L/V_A$ value.*
3. Decrease $D_L$ in conjunction with a normal, increased, or even slightly decreased $V_A$. *This produces a decreased value for $D_L/V_A$.*

Table 6–14 lists the trends of $D_L/V_A$ values as they relate to conditions that affect $D_L$.

TABLE 6–14   **D$_L$/V$_A$ Trends in Response to Disorders That Affect D$_L$CO-SB**

| Near Normal D$_L$/V$_A$ | D$_L$ | | V$_A$ |
|---|---|---|---|
| Pulmonary resection | Decreased | 1 | Decreased |
| **Normal, Slightly Increased, or Slightly Decreased D$_L$/V$_A$** | **D$_L$** | | **V$_A$** |
| Asbestosis | Decreased | 2 | Decreased |
| Chronic hypersensitivity pneumonitis | Decreased | 2 | Decreased |
| Lymphangitic spread of carcinoma | Decreased | 2 | Decreased |
| Hamman-Rich disease (chronic interstitial pneumonitis) | Decreased | 2 | Decreased |
| Histiocytosis | Decreased | 2 | Decreased |
| Oxygen toxicity | Decreased | 2 | Decreased |
| Radiation-induced fibrosis | Decreased | 2 | Decreased |
| Sarcoidosis | Decreased | 2 | Decreased |
| Scleroderma lung disease | Decreased | 2 | Decreased |
| Systemic lupus erythematosus | Decreased | 2 | Decreased |
| **Increased D$_L$/V$_A$** | **D$_L$** | | **V$_A$** |
| Left-to-right cardiovascular shunt abnormalities | Increased | | Normal |
| Indigenous peoples living at high altitude | Increased | | Normal |
| Exercise | Increased | | Normal |
| Left heart failure | Increased | | Normal |
| Supine body position | Increased | | Normal |
| Early polycythemia | Increased | | Normal |
| **Decreased D$_L$/V$_A$** | **D$_L$** | | **V$_A$** |
| Anemia | Decreased | | Normal |
| Pulmonary emboli | Decreased | | Normal |
| Early collagen-vascular disorders | Decreased | | Normal |
| Early miliary tuberculosis | Decreased | | Normal |
| Early sarcoidosis | Decreased | | Normal |
| Emphysema | Decreased | | Increased |

**TABLE 6–14  (Continued)**

| | | | |
|---|---|---|---|
| Pulmonary alveolar proteinosis | Decreased | 3 | Decreased |

$1 =$ the decrease in both $D_L$ and $V_A$ is approximately equal.
$2 =$ the decrease in $D_L$ and $V_A$ may be equal or, depending on the disorder, one may decrease to a greater degree than the other.
$3 =$ the decrease in $D_L$ is greater than the decrease in $V_A$.

## Review Questions

Please use the following review questions to evaluate your learning of information from this chapter. It might be helpful to write out your answers on a sheet of paper. If you are unsure of the answers to these questions, review the chapter to reinforce your learning.

1. What is meant by the diffusing capacity of a gas, and what two factors affect diffusing capacity?
2. How is factional CO uptake measured, and how is it clinically useful?
3. What is the basic technique for performing the single-breath method test for CO diffusing capacity?
4. Relating to steady-state method tests for CO diffusing capacity,
   a. What is the basic technique for performing steady-state method tests for CO diffusing capacity?
   b. How do the deadspace-compensated techniques differ from the alveolar gas sampling technique?
5. Relating to rebreathing method tests for CO diffusing capacity,
   a. What is the basic technique for performing rebreathing method tests for CO diffusing capacity?
   b. How does the reservoir-sampling technique differ from the washout-sampling technique?
6. What are relative advantages and disadvantages for the different CO diffusing capacity tests?
7. Relating to the physical and chemical characteristics of the pulmonary diffusion pathway,
   a. What are the physical and chemical characteristics of the pulmonary diffusion pathway that can affect $D_L CO$?
   b. How can these characteristics be determined?
8. Relating to $D_L CO$-SB testing,
   a. How is a $D_L CO$-SB test performed?
   b. What are key points about the subject's activity level and the way the subject should breath during the test?
   c. What are criteria for $D_L CO$-SB test acceptability, reproducibility, and selection of data for reporting?

9. Relating to $D_LCO$ values,
   a. What factors affect a subject's predicted normal $D_LCO$ values?
   b. How can a $D_LCO$ value be adjusted to reflect a value for $D_LO_2$?
10. What conditions can cause changes in a subject's $D_LCO$ values?
11. How can relating $D_LCO$-SB values to the volume at which they are measured provide for easier differentiation of changes or pathophysiologies in the lung?

# CHAPTER SEVEN

# PREDICTED NORMAL VALUES FOR PULMONARY FUNCTION TESTS

## ——— RELATED LEARNING ———

Prior knowledge of the following related information will facilitate understanding and learning of the material in this chapter. The learner will be aided by being able to

1. Recall the concepts of pulmonary function testing covered in Chapters 2, 4, 5, and 6.

## ——— LEARNING OBJECTIVES ———

Upon successful completion of this chapter, the learner should be able to

1. State factors that affect predicted normal pulmonary function values in relation to
   a. primary characteristics
   b. secondary characteristics
2. Describe sources of predictive equations that can be used to establish normal pulmonary function values.
3. Describe the selection of predictive equations for use in a laboratory.
4. Describe procedures that can be used to establish a normal range for predicted pulmonary function values based on the
   a. percentage-range method
   b. 95% confidence limit methods

## ——— KEY TERMS ———

coefficient of variation
gender
mean value (arithmetic mean)

95% confidence limit (or interval)
normal (Gaussian) distribution
standard deviation

Assessment of pulmonary function is based on comparing a subject's test results against the predicted normal values for that subject. For example, suppose a subject's FVC measures 3.8 liters. Does this indicate that the subject's pulmonary function is normal? Or is this an abnormal value, indicating that a disorder is present? How can we know?

In this case, the results are normal if the subject is a five foot, six inch, 20-year-old female. What if, however, the subject were taller or shorter, older or younger, or male. Predicted normal pulmonary function values make it possible to determine whether a given subject's test results indicate the presence of an abnormality. Although examples in this chapter relate primarily to tests for lung volume and pulmonary mechanics, the principles covered are appropriate for use with any measure of pulmonary function.

Normal pulmonary function values are affected by the physical characteristics of the subject. For this reason, it is not possible to have a single "normal" value for each pulmonary function parameter as applied to all subjects. It is possible, however, to have certain key physical characteristics taken into account when predicting normal pulmonary function values for a given subject. This is done by building the key physical characteristics into an equation. For example, the following two equations have been developed to predict normal values for VC for adult male and female subjects.

Male Subjects $\qquad$ VC = $(0.0580 \times \text{height}) - (0.025 \times \text{age}) - 4.24$

Female Subjects $\qquad$ VC = $(0.0453 \times \text{height}) - (0.024 \times \text{age}) - 2.85$

These examples demonstrate that the primary characteristics affecting pulmonary function are the subject's height (and possibly weight), age, and **gender**. Secondary characteristics include the race/ethnic origins of the subject, the altitude at which the subject is living, and other environmental factors relating to the subject's location.

# FACTORS AFFECTING PREDICTED NORMAL VALUES

## PRIMARY CHARACTERISTICS

Among subjects of the same gender, *height* is the single greatest factor that affects pulmonary function. Taller subjects have, overall, greater pulmonary function values. This is especially true for lung volume and diffusing capacity values. The relative increases in expiratory flow rate values with greater height are not as significant.

In children, normal values are more directly related to height than to age. This is true until a height of approximately 60 inches (152 cm) is reached. After that point, the age of the subject also begins to be a factor in predicting normal values.

The *weight* of the subject is sometimes taken into consideration along with height. This is often done by using the value for the subject's *body surface area* (BSA). The equation for calculating BSA is

$$\text{BSA} = \text{Ht}^{0.725} \times \text{Wt}^{0.425} \times 0.007148$$

where the height (Ht) is in centimeters, the weight (Wt) is in kilograms, and the BSA is in square meters (m²).

The effects of weight can be seen when comparing lung volume values for adult subjects of the same height. Beginning with lesser values of normal weight for a given height, there is an increase in the lung volumes as weight increases. This increase is related to the effects of greater muscularity. As weight continues to increase beyond the normal range, however, there begins to be a decrease in lung volumes. This decrease is related to the effects of obesity.

The *age* of the subject has an effect on the normal predicted values used for pulmonary function parameters. With adult subjects, especially after the age of 25, advancing age tends to have a deteriorating effect on normal pulmonary function values. As age increases, normal values decrease for

- Lung volumes (exceptions are RV and FRC, which increase with advancing age).
- Expiratory flow rates.
- Diffusing capacity.

A complicating factor is the loss of height that normally occurs with aging. Aging alone does affect the lungs in a way that reduces pulmonary function. However, the decrease in height that normally occurs with aging also contributes to the reduction of values seen in older subjects. The precise relationship of the effects of these two factors has not been established.

The *gender* of the subject affects predicted normal pulmonary function values. Male subjects tend to demonstrate greater lung volumes, expiratory flow rates, and diffusing capacities than female subjects of the same height and age. A modifying factor should be noted, however. *When male and female subjects with the same predicted normal FVC values are compared, the female subject will have greater predicted values for expiratory flow rates.*

## SECONDARY CHARACTERISTICS

As stated earlier, there are secondary characteristics that also affect predicted values for pulmonary function. The *race* or *ethnic origin* of the subject has some effect on normal predicted values. Black and Oriental subjects tend to demonstrate smaller predicted normal values for a given height and age than subjects of European origin. For black subjects, many laboratories reduce the values that are predicted for normal lung volumes (TLC, FVC, etc.). The values are generally reduced to between 85% and 90% of the values normally predicted for subjects of European descent. It should be noted, however, that values for predicted expiratory flow rates are the same for both black and European-descent subjects who have the same predicted FVC values.

Studies continue to be done with blacks, Hispanics, Orientals, and other groups to establish predicted normal values for each group. Some studies are attempting to assess differences that may exist between groups of differing European descent (e.g., Central European, British, Scandinavian, etc.).

The effects of altitude and other environmental factors on predicted normal values for pulmonary function are not well established. Research is continuing in this area. Knowledge of the effects of *altitude* would be most beneficial to laboratories located at high altitude, especially if they test subjects who have grown up and currently live under those conditions. Historically, most studies have been performed on populations who live at low to moderate altitudes. This is reasonable since the majority of the general population lives under these conditions. For those living and being tested at high altitude, however, the use of these standard predicted normal values may lead to erroneous evaluation of a subject's pulmonary condition.

*Air pollution* and other environmental factors (e.g., rural versus urban living) may have some effect on predicted normal values. Pollution caused by high levels of "reducing"-type agents (by-products of high-sulfur coal combustion) has been documented to cause deterioration in pulmonary function. This is most true with chronic exposure to high levels of pollution. The "oxidant"-type pollution prevalent in southern California has not demonstrated the same damaging effects on pulmonary function, even with chronic exposure. The specific effects of air pollution on predicted normal pulmonary function values have not been established.

# SOURCES OF PREDICTIVE EQUATIONS FOR NORMAL PULMONARY FUNCTION VALUES

Equations for predicting "normal" pulmonary function parameters are based on the testing of populations of "normal" individuals. As with any other type of scientific research, control of the research variables is important for establishing the validity of the study's results. Variables that must be controlled with pulmonary function testing to establish normal values include the following:

- *The individuals tested.* How many individuals are to be included in the sample population? How is the population to be selected? What characteristics (history of disease, history of smoking) are controlled regarding their "normalcy"? Where, geographically, do the subjects reside, and where are the tests to be performed?
- *The test procedures.* What tests are to be performed? What commands are to be given to the subjects in performing the tests? At what specific points in the subject's breathing maneuver are the measurements begun and ended?
- *The test equipment.* What type of spirometry system is to be used? What types of calibrations and quality control procedures are to be performed with the equipment?

Over the years, many studies have been performed to test populations of "normal" subjects to establish "normal" pulmonary function values. Table 7–1 provides examples of some of these studies. Unfortunately, each study resulted in the development of a slightly different set of equations for calculating normal pulmonary function values. For example, four studies in Table 7–1 include a calculated **mean value** for $FEV_1$. This provides an example of how they differ in the determination of a normal mean value.

These differences in prediction are due largely to the fact that the research variables described earlier were not managed the same way in each study. For instance, in some

**TABLE 7-1  Examples of Studies to Establish Normal Values for Spirometric Parameters**

| | Cherniak and Raber | Schmidt et al. | Morris et al. | Knudson | Schoenberg | Crapo et al. |
|---|---|---|---|---|---|---|
| **Year Published** | 1972 | 1973 | 1971/1973 | et al. 1976 | et al. 1978 | 1981 |
| **Subjects** | | | | | | |
| Total | 1322 | 532 | 988 | 746 | 3046 | 251 |
| Age Range | 15–79 | 55–94 | 20–84 | 8–90 | 7–65+ | 15–91 |
| Adult Male | 782 | 295 | 471 | 128 | 256 | 125 |
| Adult Female | 382 | 237 | 517 | 321 | 569 | 126 |
| Male <20 yrs. | 88 | 0 | 0 | 163 | 1073 | Minimal |
| Female <20 yrs. | 70 | 0 | 0 | 134 | 1148 | Minimal |
| Smokers included? | No | Yes | No | No | No, except for some black males | No |
| **Location** | | | | | | |
| Environment | Mixed | Urban | Rural | Urban | Mixed | Urban |
| Altitude | 230 m | 1400 m | <150 m | 730 m | sea level | 1400 m |
| **Procedures Used** | | | | | | |
| Met ATS Specs? | NA | Yes | Yes | NA | NA | Yes |
| Equipment | WS-OL | CS-OL | SWA | PT-OL | PT-OL | CS-OL |
| Number of Trials | Best of 3 | Best of 2 | Best of 2 | Avg. Best of 5 | Avg. Best 2 of 5 | Best of 3 |
| Zero-Time Technique | MFT | K | K | BE | NA | BE |
| **Regression Equations** | | | | | | |
| Linear or Nonlinear? | Linear | Linear | Linear | Linear | Nonlinear | Linear |
| Separate for blacks | No | No | No | No | Yes | No |

**TABLE 7-1** *(Continued)*

| | Cherniak and Raber | Schmidt et al. | Morris et al. | Knudson | Schoenberg | Crapo et al. |
|---|---|---|---|---|---|---|
| **Estimate of Lower Limit for Normal Values?** | Yes | No | No | Yes | Yes | Yes |
| **Mean FEV₁ Value** | NA | NA | 3.08 liters | 2.79 liters | 2.97 liters | 3.22 liters |

**Spirometric Parameters Reported**

| | Cherniak and Raber | Schmidt et al. | Morris et al. | Knudson | Schoenberg | Crapo et al. |
|---|---|---|---|---|---|---|
| FVC | X | X | X | X | X | X |
| FEV₁ | X | X | X | X | X | X |
| FEV₁/FVC | | X | X | X | X | X |
| FEV₂ | | | | X | | X |
| FEV₃ | | | | X | | X |
| PEF | | | | X | X | |
| FEF₂₅% | X | | | X | | |
| FEF₅₀% | X | | | X | X | |
| FEF₇₅% | X | | | X | X | |
| FEF₂₅%₋₇₅% | X | X | X | X | | |
| FEF₂₀₀₋₁₂₀₀ | | X | X | X | | X |

NA = unknown or not available.
WS = wedge spirometer.
CS = 13.5 liter Collins Water-Seal spirometer.
SWS = Stead-Wells spirometer.
  P = pneumotachometer.
−OL = spirometer provided a direct on-line electrical data signal.
  BE = back-extrapolation technique.
  K = Kory technique.
MFT = minimum-flow threshold.
  ZT = zero-time technique.
*Source: Modified from J. L. Clausen, Pulmonary Function Testing Guidelines and Controversies (Orlando: Grune and Stratton, Inc., 1982).*

earlier studies, smokers were included in the group of "normal" subjects studied. Other differences may be in the equipment used for the test or in how the measurements were made.

The equations used to predict normal pulmonary function values are referred to as *regression equations*. These equations make a prediction or correlation based on a set of statistical relationships. They can be either *linear* or *nonlinear* in their mathematical relationships. Table 7–2 provides an example of each type of equation.

Linear equations are based on simple differences in gender, age, and height and offer relatively easy calculation of normal values. However, not all pulmonary function relationships are linear over the full range of normal values. Especially for children and older subjects, the relationships may be more curvilinear (nonlinear).

Nonlinear equations allow calculation of predicted normals over a wider and possibly nonlinear range. Nonlinear equations also allow the inclusion of other physical characteristics, such as weight. Some researchers feel that this may allow more specific and accurate equations to be developed. Of course, because of their complexity, nonlinear equations require the use of computers to rapidly and correctly generate predicted normal values. Additionally, because of the nature of nonlinear calculations, even a slight error in using the equation will be magnified to produce a significant error in pulmonary function value prediction.

Some research has indicated that the nonlinear equations developed to date do not significantly improve the predictability of the calculations. Therefore, use of the simpler linear equations may be appropriate until better nonlinear equations are developed.

**TABLE 7–2  Examples of Linear and Nonlinear Predictive Equations for $FEV_1$**

### Linear Equation*

$$FEV_1 = (0.1052 \times Ht) - (0.0244 \times Age) - 2.190$$

### Nonlinear Equation†

$$FEV_1 = [0.0006394 (Ht \times Wt)] + [0.7466 (In\ Age)] - [0.06385 (Wt)]$$
$$- [0.0001608 (Wt^2)] - [0.000003313 (Age \times Ht \times Wt)] - 0.05296$$

*In* = natural logarithm.
*R. O. Crapo et al. 1981. Reference Spirometric Values Using Techniques and Equipment That Meet ATS Recommendations. Am Rev Respir Dis. 123:659–64.
†J. P. Schoenberg et al. 1978. Growth and Decay of Pulmonary Function in Healthy Blacks and Whites. Respir Physiol. 3:367–93.
*Note: all heights are in units of centimeters.*

# USING PREDICTIVE EQUATIONS FOR NORMAL PULMONARY FUNCTION VALUES

## SELECTING PREDICTIVE EQUATIONS

The pulmonary function technologist has a wide variety of predictive equations from which to choose. Unfortunately, all these choices can make selection difficult for a laboratory. One option is for a laboratory to test a population of its own "normal" subjects in order to establish its own specific equations. But a project of that scope is beyond the practical ability of most laboratories.

Generally, the best option is for a laboratory to select carefully from predictive equations that are already published. Table 7–3 provides a procedure for doing so.

No single study will provide all the best equations for use in the laboratory. Predicted normals for lung volume tests may come from one study. The normal pulmonary mechanics tests and diffusion tests may be based on other studies.

The manufacturer of a laboratory's equipment may be able to suggest predictive equations that are best suited for the equipment they supply. Computer-based testing systems are generally supplied with several different options for predictive equations already available in the system programming. Some system programs even permit the operator to make modifications to the existing program equations.

## ESTABLISHING RANGES FOR NORMALCY

Pulmonary function tests are generally performed to identify subjects who have abnormalities in pulmonary function. Test results are considered abnormal if they fall outside a range of values considered normal. For example, given that the normal range for arterial blood pH is 7.35–7.45, a pH of 7.28 is abnormal because it is outside of the normal range.

The predictive equations described earlier are the first step in establishing normalcy. Using $FEV_1$ as an example, a predictive equation allows the determination of a single *normal mean value* for $FEV_1$ that is based on a subject's physical characteristics. This same value would be predicted for every subject who is the same gender, age, and height. Obviously, though, even subjects of the same gender, age, and height will not have exactly the same values for $FEV_1$. A single value for normal is too limiting for use in differentiating normal from abnormal.

A *range* of values is needed to establish normalcy. Depending on the test, pulmonary function parameters require one of two types of normal ranges. These ranges differ in how they extend above and/or below the predicted mean value and in how many **standard deviations** (SD) they extend. Measurements for parameters such as FVC, $FEV_1$, and other expiratory flow values are abnormal only if the subject's results are too far *below* (−1.65 SD) the mean normal value. For this reason, only a low value for the normal range is needed to identify the start of abnormal test results.

Conversely, TLC and RV test results can be abnormal if they are either too far *above or below* (±1.96 SD) the mean normal value. Both a high and a low normal value range are needed to establish normalcy.

---

TABLE 7–3 **Procedure for Selection of Predictive Equations**

---

1. Review available studies and select groups of predictive equations from one or more studies that have the greatest similarities to your laboratory in relation to the population studied, equipment used, and other methodology.
2. Select at least 10 and preferably 20 or more nonsmoking subjects who are normal on the basis of being free of cardiopulmonary disease. The subjects should be typical of the population test by the laboratory in terms of age, height, race, etc.
3. Perform tests on the chosen subjects. Compare the results with the normal values predicted from the selected equations.

COMPARISON THAT INDICATES THE SELECTED PREDICTIVE EQUATIONS ARE *ACCEPTABLE*:

- Predictive equations providing normals that demonstrate the smallest average differences and smallest range of differences from the test subjects are the most appropriate for use.
  *Note*: It is better to select and use a group of related equations from a single study than it is to choose individual equations from a number of different studies.

COMPARISONS THAT INDICATE THE PREDICTED EQUATIONS ARE *UNACCEPTABLE*:

- If three or more out of ten tested subjects have results that fall outside the *95% confidence limit* for the predictive equations, then all test procedure aspects should be reviewed and evaluated.
- Another, different group of subjects should then be tested.
- If, again, three or more of ten subjects fall outside of the 95% confidence limit for the predictive equations, then one of two possible problems exists. Either the testing procedures are inaccurate, or the selected predictive equations are inappropriate for use with the laboratory's population and equipment.
- The laboratory procedures should again be reviewed and a different set of predictive equations tried.

---

Since predictive equations provide only a mean normal value, some other method must be used to establish the *range* of values considered to be normal. Two such methods exist:

1. The *percentage-range method* uses a range that is 20% above and/or below the subject's predicted mean normal value (±20%).
2. The **95% confidence limits** (95% CL) method uses a range that is based on 95% of the population with normal pulmonary function. Two variations of this method are where
   a. A *constant 95% CL range* above and/or below the subject's predicted mean normal value is used. The constant 95% CL value that is selected for use is the value of

the single overall mean 95% CL found for that parameter as demonstrated by the study's entire population.

    b. A range that is based on a *coefficient of variation adjustment to the 95% CL* is used. This adjustment is made for a given subject's mean normal value.

A more detailed discussion of each method follows.

## Percentage-Range Method

The percentage-range method was developed from observations made in some of the earliest studies done to determine normal pulmonary function values. Based on the parameters measured in those studies (VC, for example), the **coefficient of variation** for the population was often found to be about 12%. In other words, one SD for the data was equal to a value of 12% of the mean normal value. As a result, using the 95% CL to establish a normal range, the low normal value for the parameter was determined as follows:

    Predicted Mean Value − (12% × 1.65 SD)

or

    Predicted Mean Value − 20%

Given these early observations, this method was later applied to establishing normal ranges for other pulmonary function parameters.

    The percentage-range method is simple and easy to use. Table 7–4 provides an example of its application. (The predictive equation for $FEV_1$ used in Table 7–4 and subsequent tables is the linear equation for $FEV_1$ from Table 7–2.) The percentage-range method is useful for establishing acceptable normal ranges for such parameters as lung volumes, FVC and $FEV_1$, and $D_LCO$ in adult subjects. Unfortunately, for forced expiratory flow pa-

### TABLE 7–4   Percentage-Range Method

| Subject | Predicted FEV$_1$ | Low Normal Value |
|---|---|---|
| 58-year-old female, 5 ft. 5 in. (165 cm) tall | 2.586 liters | Low Normal $FEV_1$ = Predicted $FEV_1$ − 20% <br> or <br> Low Normal $FEV_1$ = 2.586 liters − 0.517 liter <br> or <br> Low Normal $FEV_1$ = 2.070 liters |
| 83-year-old female, 4 ft. 10 in. (147 cm) tall | 1.333 liters | Low Normal $FEV_1$ = Predicted $FEV_1$ − 20% <br> or <br> Low Normal $FEV_1$ = 1.333 liters − 0.267 liter <br> or <br> Low Normal $FEV_1$ = 1.066 liters |

*Note: Both subjects have acceptable low normal values established for them.*

rameters ($FEF_{25\%-75\%}$, $\dot{V}_{max}$, etc.) and pediatric values, the fixed-percentage method may result in a falsely low normal value.

The fixed-percentage method results in a slightly narrower range of normal values than is established by other methods. A subject is more likely to be identified as abnormal if his or her measured value is greater and/or less than the predicted mean. When used with such parameters as lung volumes, FVC and $FEV_1$, and $D_LCO$ in adult subjects, the fixed-percentage method tends to be a *sensitive* method of establishing normalcy. This sensitivity makes it less likely that a subject with true pulmonary dysfunction will be incorrectly labeled as normal.

The more sensitive narrow range of the fixed-percentage method is good for use with screening tests that are meant to identify the early presence of pulmonary dysfunction. Conversely, though, the narrower range is also more likely to label a borderline subject who actually is normal as being abnormal. This could result in a subject being inappropriately denied employment or insurance coverage.

## 95% Confidence Limit Methods

The 95% CL method, in either of its variations, assumes that throughout a population of normal subjects, there is a statistically **normal distribution** of values above and below the mean normal value. This assumption allows the use of a 95% CL to statistically identify range of normalcy. It has not been established, however, that normal values for all pulmonary function parameters demonstrate a normal distribution.

For most subjects, the 95% CL methods tend to produce a slightly wider normal value range than the percentage-range method. Accordingly, the 95% CL methods tend to be more *specific* in identifying abnormalities. These methods are more specific in that when a subject's value is labeled as being abnormal, it is almost assured that the subject does in fact have a pulmonary dysfunction. There is less than a 5% chance that a false-abnormal interpretation will occur.

For this reason, the 95% CL range methods are well suited for tests that relate to acceptance for employment or insurance. In either of these situations, a subject may be rejected if the test results indicate an abnormality. Since false abnormal interpretations are minimized, there is a minimal chance of a normal subject being inappropriately rejected.

Because of the slightly wider ranges the 95% CL methods produce, they may not be as effective in identifying the early presence of pulmonary dysfunction. For this reason, they may be less appropriate for screening tests than the fixed-percentage method.

There are two different ways of establishing 95% CL ranges.

*Constant 95% Confidence Limit Range Method.* As can be seen in the examples in Table 7–5, this method determines a single normal value range. The resulting range is intended for application to all subjects regardless of gender, age, or height.

Some researchers have indicated that this is an acceptable method for establishing a range for normalcy. However, the range is likely to be inappropriate for subjects at extremes of age and height. Table 7–4 demonstrates this problem. As can be seen in Table 7–1, the literature for some published predictive equations provides a 95% CL value for

---

### TABLE 7–5  Constant 95% Confidence Limit Normal Range Method

With this method, a constant 95% CL value is used to establish the normal range for all test subjects, regardless of age or height. In these examples, 0.561 liters is used as the 95% CL value. This is based on 0.561 liter being the overall 95% CL value for the mean $FEV_1$ of the female subjects in the study used to establish the predictive equation.

| Subject | Predicted $FEV_1$ | Low Normal Value |
|---|---|---|
| 58-year-old female, 5 ft. 5 in. (165 cm) tall | 3.275 liters | Low Normal $FEV_1$ = Predicted $FEV_1$ − Constant 95% CL<br>or<br>Low Normal $FEV_1$ = 2.586 liters − 0.561 liter<br>or<br>Low Normal $FEV_1$ = 2.025 liters |

**Comment**—For this subject, the constant 95% CL value is 22% of her predicted $FEV_1$. It is reasonably close to the 20% value used with the percentage-range method and produces an acceptable low normal $FEV_1$ value.

| Subject | Predicted $FEV_1$ | Low Normal Value |
|---|---|---|
| 83-year-old female, 4 ft. 10 in. (147 cm) tall | 1.333 liters | Low Normal $FEV_1$ = Predicted $FEV_1$ − Constant 95% CL<br>or<br>Low Normal $FEV_1$ = 1.333 liters − 0.561 liter<br>or<br>Low Normal $FEV_1$ = 0.772 liter |

**Comment**—For this subject, the constant 95% CL value is 42% of her predicted $FEV_1$, which produces an unacceptably low normal $FEV_1$ value.

---

each parameter. A specific method for calculating the 95% CL, given a subject's specific physical characteristics, may also be included.

*Coefficient of Variation Adjustment to the 95% Confidence Limit Range Method.* Table 7–6 provides examples of how this method is used. Like the constant 95% CL method, the coefficient of variation adjustment method allows the use of a statistical basis for establishing normalcy. However, it also permits normal ranges to be adjusted for a subject's physical characteristics. As a result, subjects at extremes of age and height will

---

**TABLE 7–6  Coefficient of Variation Adjustment to the 95% Confidence Limit Normal Range Method**

---

With this method, a coefficient of variation adjustment (CoV Adj) is made to the 95% CL before it is applied to determine a subject's low normal $FEV_1$ value. This adjustment permits compensation of the low normal value range in response to the subject's actual age and height.

Depending on the data available from the study used to supply the predictive equations, either of the following two methods can be used to determine the CoV Adj

CoV Adj = (SD for the Mean $FEV_1$/Mean $FEV_1$) $\times$ 1.65

(Use 1.65 when only a low normal value is required. A value of 1.96 is used if both a high and a low normal value are required.)

CoV Adj = 95% CL for the Mean $FEV_1$/Mean $FEV_1$

In both of these equations, the SD, 95% CL, and mean $FEV_1$ are values based on the statistical data from the overall population used to establish the predictive equation.

In the following examples, 0.561 liter is the $FEV_1$ 95% CL value for the female population used to establish the predictive equation. The mean $FEV_1$ value for the same population is 2.679 liters. Using the second equation just given, the CoV Adj. that will be used in the examples is

CoV Adj = 0.561 liter/2.679

or

CoV Adj = 21%

---

| Subject | Predicted $FEV_1$ | Low Normal Value |
|---|---|---|
| 58-year-old female, 5 ft. 5 in. (165 cm) tall | 3.275 liters | Low Normal $FEV_1$ = Predicted $FEV_1$ − 21% <br> or <br> Low Normal $FEV_1$ = 2.586 liters − 0.543 liter <br> or <br> Low Normal $FEV_1$ = 2.043 liters |

---

| Subject | Predicted $FEV_1$ | Low Normal Value |
|---|---|---|
| 83-year-old female, 4 ft. 10 in. (147 cm) tall | 1.333 liters | Low Normal $FEV_1$ = Predicted $FEV_1$ − 21% <br> or <br> Low Normal $FEV_1$ = 1.333 liters − 0.280 liters <br> or <br> Low Normal $FEV_1$ = 1.053 liters |

---

Note: In both subjects, acceptable low normal values are established.

still have appropriate ranges for normalcy. In this respect, the coefficient of variation adjustment is an improvement over the constant 95% CL method.

*Selection of a Range Establishment Method.* Selection of a method for establishing a range of normal values should be based on how the data are to be used. If the primary goal for testing is to screen for early detection of disorders, the percentage-range method may be most appropriate. If testing is for documentation that may affect acceptance for insurance or employment, one of the 95% CL methods may be a better choice.

Computerized testing systems generally perform automatic identification of test results as normal or abnormal. It is important, therefore, that the system operator understand the method the system uses in making that determination.

## Review Questions

Please use the following review questions to evaluate your learning of information from this chapter. It might be helpful to write out your answers on a sheet of paper. If you are unsure of the answers to these questions, review the chapter to reinforce your learning.

1. Relating to primary characteristics that affect normal pulmonary function values:
   a. What are the primary characteristics that affect normal pulmonary function values?
   b. How do these primary characteristics affect pulmonary function values?
2. Relating to secondary characteristics that affect normal pulmonary function values,
   a. What are the secondary characteristics that affect normal pulmonary function values?
   b. How do these secondary characteristics affect pulmonary function values?
3. How are normal pulmonary function values determined?
4. What variables must be controlled when testing is done to establish normal pulmonary function values?
5. What are regression equations? How do linear equations differ from nonlinear equations?
6. What is the process that a laboratory can use to select predictive equations for use?
7. Relating to the percentage-range method for establishing a normal range for pulmonary function values:
   a. What is the basis for the percentage-range method of establishing a normal range for pulmonary function values?
   b. How is this method applied?
8. Relating to both variations of the 95% confidence limit method for establishing a normal range for pulmonary function values:
   a. What is the basis for the 95% confidence limit methods of establishing a normal range for pulmonary function values?
   b. How is the constant 95% confidence limit range method used?
   c. How does the coefficient of variation adjustment variation differ from the 95% confidence limit range variation of this method?

# CHAPTER EIGHT

# PULMONARY FUNCTION TESTING REGIMENS

## —————— RELATED LEARNING ——————

Prior knowledge of the following related information will facilitate understanding and learning of the material in this chapter. The learner will be aided by being able to

1. Recall the equipment concepts from Chapters 1 and 3.
2. Recall the concepts of pulmonary function testing covered in Chapters 2, 4, 5, and 6.
3. Relate the material in this chapter to the use of basic surgical terms.
4. Relate the material in this chapter to the basic function of the sympathetic and parasympathetic branches of the autonomic nervous system.
5. Relate the material in this chapter to the pharmacology of bronchodilator-type medications.
6. Relate the material in this chapter to the basic practices of administration of aerosolized medications.
7. Relate the material in this chapter to the significance of wheezing as an abnormal breath sound.
8. Relate the material in this chapter to basic concepts of mechanical ventilatory support and the use of positive end-expiratory pressure (PEEP).

## LEARNING OBJECTIVES

Upon successful completion of this chapter, the learner should be able to

1. Describe the assessment needed before pulmonary function testing is performed in relation to
   a. basic information and history taking
   b. physical assessment
2. Describe the administration of pulmonary function tests in relation to the
   a. procedure for test administration
   b. reporting of pulmonary function test results

3. Describe the administration of bronchodilator benefit studies in relation to the
   a. procedure for test administration
   b. evaluation of test results
4. Describe the administration of preoperative pulmonary function studies in relation to
   a. general surgical risk pulmonary function assessment
   b. assessment prior to pulmonary resection
5. Describe the administration of bronchoprovocation (methacholine challenge) studies in relation to the
   a. procedure for test administration
   b. evaluation of the study's results
   c. administration of antigen challenges
6. Describe the administration of studies for exercise-induced asthma and wheezing related to environmental triggers in relation to the
   a. procedure for test administration
   b. evaluation of test results
7. Describe the administration of studies to document impairment/disability.
8. Describe the use of pulmonary function testing for critical monitoring in relation to
   a. evaluation of spontaneous ventilatory parameters
   b. monitoring of ventilatory parameters for subjects on mechanical ventilatory support
   c. critical care blood gas monitoring

## KEY TERMS

Briggs adapter
disability
impairment
intermittent positive pressure breathing (IPPB)
metered-dose inhaler (MDI)
methacholine chloride
morbidity
mortality

pack years
parasympatholytic
parasympathomimetic
resection
small-volume nebulizer (SVN)
surgical risk
sympathomimetic
ventilatory failure

Pulmonary function testing provides for a controlled clinical evaluation of the performance of a subject's lungs and related structures. Testing can be performed as a general evaluation of the pulmonary system. Testing can also be performed in order to quantify a specific pulmonary performance parameter. This is the case with bronchodilator-benefit and bronchoprovocation studies. This chapter will review the different types of clinical pulmonary function evaluations that can be performed.

# PATIENT ASSESSMENT FOR PULMONARY FUNCTION TESTING

The first step in any pulmonary function study is to assess the patient's pulmonary system before testing. Often information for this assessment will have been gathered by a physician's examination early in the subject's care. However, it is useful to repeat this type of assessment just prior to the administration of any specific pulmonary function test. A better interpretation of test results is possible if all of the significant and most recent information on the subject's pulmonary system is available in a single report.

A general preassessment of the subject's pulmonary system includes gathering basic personal information on the subject's medical history. A physical examination of the subject's breathing and pulmonary system should also be performed. A more detailed description of these assessment procedures follows.

## BASIC INFORMATION AND HISTORY TAKING

Most often, basic information and history taking involves the use of a prepared form that ensures that all pertinent data are gathered. The form can be completed by the subject in advance of the study. It can also be completed either in part or completely through an interview process involving the technologist and the subject. Important information that must be gathered on the subject includes the following:

### Basic Information

The subject's name, age, gender, standing height in stocking feet, weight, race, and current diagnosis, if one has been made, are basic information. If at all possible, the subject's height and weight should be measured at the time the study is performed. For subjects who cannot stand or have spinal deformities, the measurement of arm span can be substituted for standing height. Arm span is measured between the tips of the middle fingers when the subject's arms are extended directly outward from each side.

### Personal Medical History

Personal medical history includes whether the subject has ever had allergies/hay fever, asthma, chest injury or surgery, recurring colds, pneumonia/recurrent lung infections, lung abscess, pleurisy, tuberculosis, lung cancer, pulmonary fibrosis, bronchiectasis, emphysema, or chronic bronchitis.

### Medications Prescribed for Lung or Heart Problems

The information gathered on medications should include the types of medications prescribed or purchased "over the counter," for what problem(s) they were or are being taken, and the dose and schedule of the medications, including when they were last taken.

## Family History

The subject's family history should include that of any immediate family member: mother, father, sister(s), and/or brother(s). Each family member's history should be described as it relates to the disorders listed earlier under the heading of "Personal Medical History."

## Smoking History

Does the subject smoke or live with a smoker? For subjects who smoke or have smoked, the following information must be gathered: age smoking began, years smoked, type(s) of tobacco or other substance smoked (e.g., cigarettes, cigar, pipe tobacco, marijuana), and past and current daily consumption. It is useful to know the brands or types of cigarettes smoked and to make a calculation of **pack years** smoked. If the subject has quit smoking, the date and reason for quitting should be recorded.

## Hobbies

A list and description of the subject's hobbies can be useful, especially if the hobbies involve the use of chemicals, art supplies, or other possibly irritating or poisonous substances.

## Pets

A list of the types and numbers of the subject's pets may show a link between the presence of a pet or pets to certain pulmonary symptoms (e.g., wheezing). It is important to know whether the pets are maintained indoors or outdoors.

## Places of Residence

A chronological history of the localities where the subject has lived can help in diagnosing certain endemic diseases (e.g., fungal disorders, such as histoplasmosis).

## Occupational History

A chronological history of the subject's occupations should include a description of the actual jobs performed. A description is more useful than simply listing job titles held by the subject. Exposure to gases, fumes, and dusts should be recorded. The length of time in each occupation should also be noted. A history of employment in farming, foundry, mining, quarrying, textiles, and other occupations can be significant in diagnosing pulmonary problems.

## History of Symptoms Associated with Pulmonary Disorders

A history of the pulmonary symptoms experienced by the subject must be recorded, including the following:

*Cough.*   When does the subject experience coughing (time of day or year)? Does coughing affect the subject's ability to breathe? Is the cough productive? If blood or sputum is produced, what is its appearance (volume, color, odor, consistency) when expectorated?

*Dyspnea.* Does the subject experience problems with dyspnea? When is the dyspnea experienced (at rest; with exertion—after what distance walked, number of stairs climbed, etc.)? Is the dyspnea positional? Does it occur only at night?

*Wheezing.* Is wheezing experienced by the subject? When does the wheezing occur (frequency, time of day or year, with exertion, cold air)? Is the wheezing linked to dyspnea that limits the subject's ability to perform certain tasks?

## Present Complaints or Concerns for Breathing

Any current difficulties that the subject may have with breathing should be recorded, including coughing, dyspnea, and/or wheezing.

## PHYSICAL ASSESSMENT

Physical assessment should include at least observation of the subject, vital signs, auscultation, and the results of X-ray examination if they are available. Each component of the physical assessment is described here.

## Observation of the Subject

The shape and configuration of the subject's thorax should be observed for a barrel chest, spinal deformities, or other thoracic abnormalities. The subject's posture and body position should be noted. Are the subject's shoulders fixed and upper torso leaning forward to assist in breathing?

The pattern and effort of the subject's breathing should be noted. Is there prolonged expiration, labored breathing at rest, inability to speak in complete sentences, use of accessory muscles, paradoxical movement of thorax and abdomen during breathing, or the use of pursed lips during expiration?

Noticeable wheezing or strider, cyanosis (central and/or peripheral), digital clubbing, signs of cor pulmonale (distended neck veins, edema in dependent limbs), and the level of cooperativeness demonstrated by the subject should be recorded.

## Vital Signs

The subject's pulse, respiratory rate, and blood pressure at the time of testing should be measured and recorded.

## Auscultation

The subject should be auscultated, and any abnormalities in the subject's breath sounds should be recorded. With adventitious sounds, such as wheezing, rhonchi, and/or crackles, the intensity, location, and relation of the sounds to the breathing cycle should be noted.

## Results of X-Ray Examination

If X-ray reports are available, significant information from the reports should be noted. This could include such things as abnormal densities in the lung fields; lung hyperinflation; loss of vascular markings; presence of bullae; presence of flattened diaphragm; increases in the retrosternal air space, sternophrenic angle, and posterior-anterior diameter; or evidence of cardiac abnormalities or cor pulmonale.

# GENERAL ADMINISTRATION OF PULMONARY FUNCTION TESTS

A pulmonary function test can be performed as an individual test, or it can be performed as part of a larger study of the subject's pulmonary performance. Regardless, there are certain things that go into making the administration of any test more successful. Three key factors are

- The skill of the technologist administering the test.
- The accuracy of the test equipment.
- The understanding, cooperation, and ability to follow instructions demonstrated by the subject.

The first of these factors can have a significant effect on the quality of the latter two.

In order to be able to work effectively with the subject, the technologist should demonstrate certain personal qualities. These include a combination of concern and forcefulness along with patience, supportiveness, persistence, and humor. Firmness may be necessary with subjects who are less cooperative.

Most subjects are cooperative and interested in having successful tests performed. A lack of cooperation may be intentional, or it may be due to the subject having difficulty in comprehending what is required.

## PROCEDURE FOR TEST ADMINISTRATION

The procedure for any test can be broken down into the steps of preparation and actual test administration.

### Preparation

As preparation for participating in any type of pulmonary function test, the subject should avoid wearing items of apparel that are tight or restrictive (necktie, buttoned shirt collar, tight belt, tight brassiere or girdle). Any restrictive clothing worn at the time of the test should be loosened or removed.

The laboratory must place a clean and disinfected or a new disposable mouthpiece on the measuring system prior to testing. Depending on the system's design and manufacturer's recommendations, other system parts may need to be replaced or cleaned between subjects.

### Test Administration

FVC tests can be performed with the subject either seated or standing. The position used for a given subject should be noted in the test report. The subject must be seated for lung volume, $D_L CO$, and any other types of tests.

Clear and simple instructions must be given to the subject. It is often helpful to explain to the subject what the test is designed to measure. A demonstration by the technologist of how the subject is to breathe can be especially helpful for effort-dependent tests, such as the FVC.

Use of nose clips by the subject is recommended for most tests. Nose clips are required if a closed measuring system is used and when tidal breathing and a maximal inspiration must be performed on the system prior to an FVC maneuver.

The mouthpiece should be positioned so that the subject's chin is slightly elevated and the neck extended. Once the mouthpiece is in the subject's mouth, the technologist must check to make sure that there are no leaks present. Dentures may have to be removed in order for the subject to use the mouthpiece effectively.

The test or tests to be performed should be administered as described in the previous chapters. Coaching of the subject during the test is very important, especially with effort-dependent tests. Coaching should be firm, enthusiastic, and encouraging.

Once the test is administered, its results should be evaluated. Subject effort and cooperation are the primary sources of error for effort-dependent tests (e.g., FVC). Error is demonstrated by poor reproducibility of results from repeated tests. For subjects with hyperreactive airways, the best results may be on a well-performed first test. Later test results may be poor due to bronchospasm triggered by a maximal, TLC-level inspiration.

## REPORTING PULMONARY FUNCTION TEST RESULTS

Every laboratory should have a standardized method for reporting pulmonary function test results. All pertinent information should be included when pulmonary assessment data are submitted to a physician for interpretation. Included should be the subject's basic personal information, medical history, and physical assessment data plus the data from specific pulmonary function tests. Figure 8–1 provides an example of a test-data reporting form. As can be seen, the general pattern is to report the subject's actual results, the subject's predicted values, and the percent of the predicted value that the subject's results represented for each parameter of a test. If a computer-generated interpretation of the test results is included on the report, the origin of the interpretation should be clearly indicated.

Important clinical decisions are based on interpretations of the test data. For this reason, questionable test results should not be reported. The interpreting physician must be notified of any concerns that the technologist has as to the quality of the test results. If, under these conditions, the results are reported as final, a notation should be included regarding the concerns for the test.

A notation should be made on the report if population-specific predictive equations (e.g., adjustment for race or ethnic origin) were used. This is most important when the predictive equations used differ from the ones routinely used by the laboratory. If "corrections" to the raw data from tests are made (Hb and HbCO corrections for $D_LCO$ tests), both the raw data and the corrected data should be included.

When reporting the results of a test, it is helpful to make reference to any previous tests performed on that subject. This will allow the test interpreter to note any changes in the subject's pulmonary function and the degree to which the changes have occurred. Historical comparisons allow for assessment of how rapidly a specific pulmonary parameter is deteriorating.

SWEDISHAMERICAN HOSPITAL
ROCKFORD, ILLINOIS
DEPARTMENT OF PULMONARY SERVICES

Name:                                              ID:                    Date:
Race: Caucasian          Height: 71 in             Weight: 175.0 lbs
Room: O.P.               BSA: 1.99                  Age: 75 yr
Dr. :                                                                     Sex: M

                              Technician:

Diagnosis: CA ESOPHAGEAL


Years quit: 13.0     Pack Years: 25.0     Packs/Day: 1.00
Dyspnea History: After severe exertion
Cough: Productive      Wheeze: Rare

|  | | PRE - BRONCH | | | POST - BRONCH | | |
|---|---|---|---|---|---|---|---|
| **LUNG MECHANICS** | | Actual | Pred. | %Pred. | Actual | %Pred. | %Chng |
| FVC | (L) | 2.67 | 4.20 | 64 | 3.29 | 78 | 23 |
| FEV1 | (L) | 1.46 | 3.29 | 44 | 1.76 | 53 | 21 |
| FEV1/FVC | (%) | 55 | 78 | | 53 | | -2 |
| FEF 25% | (L/sec) | 1.91 | 6.79 | 28 | 2.11 | 31 | 10 |
| FEF 50% | (L/sec) | 0.79 | 3.68 | 21 | 0.84 | 23 | 6 |
| FEF 75% | (L/sec) | 0.23 | 1.03 | 22 | 0.26 | 25 | 13 |
| FEF MAX | (L/sec) | 4.28 | 7.42 | 58 | 5.03 | 68 | 18 |
| FEF 25-75% | (L/sec) | 0.63 | 3.20 | 20 | 0.67 | 21 | 6 |
| FEF 75-85% | (L/sec) | 0.17 | | | 0.19 | | 12 |
| | | | | | | | |
| FIVC | (L) | 2.69 | 4.25 | 63 | 3.28 | 77 | 22 |
| FIF 50% | (L/sec) | 3.42 | | | 2.43 | | -29 |
| FEF 50%/FIF 50% | | 0.23 | .9-1.0 | | 0.34 | | 48 |
| **LUNG VOLUMES** | | Actual | Pred. | %Pred. | Actual | %Pred. | %Chng |
| SVC | (L) | 2.89 | 4.20 | 69 | | | |
| IC | (L) | 2.22 | 3.35 | 66 | | | |
| ERV | (L) | 0.67 | 0.86 | 78 | | | |
| TGV (Pleth) | (L) | 4.11 | 3.90 | 105 | | | |
| RV (Pleth) | (L) | 3.44 | 2.61 | 132 | | | |
| TLC (Pleth) | (L) | 6.33 | 7.24 | 87 | | | |
| RV/TLC (Pleth) | (%) | 54 | 36 | | | | |
| Raw | (cmH2O/L/s) | 16.55 | < 2.00 | 957 | | | |
| Gaw | (L/sec/cmH2O) | 0.06 | > 0.50 | | | | |
| sGaw | (sec/cmH2O*L^2) | 0.01 | > 0.21 | | | | |

|  | PRE - BRONCH | | | POST - BRONCH | | |
|---|---|---|---|---|---|---|
| **LUNG DIFFUSION** | Actual | Pred. | %Pred. | Actual | %Pred. | %Chng. |
| DLCOunc (ml/min/mmHg) | 15.65 | 33.68 | 46 | | | |
| ALVEOLAR VOLUME (L) | 5.18 | 7.24 | 72 | | | |
| DL/VA (ml/min/mmHg/L) | 3.02 | 6.47 | 47 | | | |

**Figure 8–1** *Example of a pulmonary function testing report form generated by computer.*

SWEDISHAMERICAN HOSPITAL
ROCKFORD, ILLINOIS
DEPARTMENT OF PULMONARY SERVICES

Name:                                    Height: 71 in          ID:                  Date:
Race: Caucasian                          BSA: 1.99              Weight: 175.0 lbs
Room: O.P.                                                      Age: 75 yr           Sex: M
Dr. :                                         Technician:

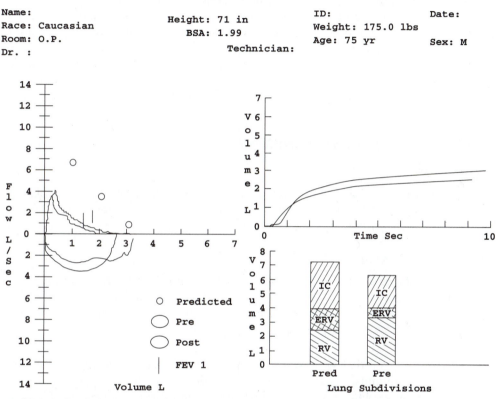

Before and after bronchodilator spirometry reveal evidence for moderate to
severe obstructive ventilatory defect with mild reversability acutely
following the inhalation of nebulized bronchodilator. The lung volumes
confirm obstructive ventilatory defect with elevation of residual volume
to 132% of predicted normal and airways resistance nearly 10 times predicted
normal. Diffusion capacity is markedly reduced indicative of loss of
functional alveolar capillary membrane units in the absence of anemia.

Impression: Moderate to severe obstructive pulmonary disease probably
primarily emphysematous in nature; but with some reversability likely
secondary to bronchospasm. He is at high risk for post-operative respiratory
complications following upper abdominal and/or thoracic surgery.

MEDICAL DIRECTOR
PULMONARY SERVICES

**Figure 8–1** (*Continued*).

# BRONCHODILATOR-BENEFIT STUDIES

Bronchodilator-benefit studies are useful when considering, planning, or evaluating the therapeutic administration of bronchodilator therapy. A study is indicated any time there is clinical evidence that an individual has abnormally reactive airways. $FEV_{1\%}$ values of ≤70% can indicate the need to evaluate a subject's potential benefit from bronchodilator therapy. This ≤70% cutoff is a less useful indicator in older subjects and in subjects who have a combination of a slightly increased FVC value and a slightly reduced $FEV_1$ value. A history of wheezing and dyspnea can also indicate the need for a bronchodilator-benefit study.

## PROCEDURE FOR TEST ADMINISTRATION

### Preparation

Prior to the study, the subject should abstain from using medications that have been prescribed to manage bronchospasm. The length of abstinence varies, depending on the type of medication in use. Guidelines are presented in Table 8–1.

### Test Administration

There are three stages to administration of a bronchodilator-benefit study: administration of a pre-test, administration of the bronchodilator being evaluated, and administration of a post-test to measure any changes from the pre-test that may have resulted from use of the bronchodilator. Each of these stages will be described.

*Pretest.*    Generally a broad series of pulmonary function tests are performed before the bronchodilator is administered. The tests can include spirometry for lung volumes and pulmonary mechanics, FRC and TLC determination, and diffusing capacity. These tests provide a baseline of values against which the response to bronchodilators can be evaluated.

**TABLE 8–1   Guidelines for Abstaining from Bronchoactive Medications Prior to Administration of Bronchodilator-Benefit Study**

1. Eight hours' abstinence from medium-duration sympathomimetic bronchodilators.
2. Twelve hours' abstinence from long-duration sympathomimetic and methylxanthine bronchodilators.
3. Twenty-four hours' abstinence from cromolyn sodium and nedocromil sodium.

The subject can continue to take prednisone and other corticosteroids as long as the prescribed maintenance dose is not exceeded.

*Bronchodilator Administration.* A bronchodilator is administered to the subject after the baseline pulmonary function tests have been performed. Usually a **sympathomimetic** bronchodilator is used. However, the effectiveness of any bronchodilator can be measured by this procedure. Some subjects may, by past medical history, be at risk for developing cardiovascular side effects after receiving a sympathomimetic bronchodilator. If the risk exists, the subject's pulse and blood pressure should be monitored regularly before, during, and after the bronchodilator administration and retest procedure.

The bronchodilator can be administered by use of either a **small-volume nebulizer** (SVN) or a **metered-dose inhaler** (MDI). An **intermittent positive pressure breathing** (IPPB) device could be used if indicated, but it should not be used as a general practice of the laboratory. MDIs are probably the administration system of choice. The dose administered by this method is more reproducible than by the other methods, especially if a reservoir system is used.

It is important that proper guidelines for aerosolized medication administration be followed. Key points of concern include

- An appropriate breathing pattern should be used by the subject during the aerosol's administration (a slow, deep inspiration with an end-inspiratory pause of three to five seconds).
- If an MDI is used, there should be a delay of at least two minutes between "puffs."

Once the bronchodilator has been administered, there should be a delay before the post-administration tests are performed. A delay of 10–15 minutes is appropriate for sympathomimetic bronchodilators. **Parasympatholytic** bronchodilators may require a post-administration delay of as long as 45–60 minutes.

*Retest.* Retesting is performed after a sufficient amount of time has passed after the bronchodilator's administration. Pulmonary mechanics tests (e.g., FVC) are most often repeated for use as indicators of a subject's response to bronchodilator therapy. Parameters such as $FEV_1$ and $FEF_{25\%-75\%}$ provide excellent indicators of bronchodilator response. $FEV_1$ values are especially useful because of their high degree of reproducibility. $\Delta V_{max\ 50}$ and $SG_{aw}$ values can also be used. If desired, $D_LCO$ testing can be repeated. $D_LCO$ values can demonstrate a response to bronchodilator therapy and thus can be used as an indicator of therapeutic benefit.

## EVALUATION OF TEST RESULTS

Pulmonary disorders that involve the smooth muscle tissue of the bronchial and, especially, bronchiolar airways (e.g., asthma) are responsive to bronchodilator therapy. A subject's response to bronchodilator therapy can be demonstrated in a variety of different ways. Increases and improvement in pulmonary mechanics and other values are significant.

A 15–20% or greater increase in expiratory flow rates indicates a positive response to the administration of the bronchodilator. Significant air flow improvements (greater than 50%) can occur. Table 8–2 demonstrates how this determination is made. With this method,

---

**TABLE 8–2  Calculation of Percent Change for Bronchodilator-Benefit Studies**

---

$FEV_1$ is the pulmonary function parameter used for this example. Other parameters can have their percent change calculated in the same manner.

$$\%FEV_1 \text{ Change} = \frac{\text{Post-Test } FEV_1 - \text{Pre-Test } FEV_1}{\text{Pre-test } FEV_1} \times 100$$

For example, where a subject demonstrates the following

    Pre-test $FEV_1$ = 2.470 liters

    Post-Test $FEV_1$ = 2.890 liters

the percent change is calculated as being

$$\%FEV_1 \text{ Change} = \frac{2.890 \text{ liters} - 2.470 \text{ liters}}{2.470 \text{ liters}} \times 100 = 17\% \text{ Change}$$

---

a post-test value that is worse (less) than the corresponding pre-test value would result in a negative solution to the calculation. Although this example is based on using $FEV_1$ as the test standard, the same method can be used to assess the amount of change in other measured parameters.

With subjects who respond to bronchodilators, any measured increase in VC is usually a result of a corresponding decrease in RV values. If the volume of the subject's FVC increases by a greater amount than the increase in $FEV_1$ volume, it can result in a worsening of the $FEV_{1\%}$. In this situation, because improvements were actually demonstrated in both FVC and $FEV_1$, this decrease in $FEV_{1\%}$ is misleading. Therefore, changes in $FEV_{1\%}$ with bronchodilator-benefit studies should be evaluated carefully.

After bronchodilator therapy, it is possible for a subject to demonstrate a significant improvement in expiratory flow rate values without a significant change in the value for FVC. This type of test result still indicates a positive response to bronchodilator therapy.

In some cases, the subject will have no change in measured test values but will have a subjective improvement in symptoms (e.g., less dyspnea). This symptomatic improvement could be due to a redistribution of lung volume compartments or improvements in diffusing capacity or ventilation/perfusion relationships.

It is possible for a subject to demonstrate little or no improvement of any kind after bronchodilator administration. There are different reasons why this might occur:

- Poor inspiratory effort and aerosol deposition during bronchodilator administration may result in too little medication reaching the airways to produce a therapeutic benefit.
- The subject may simply have airways that are not affected by the type or dose of bronchodilator that was administered.

- If the bronchospasm is episodic, the subject may not have been experiencing acute bronchospasm at the time of the test.

A limited measured improvement in pulmonary mechanics (less than 15%) during the study does not automatically eliminate the possibility of a bronchodilator being prescribed for the subject. This is especially true if the subject experienced symptomatic relief or an increase in exercise tolerance during the study. An initial administration of a bronchodilator may not produce a significant response. However, experience has shown that, over time, a greater responsiveness can develop. For this reason, bronchodilators are often prescribed despite poor initial results. Follow-up studies can be performed to identify a greater responsiveness at a later time.

It should be noted that $PaO_2$ levels can deteriorate as a result of sympathomimetic bronchodilator administration. This is because of the generalized beta response that occurs within the lungs. The response causes relaxation in the smooth muscle tissue of both the airways and the pulmonary vasculature. As a result, both the airways and the vasculature can undergo dilation. With this dual dilation response, the increase in circulation within the lungs can sometimes be greater than the corresponding increase in ventilation. The result is a mismatching of ventilation and perfusion that produces the drop in $PaO_2$.

Other options are available when bronchodilator-benefit test results fail to clearly indicate that the subject has abnormally reactive airways. Bronchoprovocation testing can be performed. A study for exercise-induced asthma can also be performed. These tests can be used to further identify the nature and degree of a subject's airway reactivity.

# PREOPERATIVE PULMONARY FUNCTION STUDIES

Preoperative evaluation is important to ensuring a patient's survival and well-being after surgery and postoperative care. It is used to discover and appraise the significance of any preexisting pulmonary dysfunction. Specifically, the purposes of preoperative testing are

1. To assess the risk of **morbidity** and/or **mortality** associated with a surgical procedure for a particular patient.
2. To predict postoperative pulmonary function for patients who are being evaluated for possible lobectomy or pneumonectomy.
3. To plan the patient's care, including preparation and preoperative therapeutics, management of anesthesia during surgery, and postoperative therapeutics.

Preoperative evaluation procedures include history taking and physical examination, pulmonary function testing, electrocardiograms, and chest X rays.

Not all surgical candidates require an extensive presurgical assessment. The need for assessment is based on both the patient's preoperative physical status and the nature of the surgical procedure to be performed. Table 8–3 lists patient characteristics that would indicate the need for preoperative evaluation of postoperative pulmonary risk. Patients

---

### TABLE 8–3   Indications for Preoperative Pulmonary Function Studies

---

#### Absolute Indications

---

Patients who must always undergo preoperative pulmonary function studies include those with

1. A history of smoking.
2. Active symptoms of a pulmonary disorder (dyspnea and/or cough and sputum production).
3. Abnormalities identified during physical assessment procedures (e.g., abnormal chest X ray, breathing rate or pattern, breath sounds, etc.).

---

#### Conditional Indications

---

Patients who may be considered to undergo preoperative pulmonary function studies include those with

1. Evidence of current or recent pulmonary infections or a significant history of pulmonary infections.
2. Morbid obesity.
3. Evidence of problems with debilitation or malnutrition.
4. Advanced age (generally 70 years old or older).

---

scheduled to receive *thoracic and/or abdominal surgical procedures* are most often assessed. These patients have a greater risk of postoperative pulmonary complications associated with procedures performed on these regions of the body.

Tests that are useful for making a general assessment of preoperative pulmonary function include pulmonary mechanics tests, bronchodilator-benefit studies, blood gas analysis, and possibly cardiopulmonary stress testing. Tests additionally helpful for prelobectomy or pneumonectomy patients are perfusion and ventilation/perfusion scans and pulmonary artery occlusion pressure tests. A discussion of the role of each of these tests in preoperative assessment follows.

## Pulmonary Function Assessment for General Surgical Risk

Table 8–4 provides guidelines for interpreting pulmonary function assessment studies for general **surgical risk**.

## Pulmonary Mechanics Tests

Individuals with obstructive pulmonary disorders experience a greater risk of postoperative morbidity and mortality. As was described in Chapter 2, FVC and MVV tests are both successful in identifying such patients. Therefore, simple preoperative FVC (FVC, $FEV_1$ and $FEF_{25\%-75\%}$) and MVV screening tests can be used to identify a significant population of patients who are at risk.

**TABLE 8–4  Interpretation Guidelines for General Preoperative Pulmonary Function Studies**

| Test Procedure | Increased Postoperative Risk Demonstrated | Significant Preoperative Risk Demonstrated |
|---|---|---|
| FVC | <50% of Predicted | <1.5 liters |
| FEV$_1$ | <2.0 liter or <50% of Predicted | <1.0 liter |
| FEF$_{25\%-75\%}$ | <50% of Predicted | NA |
| MVV | NA | <50 l/min or <50% of Predicted |
| PaCO$_2$ | NA | >45 mm Hg |

*NA = no guideline for interpretation is available.*

Any subject demonstrating a below normal preoperative FVC value, regardless of the cause, is at an increased surgical risk. Postoperatively, VC values will be reduced further as a result of anesthesia, pain, and so on. When this VC reduction is combined with a preoperative reduction, the patient can be left with a severe postoperative impairment of cough function.

The MVV test offers a general screening for potential sources of postoperative pulmonary complications. Because of the nature of the test, MVV results can be affected by disorders involving either ventilatory muscle function or airway function or both. It can also be affected by disorders of the lung parenchyma, chest wall, or abdomen. The degree of subject cooperation will also be demonstrated. Since any of these factors can contribute to the likelihood of postoperative problems, MVV is useful for initial preoperative screening. Further testing may be required for a more specific evaluation of what produced poor MVV test results.

## Bronchodilator-Benefit Studies

Bronchodilator-benefit studies can be useful in preoperative patients who have demonstrated obstructive disorders. This is true both for patients who have had a history of the disorder and for patients who had the problem detected more recently through FVC and/or MVV screening. If the bronchodilator-benefit study shows significant obstructive reversibility, perioperative administration of bronchodilators may be accepted as reducing surgical risk.

For any patient, good bronchopulmonary hygiene is important to minimize surgery-related pulmonary complications. This is especially true for subjects with obstructive disorders. Therapeutic pre- and postoperative use of bronchodilators can improve bronchopulmonary hygiene and thereby reduce surgical risk for these patients.

## Arterial Blood Gas Analysis

PaCO$_2$ and PaO$_2$ values can be important tools in evaluating surgical risk in patients who are documented as having a pulmonary disorder. The PaCO$_2$ value is especially helpful. The risk of postoperative morbidity and mortality increases significantly when PaCO$_2$ values of $\geq 45$ mm Hg are demonstrated. Many patients with obstructive disorders have $PaCO_2$ levels of 45 mm Hg or greater.

$PaO_2$ values have a less specific correlation with surgical risk. However, most subjects who have poor results on spirometry tests also demonstrate reduced $PaO_2$ values. There can be a postoperative improvement in $PaO_2$ values in patients who undergo lung **resection** surgery if the portion of lung removed was a significant source of preoperative ventilation/perfusion mismatching.

## Cardiopulmonary Stress Testing

Cardiopulmonary stress testing will be covered in greater detail later in this book. It can be stated at this time, though, that stress testing can play a role in preoperative assessment. However, it is not used routinely for screening to identify patients who may be a surgical risk. For a subject who has already demonstrated a pulmonary disorder, inability to tolerate even moderate exercise levels indicates that a significant surgical risk may be present.

# ASSESSMENT PRIOR TO PULMONARY RESECTION

Having a whole lung or portion of a lung removed will cause some degree of reduction of pulmonary function. Individuals with normal preoperative lung function generally tolerate this reduction well. Unfortunately, many of the patients who are considered for this type of procedure already have diminished lung function. Certain types of preoperative studies are especially useful in assessing the surgical risk of patients who are going to undergo pulmonary resection procedures. Table 8–5 provides guidelines for the interpretation of assessment studies performed prior to pulmonary resection.

## Perfusion and Ventilation/Perfusion Scans

Both perfusion and ventilation/perfusion scans can be used in pulmonary resection and pneumonectomy preoperative assessment. It should be noted, however, that a perfusion scan alone generally provides a useful assessment.

The purpose for the scan is to evaluate the amount of functioning pulmonary tissue that will remain after the resection or pneumonectomy. The results of the perfusion scan

**TABLE 8–5  Interpretation Guidelines for Pulmonary Function Studies Performed Prior to Pulmonary Resection Surgery**

| Test Procedure | Significant Preoperative Risk Demonstrated |
| --- | --- |
| $FEV_1$ | <2.0 liters |
| MVV | <50 l/min or <50% of Predicted |
| Predicted Postoperative $FEV_1$ | <0.8 liter |
| PAOP | >35 mm Hg |

can be quantified by determining regional percentages of perfusion. This provides a basis for judging the amount of functioning lung that will remain after removal of a particular portion of lung.

The results of determining the regional percentages of perfusion can be linked to preoperative $FEV_1$ values as a method of estimating a postoperative $FEV_1$ value by the following equation:

Postoperative $FEV_1$ = Preoperative $FEV_1$ × %Remaining Perfused Lung

where the %Remaining Perfused Lung is the percentage of the lung tissue that will remain after surgery that has adequate perfusion to maintain gas exchange.

As seen in Table 8–5, a poor estimated postoperative $FEV_1$ value helps to indicate a poor risk for pulmonary resection surgery.

## Pulmonary Artery Occlusion Pressure

Individuals who undergo a pneumonectomy procedure are at risk for developing postoperative pulmonary hypertension. This is because of how the pulmonary circulation is redirected as a result of the surgery. Postoperatively, all pulmonary blood flow is accepted by the one remaining lung. With some individuals, this can place an excessive burden on the pulmonary circulation and right ventricle. If pulmonary hypertension occurs postoperatively, it can lead to the development of cor pulmonale.

Measurement of *pulmonary artery occlusion pressure* (PAOP) can be used to evaluate the risk of postpneumonectomy pulmonary hypertension. The study is performed by having a balloon-tipped catheter directed into the pulmonary artery of the lung to be resected. The balloon is inflated and circulation is temporarily blocked from entering that lung. This simulates the redirection of blood into the good lung that would occur after the pneumonectomy. The blood pressure in the pulmonary artery supplying the good lung is then measured and is accepted as being the PAOP.

At the time the PAOP is being measured, an arterial blood gas sample can also be taken and analyzed. The $PaO_2$ of this blood will approximate the $PaO_2$ the patient will experience after the pneumonectomy procedure.

# BRONCHOPROVOCATION (METHACHOLINE CHALLENGE) STUDIES

Bronchoprovocation studies are used to determine objectively whether a subject has a disorder of airway hyperreactivity. Diagnosing airway hyperreactivity can be difficult. There are some subjects who have a history of periodic symptoms (episodic wheezing, etc.) that suggests a hyperreactive, bronchoconstrictive condition exists. Of course, since these symptoms are periodic, the subjects may demonstrate nearly normal results at the time of testing for pulmonary mechanics and bronchodilator benefit. Bronchoprovocation studies overcome this difficulty.

Bronchoprovocation studies, quite simply, are based on having the subject breathe a substance that will cause bronchoconstriction. In normal subjects, the degree of bronchoconstriction will be limited. In subjects who have hyperreactive airways, there will be a much greater response to the substance.

**Methacholine chloride** and histamine are both bronchoactive substances used for bronchoprovocation testing. The one most commonly used is methacholine chloride, a drug with **parasympathomimetic** properties. Delivered to the airways by aerosol, it causes a parasympathomimetic response in the airways—bronchoconstriction.

Beginning with a very small dose, a series of progressively larger doses is given. Following each dose, pulmonary mechanics tests are performed. If at some dose there is a significant decrease in the test parameter value, it is considered a positive test for airway hyperreactivity. For histamine, the maximum dose administered is 10 mg/ml; for methacholine the maximum is 25 mg/ml. With both substances, normal subjects can tolerate doses at these levels without developing a significant reduction in pulmonary function.

$FEV_1$ is most often used as the test parameter for bronchoprovocation studies. It is a simple to measure and very reproducible parameter. A 20% decrease in $FEV_1$ is considered positive for indicating that the subject has hyperreactive airways. Other parameters can be used, however. For $FEF_{25\%-75\%}$, $FEF_{50\%}$, and $FEF_{max}$, a 25% reduction is significant. For $SG_{aw}$, a 35% reduction is significant.

As will be discussed later, a similar study can be performed to evaluate a subject's reaction to the aerosolized administration of a specific antigen. This study can be used to relate the development of bronchospasm or hypersensitivity pneumonitis in the event of exposure to the antigen.

It is important to note that, because of the type of reaction these substances are intended to produce, *resuscitation equipment and medications with effects that are antagonistic to the provocative test agents must be kept on hand in the laboratory.* Though rare, it is possible for a subject to have a life-threatening bronchospastic reaction to an agent.

## PROCEDURE FOR TEST ADMINISTRATION

### Preparation

A subject who is considered for a bronchoprovocation study should be asymptomatic for wheezing or other signs of a bronchoconstrictive problem. The subject should currently be capable of performing an $FEV_1$ that is at least 80% of her or his best previous test value. A baseline test should be performed to ensure that the subject's current capabilities are at an acceptable level.

As with the bronchodilator-benefit study, the subject should abstain from using medications that have been prescribed to manage bronchospasm. The length of abstinence varies, depending on the type of medication in question. Table 8–6 provides some guidelines for abstinence.

### Test Administration

During the study, the subject will be given a series of progressively more concentrated doses of methacholine chloride. Table 8–7 provides an accepted series of methacholine doses. The methacholine chloride used can be prepared in advance from 25 mg/ml stock. Most dose mixtures are relatively stable and can be stored for up to two weeks if refrig-

**TABLE 8–6  Guidelines for Abstinence Prior to Administration of a Bronchoprovocation Study**

1. Eight hours' abstinence from medium-duration sympathomimetic bronchodilators (metaproterenol).
2. Twelve hours' abstinence from use of methylxanthines and long-duration sympathomimetic (terbutaline and salbutamol) bronchodilators.
3. Twelve hours' abstinence from use of prednisone and other corticosteroids.
4. Forty-eight hours' abstinence from sustained-release methylxanthines.
5. Forty-eight hours' abstinence from use of cromolyn sodium.
6. Forty-eight hours' abstinence from antihistamines (especially if the test is for an antigen reaction).
7. Significant exercise and exposure to cold air should be avoided within two hours of the study.
8. Smoke and smoking should be avoided for at least six hours before the study.
9. Stimulants such as coffee, tea, cola drinks, and chocolate should be avoided for at least six hours prior to the study.

erated. The smallest doses (0.075 mg/ml or less) are less stable and if possible should be mixed just prior to use.

Other series' dose values can be used as long as they remain within certain parameters. The initial small dose should be approximately 0.1 mg/ml and the largest dose no greater than 25 mg/ml. There should be at least five intermediate doses between the smallest and largest doses used. With a total of at least seven stages of doses, it is generally

**TABLE 8–7  Dilution and Cumulative Dose Schedule for a Bronchoprovocation Study**

| Methacholine Concentration (MG/ML) | Number of Breaths | Cumulative Dose Units (CDU) | Time Between Dose and Retest (Minutes) | Cumulative Test Time (Minutes) | Cumulative PD$_{20\%}$ FEV$_1$ (CDU/MIN) |
|---|---|---|---|---|---|
| 0.075 | 5 | 0.375 | 3 | 3 | 0.375 units/3 min |
| 0.15 | 5 | 1.125 | 3 | 6 | 1.125 units/6 min |
| 0.31 | 5 | 2.68 | 3 | 9 | 2.68 units/9 min |
| 0.62 | 5 | 5.78 | 3 | 12 | 5.78 units/12 min |
| 1.25 | 5 | 12.00 | 3 | 15 | 12.00 units/15 min |
| 2.50 | 5 | 24.50 | 3 | 18 | 24.50 units/18 min |
| 5.00 | 5 | 49.50 | 3 | 21 | 49.50 units/21 min |
| 10.00 | 5 | 99.50 | 3 | 24 | 99.50 units/24 min |
| 25.00 | 5 | 225.00 | 3 | 27 | 225.00 units/27 min |

possible to reach a dose that produces a positive reaction without producing serious breathing difficulty for the subject.

Care must be taken when administering the aerosolized methacholine. At each dose level, one milliliter of the agent must be inhaled by the subject over five inspirations. A standard small-volume reservoir nebulizer can be used. However, this device may not provide for the controlled administration that is required for this type of study.

For greater control of the dose, a *dosimeter* should be used to control the nebulizer system. A dosimeter is a type of metered-dose delivery system. It is comprised of a breath-triggered solenoid valve and a timing circuit that can regulate the flow of gas to a good quality nebulizer. The dosimeter can be triggered automatically by a flow sensor near the subject's mouth or manually by the technologist. It then provides a controlled flow to the nebulizer only during the subject's inspiration. As a result, very reproducible individual doses from the nebulizer's contents can be administered with great precision. Use of a dosimeter can also minimize environmental exposure to the methacholine chloride. In addition to being of general importance, this is of special importance to technologists who themselves experience asthma or otherwise hyperreactive airways.

The first step in the test is performing the baseline $FEV_1$ measurement. As stated earlier, the result of the test should be at least 80% of the best previous $FEV_1$ test result. After the baseline $FEV_1$ test is performed, the first aerosol administration can be performed.

The first aerosol administration is of a neutral control agent, usually normal saline. Five slow, maximally deep inspirations from the FRC level should be taken from the aerosol. There should be an end-inspiratory hold of three to five seconds at the end of each inspiration. This same breathing pattern should be used with all later aerosol administrations.

Three minutes after the aerosol administration, an FVC test is performed. The $FEV_1$ measured from this test will serve as the *control $FEV_1$ value* ($FEV_1$-C) for the study. In order for the study to continue, the $FEV_1$-C value must be acceptable. It must be at least 90% of the initial *baseline* value measured earlier.

Individuals with very highly reactive airways may have a >20% reduction in $FEV_1$ at this point. This is considered to be a positive test for airway hyperreactivity, even if the first actual dose of methacholine was never administered.

If the value of the $FEV_1$-C is acceptable, then five breaths of the first, smallest dose of methacholine are administered. Three minutes later, an FVC test is again performed, and the test's $FEV_1$ ($FEV_1$-T) is evaluated. The $FEV_1$-T's percent of decrease from the $FEV_1$-C (%$FEV_1$-T Decrease) can be determined by the following equation:

$$\%FEV_1\text{-T Decrease} = \frac{FEV_1\text{-C} - FEV_1\text{-T}}{FEV_1\text{-C}} \times 100$$

Once the %$FEV_1$-T Decrease is calculated, there are three possible outcomes:

1. The $FEV_1$-T is clearly reduced to a value that is more than 20% below the $FEV_1$-C value. This constitutes a *positive* reaction to the methacholine. In order to confirm that this is a positive response, the $FEV_1$ test is repeated six minutes after the administration of that dose. This is just to ensure that the test was truly positive instead of just demonstrating a variability in the pre- and postadministration maneuvers. Typi-

cally, the $FEV_1$ will still be reduced by approximately the same percentage in confirmation of the positive response. If it is not, the result is considered *borderline* and is managed in the manner described shortly.

2. The $FEV_1$-T is reduced to a value that is nearly 20% below the $FEV_1$-C value but without representing a clearly positive test. This is a *borderline* reaction. In this case, the next dose of methacholine is administered, but possibly not for a total of five breaths. The $FEV_1$ test is repeated three minutes after the dose.

3. The $FEV_1$-T is clearly not reduced to a value that is 20% below the $FEV_1$-C value. This represents a *negative* reaction. In this case, the study should continue with the administration of five inhalations of the next greater dose of methacholine and a repeat of the $FEV_1$ test. The series of doses is continued until a positive response is demonstrated. *If the largest dose (25 mg/ml) is administered and the results are still negative, the subject is demonstrated as not having hyperreactive airways.*

The study is ended once the subject demonstrates a clearly positive reaction or the maximum dose is achieved without a positive reaction. It is important that the subject be observed and questioned at each stage of the test in order to determine whether any subjective indications for bronchospasm are present. These indications may include the subject describing feelings of dyspnea and/or tightness in the chest. Auscultation of the subject can also be helpful in assessing the rapid onset of bronchospasm.

If the subject does demonstrate a positive reaction during the study, an aerosolized bronchodilator agent must immediately be administered. A follow-up FVC test must be performed once the bronchodilator has been given time to work. The follow-up FVC test is to document that the subject has returned to normal pre-test pulmonary function levels. Without the bronchodilator, a subject can generally return to normal function in 30–90 minutes. Even with the administration of a bronchodilator, the subject should be observed for at least this amount of time before being dismissed from the laboratory.

## Evaluation of the Study Results

The dose at which a positive 20% reduction in $FEV_1$ is demonstrated is considered the *provocative dose* ($PD_{20\%}FEV_1$). This dose can be reported in the results of the study. A more specific way of reporting the $PD_{20\%}FEV_1$ is as a *cumulative value*.

The first step in assigning a cumulative value to the $PD_{20\%}FEV_1$ is to determine the number of *cumulative dose units* (CDUs) of methacholine that have been administered:

$$CDU = (\text{1st dose conc.} \times 5 \text{ breaths}) + (\text{2nd dose conc.} \times 5 \text{ breaths})$$
$$+ (\text{3rd dose conc.} \times 5 \text{ breaths}) \ldots$$

This calculation continues up to the dose that produced a positive reaction.

Table 8–7 provides the CDU for each stage of the test. The final step in determining a cumulative value for $PD_{20\%}FEV_1$ is to report the CDU value as a function of the cumulative minutes of time needed to produce the response. Again, Table 8–7 provides an example of cumulative time values. As can be seen in Table 8–7, an example of final cumulative value for a positive bronchoprovocation test is

$$PD_{20\%}FEV_1 = 5.78 \text{ CDUs}/12 \text{ minutes}$$

The final report for a bronchoprovocation study should include

- The provocative substance used.
- Whether the study provided positive or negative results.

If the study results were positive,

- The nature of the subject's positive reaction.
- The test parameter(s) that was (were) monitored.
- The last actual measured test parameter value and the value for the $PD_{20\%}$ value for that test parameter ($PD_{20\%}FEV_1$, for example).

## ANTIGEN CHALLENGES

Bronchoprovocation challenges can also be performed to measure a subject's reaction to a specific antigen. There are significant differences between how histamine/methacholine challenges and antigen challenges are performed.

One difference is that the initial low dose of an antigen must be tailored to what the subject is most likely going to be able to tolerate. This is done by having intradermal (cutaneous) testing done prior to the aerosol administration challenge. The dose that produces a 6–8 mm wheal on the skin is generally used as the initial aerosolized dose of the antigen.

There must be a wait of 10 minutes between the administration of a dose of the antigen and the corresponding $FEV_1$ measurement. Also, if a positive (greater than 20%) reduction in $FEV_1$ is demonstrated, there is a wait of an additional 10 minutes before the confirmation $FEV_1$ is measured.

A late reaction to the antigen can develop in subjects who have a positive reaction during the study. The delayed reaction will be gradual in onset and may be exhibited as either bronchospasm or as hypersensitivity pneumonitis. Typically, it will happen within 4–10 hours after the study. If allowed to continue, the reaction could lead to bronchospasms that respond poorly to bronchodilators and can result in status asthmaticus. For this reason, *subjects who demonstrate positive antigen challenge results must be monitored for 24 hours after the test.* During the first 8–12 hours of monitoring, hourly pulmonary assessment must be performed to note any deterioration in function.

Severe reactions are more likely with antigen studies than with histamine/methacholine studies. Because of the resulting need for 24 hours of monitoring, antigen studies should be limited to institutions where proper care and monitoring can be provided.

## STUDIES FOR EXERCISE-INDUCED ASTHMA

Some individuals experience bronchospasm in association with exercise. Although the bronchospasm can occur during the exercise, it is much more likely to occur immediately after the exercise is ended.

Cooling of the respiratory tract mucosa is thought to be the primary triggering mechanism for *exercise-induced asthma.* The increases in ventilation that occur during exercise are responsible for the loss of heat from the mucosa of the respiratory tract. The heat loss is proportional to the level of ventilation—greater ventilation results in greater heat loss.

Both heat exchange and evaporation from the mucosa to the inspired air occur during breathing. Together, they contribute to mucosal heat loss. Of the two processes, evaporation from the mucosa is the more significant mechanism. At any level of ventilation, a subject is more likely to have a bronchospastic reaction to breathing cold, dry air. Bronchospasm is also possible from breathing warm, moist air during exercise but is less likely.

Studies for exercise-induced asthma are designed to evaluate the amount of bronchospasm that may occur in a subject as a result of vigorous exercise. Table 8–8 lists the types of subjects who can benefit from testing for exercise-induced asthma.

In implementing the study, the subject is asked to perform controlled, vigorous exercise. Ideally, having the subject breathe cold, dry air during the exercise would be beneficial to the study. Because of the difficulty in cleanly and conveniently supplying such air, room air breathing is used instead. After the exercise, tests are performed to determine whether there has been a bronchospastic reaction to the exercise.

## PROCEDURE FOR TEST ADMINISTRATION

### Preparation

An assessment must be done to evaluate the appropriateness of having the subject perform vigorous exercise. History taking, physical evaluation, electrocardiography, and other studies can be useful in determining whether the subject will tolerate the required levels of exercise.

Subjects who are found to currently be symptomatic for bronchospasm may not need to have the exercise-induced study performed. The fact that they are symptomatic already indicates that they have a problem with airway hyperreactivity.

In advance of the study, the subject should follow the same guidelines for abstaining from medications as were presented for bronchoprovocation studies in Table 8–6. A baseline pulmonary mechanics test should be performed. The test results must demonstrate that the subject's current capabilities are at least 80% of the past best values. Additionally, the subject's value for $FEV_1$ must be at least 65% of her or his predicted value. The

---

**TABLE 8–8  Indications for Exercise-Induced Bronchospasm Studies**

Subjects who may benefit from exercise-induced bronchospasm studies include those with

1. A history of dyspnea with exertion, but where past routine tests have demonstrated normal results.
2. Complaints of asthma-like symptoms, but where past bronchoprovocation testing has demonstrated negative or questionable results.
3. A diagnosis of asthma in someone considering participating in athletics.
4. Known exercise-induced bronchospasm, but where further study could be done to evaluate the effectiveness of prescribed therapy.

values for ambient barometric pressure, air temperature, and humidity should also be recorded because of their possible effect on airway muscle tone.

## Test Administration

Once the pre-study preparation is completed, the active portion of the study can begin. The subject must perform exercise to a level that is likely to produce a bronchospastic response. A device such as a treadmill or cycle ergometer can be used to provide challenging exercise for the subject. (These devices will be covered in greater detail in the section of the book on exercise testing.) Having the subject wear nose clips during the exercise will eliminate the "air-conditioning" function of the nose. This increases the thermal stress on the airway mucosa and the likelihood of the subject developing bronchospasm.

The subject must be monitored carefully during the exercise. Monitoring should include both ECG and blood pressure. The subject must be observed and questioned regarding his or her tolerance of the exercise.

The initial exercising should be at a low-intensity level for approximately one to two minutes. This will permit the technologist to evaluate the subject's cardiovascular and ventilatory response to the exercise. An extended warmup period should be avoided, however. Prolonged warmup could result in physiologic responses that protect the airways and minimize the possible bronchospastic response.

If the low-intensity exercise is tolerated, the subject must then perform more vigorous exercise for a period of six to eight minutes. The exercise must be of an intensity that raises the subject's heart rate to 85% of the predicted maximum for that subject. A simple method for calculating a subject's maximum heart rate is

Maximum Heart Rate = 220 − Subject's Age

After no more than eight minutes of the exercise, the subject should stop exercising. Pulmonary mechanics tests are then performed one to two minutes after the exercise has been ended. $FEV_1$ is generally used as a measure of the bronchospastic response to exercise. $SG_{aw}$ can also be used, however. The test chosen should be performed twice, with the greater of the two values being recorded for reporting. Testing should be repeated at intervals of five minutes after the initial pulmonary mechanics test.

There are two possible outcomes to the repeat testing:

1. A decrease in test values is demonstrated. The maximum decreases will occur in the first 5–10 minutes after the exercise is ended. Recovery and a return of the values to baseline levels generally occurs approximately 20–40 minutes after the exercise has ended.
2. No significant change is demonstrated in the test values.

The testing should be continued at five-minute intervals until

1. Values that decreased after the exercise have returned to baseline levels

*or*

2. Values have continued to remain unchanged from baseline for at least 30 minutes after the cessation of the exercise.

If the study must be repeated because of questionable results, there should be a wait of at least two hours. The buildup of catecholamines in the body from the exercise could result in there being a lesser response to a follow-up test.

## EVALUATION OF TEST RESULTS

The key measured test value for evaluation is the low value to which the $FEV_1$ (or $SG_{aw}$) decreased as a result of the exercise. To be most useful, the amount of $FEV_1$ deterioration can be related to the baseline value. This provides a value for the exercise-induced change (decrease) in $FEV_1$ (EI$\Delta$ $FEV_1$%). Table 8–9 provides an example of how this value is calculated. It also presents other, related calculations that can be performed.

---

**TABLE 8–9   Calculations for Exercise-Induced Bronchospasm Studies**

---

### Calculation of EI% $\Delta FEV_1$

---

$$EI\% \Delta FEV_1 = \frac{B\text{-}FEV_1 - LPE\text{-}FEV_1}{B\text{-}FEV_1} \times 100$$

For a subject who has a baseline B-$FEV_1$ of 4.56 liters and an LPE-$FEV_1$ of 3.59 liters,

$$EI\% \Delta FEV_1 = \frac{4.56 \text{ liters} - 3.59 \text{ liters}}{4.56 \text{ liters}} \times 100$$

$$EI\% \Delta FEV_1 = 21\%$$

---

### Other Useful Calculations

---

The amount that the postexercise $FEV_1$ is reduced from the baseline $FEV_1$, expressed as a percentage of subject's predicted $FEV_1$

$$EI\ \Delta FEV_1 \text{ as a percent of the P-}FEV_1 = \frac{B\text{-}FEV_1 - LPE\text{-}FEV_1}{P\text{-}FEV_1} \times 100$$

The post-exercise $FEV_1$ expressed as a percent of the subject's predicted $FEV_1$, follows:

$$LPE\text{-}FEV_1 \text{ as a percent of the P-}FEV_1 = \frac{LPE\text{-}FEV_1}{P\text{-}FEV_1} \times 100$$

B-$FEV_1$ = Baseline $FEV_1$.
LPE-$FEV_1$ = Lowest post-exercise $FEV_1$.
P-$FEV_1$ = Predicted $FEV_1$ for subject.

---

An EIΔ $FEV_1$% value of 20% or greater is considered significant. This value indicates that exercise is clearly a triggering mechanism for bronchospasm in the subject. However, a value of less than 20% does not eliminate the possibility of an exercise-induced bronchospasm problem for the subject. It could be that, despite the exercise, the ambient conditions of temperature and humidity in the laboratory were not sufficient to trigger the bronchospasm. The subject may still have symptomatic problems with bronchospasm at other times under other conditions.

## VARIATIONS ON STUDIES FOR EXERCISE-INDUCED ASTHMA

There are variations on the studies performed for exercise-induced asthma that can be clinically useful. The basic principle is the same—to identify the degree of bronchoreactivity to a suspected trigger. Two examples of environmental triggers that might be studied are

- Cold air exposure.
- Workplace or other physical environmental exposure.

Cold air exposure can certainly be a trigger for known asthmatics. However, even subjects with no established history of asthma may periodically complain of wheezing under cold air conditions. Exertion may play a role in the reaction. Cold air testing can be helpful in documenting and quantitating this problem.

Some subjects complain of wheezing related to a specific physical environment—work-related, home-related, school-related, for example. The reaction may be due to environmental allergens, chemicals, or other substances. Before extensive investigation is done to identify the specific trigger-substance, it may be helpful to identify the environment(s) where the problem is greatest. The procedure is the same as for studies on exercise-induced asthma:

1. A pre-test is performed at a time when the subject is asymptomatic.
2. The subject is exposed to the suspected trigger (cold air with or without exertion, the workplace, some other suspected physical environment). The conditions (location and duration of exposure to the environment) should follow as closely as possible the circumstances where the subject has identified wheezing to be triggered in the past.
3. A post-test is performed.
4. The results of pre- and post-testing are compared. As with exercise testing, a decrease in the $FEV_1$ of more than 20% from the pre-test to the post-test is significant.

Most laboratories can provide circumstances allowing cold air exposure studies to be performed. However, testing for reaction to a specific physical environment presents the following problems:

- There may need to be a prolonged exposure time in the physical environment before more subtle, persistent environmental triggers produce a clinically troubling reaction.

- The location and circumstances of the physical environment to be studied may make it difficult for the laboratory to perform appropriate and timely pre- and post-tests.
- The study may succeed in identifying the physical environment that triggers bronchospasm but not in identifying the specific trigger within that environment. Additional evaluation of the environment will need to be performed.

Because of these problems, a significant history of problems and a strong suspicion of the environment should exist before a study is considered.

# STUDIES TO DOCUMENT IMPAIRMENT/DISABILITY

A significant physical impairment can result in an individual being disabled from performing work-related tasks. Although there is a close relationship between impairment and disability, it is important to note that the two are significantly different.

- **Impairment** is a state that results from an anatomic or functional abnormality. The abnormality is one where *medical evaluation* identifies a *measurable*, clinically significant change in body function. An impairment is considered permanent if it persists for a significant period of time (for example, a year or more after maximum treatment and rehabilitation has been achieved). An impairment may or may not result in a work-related disability.
- **Disability** is an *administrative* or *legal* judgment of an individual's ability to perform certain tasks, generally work-related. Disability is often caused by a physical impairment. However, factors such as age, education, mental health, and requirements of employment are also important. A disability is considered permanent if the individual cannot be expected to significantly improve his or her performance levels.

A pulmonary function impairment may or may not create a disability. Pulmonary assessment and function studies can be used to identify and document the existence of such an impairment. The results of these studies, added to other information on the subject, can lead to a judgment regarding disability.

Pulmonary evaluation for determination of disability should be thorough. The evaluation must be complete enough for an impartial administrative or legal evaluator to decide whether the subject is sufficiently impaired to be judged disabled. Basic patient information and history taking, physical assessment, and certain specific pulmonary function studies must all be performed as a part of the evaluation. In some situations, blood gas measurements may also be included in the impairment/disability assessment.

Figure 8–2 shows a chart that outlines and organizes the pulmonary evaluation required. Information is obtained from the subject and a physical assessment performed before specific pulmonary function tests are performed. The actual testing in the study begins with a simple, relatively easy to perform test, the FVC. From there, each step in

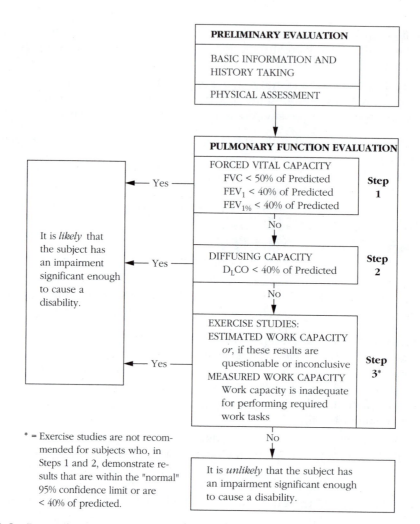

**Figure 8–2** *Process for administration of an exercised-induced bronchospasm study.*

the study involves a more complex type of test. An explanation of the key points in an impairment/disability study follows.

## BASIC INFORMATION AND HISTORY TAKING

Gathering information from the patient is an important part of evaluation for impairment and disability. The earlier section in this chapter, "Patient Assessment for Pulmonary Function Testing" (under the subhead of "Basic Information and History Taking"), provides a description of the information that must be gathered.

## PHYSICAL ASSESSMENT

A physical assessment of the subject must be performed before pulmonary function studies are done. This will not only provide information for the disability evaluation but will also indicate any limitations to the pulmonary function studies that are to be performed. The earlier section in this chapter, "Patient Assessment for Pulmonary Function Testing" (under the subhead of "Physical Assessment"), provides a description of the assessment that must be performed.

## PULMONARY FUNCTION EVALUATION

The subject undergoing testing is someone who has complained of difficulty in breathing during the performance of work-related tasks. Pulmonary function studies can provide an objective measurement of the subject's pulmonary impairment. This will help to determine how likely it is that the subject has breathing difficulties serious enough to affect work performance.

If at all possible, the subject should be in optimum health for her or his condition at the time that the tests in the study are performed. If wheezing or other evidence of bronchospasm is present, the tests should be repeated after a bronchodilator has been administered.

There are two possible outcomes to having these tests performed:

1. A severe impairment will be demonstrated by the tests. This impairment, once identified, will contribute significantly to the determination of a disability.
2. A severe impairment will not be demonstrated. This makes it less likely that a judgment of disability caused by poor pulmonary function will be made.

At each stage of the study, if a severe impairment is indicated by the test results, no further testing needs to be performed. The study is over. It is only when a test's results are negative or questionable that the study must continue to the next stage. It is important to note that a subject who demonstrates medical contraindications to exercise studies (cardiopulmonary stress testing) should not undergo Step 3 of the study. A more complete explanation of cardiopulmonary stress testing and its significance will be provided later in this book.

## ARTERIAL BLOOD GAS MEASUREMENTS

Blood gas studies are not required as a part of impairment/disability evaluation but in some situations they may be desired. Provided that the subject has a history of receiving optimum medical therapy, an impairment is demonstrated if

1. The resting $PaO_2$ is less than 55 mm Hg while the subject is breathing room air.
2. The resting $PaO_2$ is less than 60 mm Hg while the subject is breathing room air together with one or more of the following additional hypoxemia-related criteria:
   a. Pulmonary hypertension has been demonstrated by cardiac catheterization.
   b. Cor pulmonale is demonstrated by electrocardiogram and chest X ray findings.

c. Increasing hypoxemia is demonstrated during exercise (treadmill, for more than six minutes at 2 mph and 0% grade).
d. Erythrocytosis is demonstrated by a complete blood count.

## ADDITIONAL CONSIDERATIONS WHEN EVALUATING PULMONARY IMPAIRMENT/DISABILITY

Other factors to be considered when interpreting and reporting the results of an evaluation of impairment/disability include

- Lack of subject cooperation during the evaluation.
- Well-documented history of regular emergency treatment for serious problems with asthma.
- Failure to receive commonly accepted therapy for the problem that is documented.
- Coexisting disorder(s) compounding the effects of a pulmonary disorder that considered alone would not be enough to produce a disability.
- Deconditioned state whereas greater efforts toward conditioning would result in the measured impairment being less likely to produce a disability.
- Advanced age (beyond retirement age).
- Disability caused by a problem that may not provide for an easily measurable impairment (e.g., tuberculosis, bronchiectasis, sleep apnea/alveolar hypoventilation syndrome).

# CRITICAL CARE MONITORING

Pulmonary function testing in the critical care setting is generally to evaluate

- The level of spontaneous ventilation a subject is capable of sustaining.
- Pulmonary compliance and airway resistance values demonstrated by subjects on mechanical ventilatory support.
- The effects of either spontaneous or mechanical ventilation on blood gas values.

Some of these topics were discussed earlier in the book in the context of testing performed in the laboratory. The discussion will now be in reference specifically to how these tests are modified and performed in the critical care setting.

## EVALUATION OF SPONTANEOUS VENTILATORY PARAMETERS

Monitoring of spontaneous ventilation in the critical care setting is for subjects who are

1. At risk for developing **ventilatory failure**. This is done to determine whether a need for mechanical ventilatory support is indicated.

2. Currently on mechanical ventilatory support. This is
   - for subjects who appear to lack any spontaneous effort to breathe, to document, in fact, that there is or continues to be no spontaneous breathing effort.
   - for subjects who do demonstrate spontaneous breathing efforts, to evaluate the possibility that weaning may begin.
3. Currently being weaned from mechanical ventilatory support.

Subjects who are at risk for developing ventilatory failure or who are in the process of being weaned from ventilatory support (numbers 1 and 3) require the most frequent monitoring. Minimally, they should have serial measurements made every four hours. In some instances, more frequent measurements may be appropriate.

Subjects who are on ventilatory support (number 2) can be evaluated less frequently. They should, minimally, be evaluated once a day. Performing checks every eight hours would not be excessive, however.

## Monitoring of Spontaneous Volumes

Values for a subject's spontaneous breathing volumes can be measured at the critical care bedside.

*Equipment Used.* A hand-held primary volume or flow-sensing spirometer can be used at the bedside to monitor spontaneous breathing volumes. The spirometer should be attached to the exhalation side of a one-way breathing valve system. This is done in order to measure only exhaled volumes and to avoid having the subject breathe back and forth through the spirometer.

A low-deadspace-volume, one-way valve system should be selected. Using a one-way valve system with greater than 100 ml deadspace to measure tidal volumes less than 200 ml can result in $CO_2$ retention for the subject. $CO_2$ retention can produce greater discomfort and will trigger the subject to use tidal volumes larger than normal.

Conversely, care should be taken if one-way valve deadspace reductions are taken to an extreme. This can produce an increase in breathing resistance for the subject. Simple disposable models, based on adding one-way valves to a **Briggs adapter**, are available and can be used quite satisfactorily.

The appliance used for connection between the subject and the valve/spirometer system depends on the condition of the subject. An alert, nonintubated subject can make use of a mouthpiece and nose clips. For an unconscious subject, measurements can be made by using a resuscitation/anesthesia-type mask. Intubated subjects, whether conscious or not, can be connected directly to the Briggs adapter/one-way valve system.

Subjects who are receiving continuous oxygen therapy may need to have supplementary oxygen supplied during the measurement of spontaneous volumes. The oxygen can be supplied to a tubelike reservoir on the inspiratory side of the one-way valve system that is being used. *Care must be taken to ensure that the oxygen flow does not pass directly through to the expiratory side of the one-way valve system and falsely increase the volumes that are measured.*

*Measurement of Vital Capacity.* A nonforced VC can be measured with most alert, co-operative subjects. First the subject is connected to the one-way valve/spirometer system. The subject should then be given a few moments to breathe on the system and become accustomed to it. Once ready, the subject should be coached to inhale to the TLC level and then make an *unforced* exhalation down to the RV level. This test should be repeated at least once more, and the largest VC value demonstrated is the one that should be recorded.

*Measurement of Minute Ventilation, Respiratory Rate, and Tidal Volume.* Generally direct measurements are made of exhaled minute ventilation ($\dot{V}_E$) and respiratory rate (f). Once these values are available, an average value for tidal volume ($V_T$) can be determined by dividing the $\dot{V}_E$ value by the value for f during the minute of measurement.

$$\text{Average } V_T = \frac{\dot{V}_E}{f}$$

For $\dot{V}_E$ measurement, the subject must be connected to a one-way valve/spirometer system and given a few moments to establish a regular breathing pattern. Once regular breathing is established, exhaled volumes must be cumulatively measured for one minute. During the minute of volume measurement, the f (number of collected exhalations) must be counted. Given values for $\dot{V}_E$ and f, an average value for $V_T$ can be determined.

Subjects who have been removed from ventilatory support in order for the $\dot{V}_E$ measurement to be made may not tolerate spontaneous breathing for a full minute. These subjects generally demonstrate rapid respiratory rates and small $V_T$s. Direct measurement of $\dot{V}_E$ is not possible in this situation, but it is possible to determine an average value for $V_T$. This is done by cumulatively measuring the subject's exhaled volumes for 10 breaths. Once the exhaled volumes have been measured, the average $V_T$ is determined by taking the cumulative exhaled volume (in liters) and moving the decimal point two places to the right. This gives an average value for $V_T$ in milliliters. For example, 3.15 liters *cumulative exhaled volume indicates an average $V_T$ of* 315 ml.

*Measurement of Maximum Voluntary Ventilation.* A crude measurement of *maximum voluntary ventilation* (MVV) can be accomplished at the critical-care bedside using the one-way valve/spirometer system described earlier. This is done by connecting the subject to the system, permitting the subject a few moments to become accustomed to breathing on it, and then coaching her or him to perform an MVV effort. The volume collection measurement should if possible be made for 10 seconds. Once a 10-second cumulative volume value has been measured, it must be multiplied by 6 in order to determine a value for MVV.

Realistically, many critical care subjects will not be able to successfully perform this test and produce useful results. It is important that the technologist evaluate the level of the subject's cooperation and effort during the test. If the subject's understanding and cooperation appear to have been poor, the results should not be used.

*Inductive Plethysmography.* Inductive plethysmography can be used to measure values for spontaneous tidal volume and respiratory rate in the critical care setting. There are benefits and drawbacks, however. Inductive plethysmography does permit the measuring of ventilation volumes without the need to make a connection to the subject's airway. Unfortunately, in order for it to provide accurate volume measurements, frequent and difficult calibration procedures need to be performed. This is made especially difficult because of the effects of body position changes that are needed for a critical care patient.

*Monitoring of Spontaneous Volumes for Subjects on Mechanical Ventilatory Support.* Subjects who are receiving mechanical ventilation can be disconnected from the ventilator in order to have spontaneous volumes measured. If this is done, however, the subject must be carefully monitored during the time off support. This is to ensure that the subject does not experience significant physiological stress before being returned to support by the ventilator. The subject must immediately be returned to support as soon as measurements have been completed and between retests.

Another approach is to leave the subject connected to the ventilator and to use the ventilator's spirometer system to measure spontaneous volumes. Values for VC, $\dot{V}_E$, an average value for $V_T$, and MVV can be measured in this manner. Most modern ventilators can permit this to be done. The manufacturer of a ventilator may have to be consulted as to how on-ventilator spontaneous volume measurement can be accomplished with their particular system.

There is a possible problem with this method. The demand system that some ventilators use to supply inspiratory gas for spontaneous breathing can increase the subject's work of breathing. This increase may be to a level that is greater than would be experienced if the subject were actually disconnected from the ventilator. Such a resistance to breathing can rapidly fatigue the subject and affect the results of measurement.

## Monitoring Spontaneous Pressures

Both *maximum inspiratory pressure* (MIP) and *maximum expiratory pressure* (MEP) can be measured in the critical care setting as follows:

*Measurement of Maximum Inspiratory Pressure.* A simple bedside device for measuring MIP can be constructed by using a one-way valve system and pressure manometer. The manometer should be connected to the *inspiratory* side of the valve system. This arrangement does not include a leak tube, as we described in Chapter 2, to minimize the effects of the cheek muscles. However, since many critical-care subjects make use of artificial airways, the lack of a leak tube should not present a problem.

With this arrangement, inspiratory efforts that are made do not provide the subject with an inspiratory volume. Instead, each inspiratory effort is registered as a negative pressure on the manometer. This is because the manometer is connected to the inspiratory port on the valve. Each expiratory effort takes the subject further down to the RV level. As a result of using this valve/manometer system arrangement, the subject will eventually demonstrate an MIP at or near RV over a series of breathing cycles. The most negative pressure generated by the subject should be recorded.

The subject does not have to be conscious when MIP is measured in this manner. Even an unconscious subject will eventually demonstrate an MIP value when spontaneously breathing on this one-way valve/manometer system. A note of caution, however: *A subject must not be left connected and breathing on this device for more than 15 seconds before being disconnected and permitted to breath comfortably again.* Most subjects should demonstrate an acceptable value for MIP within less than 15 seconds.

*Measurement of Maximum Expiratory Pressure.* Maximum expiratory pressure can be measured by changing the arrangement of the one-way valve/manometer system. The manometer should be connected to the *expiratory* side of the valve system. Now the subject can inhale air and then forcefully exhale against the manometer. MEP can only be measured with an alert, cooperative subject. The greatest value is the one that should be recorded.

## Clinical Significance of Spontaneous Volume and Pressure Measurements

Measurements of spontaneous volumes and pressures can be useful in managing patients in the critical care setting. This is especially true for patients who may require, are receiving, or are being weaned from mechanical ventilatory support.

*Clinical Significance of Spontaneous Volume Measurements.* The measurement of VC demonstrates what a subject is capable of doing with a maximal effort. Generally, subjects who demonstrated poor VC values will easily experience breathing fatigue, especially when stressed. They will also have poor cough efforts. VC values of less than 15 ml/kg may indicate a need for mechanical ventilatory support.

Values for $\dot{V}_E$ are most useful when they are interpreted in relation to $PaCO_2$ values. In normal individuals, there is an inverse balance between the levels of ventilation that are maintained and the $PaCO_2$ levels that result. Increases in ventilation cause decreases in $PaCO_2$ values, and decreases in ventilation cause increases in $PaCO_2$ values.

In subjects with abnormalities, the relationship between ventilation and $PaCO_2$ may not be this straightforward. There are two ways in which the relationship between ventilation and $PaCO_2$ values can become out of balance:

1. Normal or elevated $PaCO_2$ values may exist despite elevated levels of ventilation ($\dot{V}_E$ greater than normal). This type of abnormality is caused by increases in physiologic deadspace. The increased ventilation represents an attempt to compensate for the increased deadspace volume.
2. Elevated $PaCO_2$ values that coincide with reduced levels of ventilation ($\dot{V}_E$ less than normal). This type of abnormality is caused by ventilatory failure resulting from neuromuscular disorders, central nervous system disorders or depression, musculoskeletal disorders, or obstructive pulmonary disorders.

Obviously, given these relationships, care must be taken when making clinical interpretations based on changes in $\dot{V}_E$ values. The subject's $PaCO_2$ should also be evaluated to help assess its relationship to the subject's $\dot{V}_E$.

The $V_T$ and f a subject uses to maintain ventilation are also of clinical significance. When small $V_T$s are used, a larger proportion of each breath's $V_T$ is deadspace volume. Therefore, *fast respiratory rates and a larger than normal $\dot{V}_E$ are required to maintain a normal* *level of alveolar ventilation and acceptable PaCO2 values.* This is why subjects with $V_T$ values less than 300 ml may have difficulty remaining off mechanical ventilatory support. Because of their smaller tidal volumes, they must perform considerable ventilatory work in order to maintain adequate $PaCO_2$ levels.

The values for spontaneous VC and $V_T$ provide a basis for evaluating a subject's *ventilatory reserve* (VR) by the following equation:

$$VR = 100 - \left( \frac{V_T}{\dot{V}_E \times 100} \right)$$

Given normal values for VC (50–70 ml/kg) and $V_T$ (6–7 ml/kg), the normal value for VR is approximately 90%. This means that the work normally performed with breathing is less than 10% of the total work that a person is capable of performing. A VR of less than 50% is clinically significant. This means that the $V_T$ needed by the subject to maintain acceptable $PaCO_2$ levels is more than half of his or her total capability to move an air volume. A subject breathing under these conditions is at risk for developing ventilatory fatigue. Weaning a subject from mechanical ventilatory support is difficult and unlikely when VR is less than 50 percent.

*Clinical Significance of Spontaneous Pressure Measurements.* MIP is useful because it correlates well with VC values. A subject who can generate an MIP of at least −20 cm $H_2O$ within 20 seconds of effort generally has a corresponding VC value of at least 15 ml/kg. MIP can be monitored regardless of whether or not a subject is conscious and cooperative. As stated earlier, VC measurements are limited to conscious, cooperative subjects. Generally, MIP values of less than 20 cm $H_2O$ may indicate a need for mechanical ventilatory support.

MEP values relate directly to a subject's ability to cough. A subject who has the ability to generate an MEP greater than 40 cm $H_2O$ should have at least an acceptable ability to generate a cough.

## Monitoring Forced Expiratory Volumes and Flow Rates

Forced expiratory volumes and flow rates can be measured at the bedside. A smaller, screening-type spirometer system can be used. The screener system must meet the American Thoracic Society standards described in Appendix C.

The FVC tests performed at the bedside and related data are most often used for assessing surgical risk and for monitoring the effects of therapy, especially for obstructive disorders such as asthma.

## MONITORING VENTILATORY PARAMETERS FOR SUBJECTS ON MECHANICAL VENTILATORY SUPPORT

Approximate values for pulmonary compliance and airway resistance can be determined for subjects on mechanical ventilatory support.

## Pulmonary Compliance

For subjects on mechanical ventilatory support, values for *static compliance* ($C_{St}$) and *dynamic compliance* ($C_{Dyn}$) can be determined (Table 8–10). $P_I$ and $P_{Plat}$ pressure values from at least three breaths should be checked and recorded. The mean of these values should be used in calculating $C_{St}$ and $C_{Dyn}$. When corresponding $C_{St}$ and $C_{Dyn}$ values are determined for a subject, $C_{St}$ will always have a greater numerical value than $C_{Dyn}$.

The value for the subject's PEEP level is subtracted from the inspiratory pressure value ($P_I$ or $P_{Plat}$) used in the equations. This is because calculations for compliance are based

---

### TABLE 8–10  Calculation of $C_{st}$ and $C_{Dyn}$

---

$C_{st}$ is calculated by use of the following equation:

$$C_{st} = \frac{V_{Tact}}{P_{Plat} - PEEP}$$

$C_{Dyn}$ is calculated by use of the following equation:

$$C_{Dyn} = \frac{V_{Tact}}{P_I - PEEP}$$

where

$V_{Tact}$ = the tidal volume that actually entered and ventilated the subject. See below for an explanation of how this volume is determined.

$P_{Plat}$ = the inflation hold/plateau pressure where the inflation hold was for at least 0.5–2.0 seconds.

$P_I$ = the peak pressure achieved during inspiration.

$PEEP$ = positive end-expiratory pressure.

$V_{Tact}$ is calculated by use of the following equation:

$$V_{Tact} = V_{Tmeas} - SVL$$

where

$V_{Tmeas}$ = the $V_T$ measured as it is exhaled from the ventilator circuit.

$SVL$ = the system volume loss. This is the amount of the inspiratory $V_T$ delivered by the ventilator that remains compressed within the circuit during inspiration instead of entering the patient.

$SVL$ is determined by

$$SVL = (P_I - PEEP) \times C_{Sys}$$

where

$C_{Sys}$ = the compliance/gas compression factor for the ventilator circuit system.

on the *change* in pressure that occurs during the inspiratory phase of ventilation. This is the difference between the baseline (PEEP) pressure value and either the $P_I$ or $P_{Plat}$ value.

It is important to note that the $V_{Tact}$ used in the calculations excludes the volume of gas delivered by the ventilator that is compressed within the ventilator circuit during the inspiratory phase (SVL). Although this volume of gas is a part of the "exhaled" volume that is measured coming out of the expiration valve of the circuit, it is not a volume that entered the subject during inspiration. Therefore, it should not be included in the calculation of either $C_{St}$ or $C_{Dyn}$. Calculation of pulmonary compliance should be based only on volumes of air that actually ventilate the subject.

An approximate value of 3 ml/cm $H_2O$ can be used for $C_{Sys}$ in the calculation of SVL. The actual value for $C_{Sys}$ for a given subject is dependent on the physical characteristics of the ventilator and circuit system used. The values for $C_{Sys}$ and SVL are important to evaluating how well a subject is being ventilated by a mechanical ventilator. They show that, for a given constant "exhaled" $V_T$, as a subject's inspiratory pressures increase, more of the $V_T$ delivered by the ventilator remains compressed in the breathing circuit during inspiration. As a result, less volume actually enters and ventilates the subject's lungs.

There is a problem with determination of a value for $C_{St}$. The subject must be *relaxed* during the inflation hold period in order for an accurate $P_{Plat}$ measurement to be made. Many patients are not capable of doing this. Because of ventilatory efforts made by the subject during the inflation hold period, a falsely low or high plateau pressure may be recorded. Careful observations should be made of the subject when $P_{Plat}$ measurements are made. If the subject's ventilatory efforts make accurate measurement of $P_{Plat}$ difficult, it is possible that an acceptable value for $C_{St}$ cannot be determined.

$C_{St}$ and $C_{Dyn}$ values are only approximate measures of compliance and should not be confused with the compliance values described in Chapter 2. When monitored serially for a subject, though, values for $C_{St}$ and $C_{Dyn}$ can be useful for patient management.

Because inflation hold/plateau pressure values are used for determining $C_{St}$, $C_{St}$ is affected only by disorders that affect either thoracic or lung compliance. Conversely, since a peak inspiratory pressure is used for calculating $C_{Dyn}$, that value is affected by a greater number of factors. Its value includes and can increase and decrease correspondingly with the factors that affect $C_{St}$. However, $C_{Dyn}$ will also be affected by changes in a subject's airway resistance. This is based on how changes in airway resistance create changes in the difference between $P_{Plat}$ and $P_I$. Increases in airway resistance will produce a greater difference between $P_{Plat}$ and $P_I$. Table 8–11 presents a series of hypothetical $C_{St}$ and $C_{Dyn}$ changes.

It should be noted that changes in body position that are common to caring for critically ill patients also affect $C_{St}$ and therefore $C_{Dyn}$ values. For example, body positions that limit thoracic expansion will reduce $C_{St}$ and $C_{Dyn}$. Hence, the subject's body position should be recorded when compliance measurements are made.

Values for $C_{St}$ and $C_{Dyn}$ for normal subjects are not available. Related studies have been performed, but the results are not conclusive and cannot be applied to the general population of ventilator patients. As a yardstick for comparison, a subject with healthy lungs who is on a ventilator may have a $C_{St}$ value of 60 cm $H_2O$. The range of values, however, can be between 50 and 100 cm $H_2O$. The range is broad because the size and shape of the subject's thorax and the subject's body position all significantly affect pulmonary compliance values.

**TABLE 8–11  Hypothetical Patterns for Changes in C$_{St}$ and C$_{Dyn}$**

| Disorder | C$_{St}$ Change | C$_{Dyn}$ Change |
|---|---|---|
| Increased R$_{aw}$ | NC | ↓ |
| Decreased R$_{aw}$ | NC | ↑ |
| Increased C$_{LT}$ | ↑ | ↑ |
| Decreased C$_{LT}$ | ↓ | ↓ |
| Increased R$_{aw}$ and decreased C$_{LT}$ | ↓ | ↓ |
| Decreased R$_{aw}$ and increased C$_{LT}$ | ↑ | ↑ |
| Increased C$_{LT}$ and increased R$_{aw}$ | ↑ | NC or ↓ |
| Decreased C$_{LT}$ and decreased R$_{aw}$ | ↓ | NC or ↑ |

*NC = no change in value.*
*C$_{LT}$ = combined lung/thoracic compliance.*
  *↑ = increase in C$_{St}$ or C$_{Dyn}$.*
  *↓ = decrease in C$_{St}$ or C$_{Dyn}$.*

C$_{St}$ values of less than 25 cm H$_2$O indicate a relatively poor state of pulmonary compliance. Because of the increased work of breathing, subjects with low C$_{St}$ values may be difficult to wean from mechanical ventilatory support. C$_{St}$ values greater than 100 cm H$_2$O should be questioned. Although such values are possible in patients with emphysema, falsely low inflation hold/plateau pressure measurements can also produce excessively high C$_{St}$ values.

"Normal" C$_{Dyn}$ values generally run 10%–20% less than a subject's corresponding C$_{St}$ values. This is because, for intubated patients, the effects of airway resistance cause P$_I$ to be approximately 10%–20% greater than P$_{Plat}$. Increases in R$_{aw}$ will increase this pressure difference and reduce C$_{Dyn}$ values to even lower levels.

## Airway Resistance

Although comparisons of C$_{Dyn}$ values to C$_{St}$ values can provide an indirect evaluation of inspiratory airway resistance (R$_{aw}$) changes, it is possible to determine R$_{aw}$ more directly (Table 8–12). The problem with this calculation is in choosing a value for the inspiratory flow rate. With most ventilators, a value for inspiratory flow can be pre-set on the ventilator or determined through calculation. However, this value may not represent the subject's actual inspiratory flow rate. This problem is minimized when a single value for inspiratory flow rate or method of choosing an inspiratory flow rate value is selected and evaluation of the subject's R$_{aw}$ is based on comparisons over a series of determinations.

Although R$_{aw}$ can be calculated for any given inspiratory flow rate, it may be helpful to consistently make the measurement at a standard inspiratory flow rate. A flow rate of .5 l/sec (30 l/min), if tolerated by the subject, could be used as a standardized flow rate setting for determining a R$_{aw}$ value.

---

**TABLE 8–12  Calculation of $R_{aw}$**

---

$R_{aw}$ is calculated by use of the following equation:

$$R_{aw} = \frac{P_I - P_{Plat}}{V_I}$$

where

$P_I$ = the peak inspiratory pressure achieved during inspiration.

$P_{Plat}$ = the inflation hold/plateau pressure where the inflation hold was for at least 0.5–2.0 seconds.

$V_I$ = the end-inspiratory flow rate at the point where the $P_I$ measurement was made.

---

As with pulmonary compliance values, it is important to note that this method does not represent an accurate measurement of a subject's inspiratory $R_{aw}$. As with $C_{St}$ and $C_{Dyn}$ values, however, serial measurement of $R_{aw}$ by this method can be useful in clinical management of ventilator patients.

Establishing a "normal" $R_{aw}$ value in this manner is not possible because of subject differences in inspiratory flow rate and artificial airway size. Instead of making comparisons against a "normal," it is best if serial measurement comparisons are used in conjunction with other clinical signs of airway resistance problems in managing the patient.

## CRITICAL CARE BLOOD GAS MONITORING

Blood gas monitoring is an important part of patient management in critical care. The method(s) used for any given subject depend(s) on the disorders that are present and the appropriateness of the alternatives that are available for use. Direct measurement of blood gas values from a blood sample provides the most specific assessment of pH, $PaCO_2$, and $PO_2$. In many situations, however, use of pulse oximetry, transcutaneous $CO_2$ and/or $O_2$ monitoring, and end-tidal $CO_2$ monitoring can be appropriate.

*Review Questions*

---

Please use the following review questions to evaluate your learning of information from this chapter. It might be helpful to write out your answers on a sheet of paper. If you are unsure of the answers to these questions, review the chapter to reinforce your learning.

1. Relating to the basic information and historical information necessary for pulmonary function testing:
   a. What basic information and historical information should be gathered on a subject before pulmonary function testing?

    b. What methods of physical assessment should be performed before pulmonary function testing?

2. Relating to the administration of pulmonary function tests:
    a. What preparation should be performed before the general administration of pulmonary function tests?
    b. What actions should be taken during the test to ensure proper test administration?
    c. How should pulmonary function test results be reported?

3. Relating to bronchodilator-benefit studies:
    a. What preparation should be performed before the administration of a bronchodilator-benefit study?
    b. What actions should be taken during the study to ensure proper test administration?
    c. How should pulmonary function test results be reported?
    d. How should results of a bronchodilator-benefit study be evaluated?
    e. What percent improvement in pulmonary function is considered significant for a bronchodilator-benefit study?

4. Relating to preoperative pulmonary function studies:
    a. What are indications that preoperative pulmonary function studies may be needed?
    b. What types pulmonary function tests should be performed for pulmonary assessment of general surgical risk?
    c. How is interpretation of the test results significant to assessing surgical risk?

5. Relating to pulmonary function studies prior to pulmonary resection:
    a. What are guidelines for interpreting results of pulmonary function studies prior to pulmonary resection?
    b. How are perfusion and ventilation/perfusion scans used for pre-resection assessment?
    c. How is measurement of pulmonary artery occlusion pressure used for pre-resection assessment?

6. Relating to bronchoprovocation studies:
    a. What is the basis for performing bronchoprovocation studies?
    b. Why is methacholine chloride useful for these studies?
    c. What preparation should be performed before the administration of a bronchoprovocation study?
    d. What are guidelines for subject abstinence prior to administration of a bronchoprovocation study?
    e. What is the general dose pattern for administration of methacholine chloride during administration of a bronchoprovocation study?
    f. How is the percent of $FEV_1$-T decrease (%$FEV_1$-T Decrease) determined, and how is it significant to termination of the study?
    g. What care should be received by the subject immediately following termination of the study?
    h. How should results of a bronchoprovocation study be evaluated?

    i. How is an antigen challenge test performed, and how should results be interpreted?

    j. How should the subject be managed to allow observation for adverse reactions to an antigen study?

7. Relating to studies for exercise-induced asthma:

    a. What is the basis for performing studies for exercise-induced asthma?

    b. What preparation should be performed before the administration of a study for exercise-induced asthma?

    c. What actions should be taken during the study to ensure proper test administration?

    d. How should results of a study for exercise-induced asthma be evaluated?

    e. What are some studies that can be done to test for wheezing that relates to environmental exposure?

8. Relating to impairment/disability studies:

    a. How does impairment differ from disability?

    b. How do impairment and disability relate to pulmonary function?

    c. What basic and historical information should be gathered for pulmonary impairment/disability studies, and how is this information significant?

    d. What physical assessment should be performed for pulmonary impairment/disability studies?

    e. What pulmonary function evaluation should be performed for pulmonary impairment/disability studies?

    f. What arterial blood gas measurements should be performed for pulmonary impairment/disability studies?

    g. What are additional considerations in evaluating pulmonary impairment/disability?

9. Relating to pulmonary function testing in the critical care setting:

    a. What are the purposes of performing pulmonary function testing in the critical care setting?

    b. What are the purposes of evaluating spontaneous ventilatory parameters in the critical care setting?

    c. What spontaneous volumes are monitored in the critical care setting, and how is the monitoring performed?

    d. What spontaneous pressures are monitored in the critical care setting, and how is the monitoring performed?

    e. What is the clinical significance of spontaneous volume and pressure measurement in the critical care setting?

10. Relating to pulmonary compliance measurement for subjects on mechanical ventilation:

    a. How is pulmonary compliance measured for subjects on mechanical ventilation?

    b. How is measurement of pulmonary compliance clinically significant?

    c. How are the results of measurement of pulmonary compliance used clinically?

11. What critical care blood gas monitoring is typically performed?

# CHAPTER NINE

# PULMONARY FUNCTION TESTING FOR CHILDREN

## RELATED LEARNING

Prior knowledge of the following related information will facilitate understanding and learning of the material in this chapter. The learner will be aided by being able to

1. Recall equipment concepts covered in Chapters 1 and 3.
2. Recall the concepts of pulmonary function testing covered in Chapters 2, 4, 5, and 6.
3. Recall the concepts relating to normal pulmonary function values covered in Chapter 8.

## LEARNING OBJECTIVES

Upon successful completion of this chapter, the learner should be able to

1. Describe lung volume determination procedures used for pediatric subjects including
   a. indirect spirometry
   b. body plethysmography
2. Describe pulmonary mechanics tests used for pediatric subjects, including
   a. expiratory volumes/flow rates
   b. airway resistance
   c. compliance
3. Describe the determination of diffusing capacity for pediatric subjects.
4. Describe the selection of predicted normal pulmonary function values for pediatric subjects.

## KEY TERM

intubated

Pulmonary function testing can be used to evaluate the performance of a child's lungs and related structures. However, there are some significant differences between adult and child subjects for pulmonary function testing, namely,

- The size of the subject.
- The ability of the subject to cooperate with the requirements of the test procedures.
- The types of pulmonary function parameters tested and the availability of normal values for those parameters.

Newborns and infants are not able to cooperate at all with testing that requires a controlled response on the part of the subject. Young children (less than six years old) may provide only very limited cooperation. Older children and adolescents have a greater ability to cooperate. Yet, they may demonstrate inconsistent results on tests that require a significant level of subject cooperation or effort.

Some basic adjustments must be made in order to accommodate the pulmonary function testing of children. These include

- Smaller-volume equipment (i.e., smaller-volume spirometers and breathing circuit tubing) should be used.
- A mask or hood enclosure should be used as a patient connection for infants instead of a mouthpiece.
- An adult should participate in performing some of the tests.

Tests that can be performed with child subjects include lung volume determinations, pulmonary mechanics tests, and blood gas determinations. The tests that are performed can be used to evaluate

- The effects of premature birth and BPD on pulmonary function.
- The progress of a child's lung development.
- The diagnosis and treatment of pediatric pulmonary disorders such as asthma, cystic fibrosis, thoracic deformities (kyphoscoliosis, pectus excavatum), and so on.

# LUNG VOLUME DETERMINATIONS

Both indirect spirometry techniques (open-circuit helium dilution or closed-circuit nitrogen washout) and body plethysmography can be used in making lung volume determinations with children.

## INDIRECT SPIROMETRY

Some modifications must be made in order to adapt indirect spirometry procedures to child subjects, especially with the helium dilution technique. A smaller-volume spirometer and smaller-volume tubing should be used with indirect spirometry by helium dilution. These changes are in response to the smaller-volume FRC that is being measured.

Regardless of the procedure, valve systems with a reduced deadspace volume should be used in the breathing circuit.

## BODY PLETHYSMOGRAPHY

### Infant Plethysmography

Infant plethysmograph systems are available but are not commonly used. These are small, variable-pressure, constant-volume plethysmographs. The infant subject lies supine within the plethysmograph cabinet. The infant's head, mouth, and nose are positioned to rest against a cuffed opening in a flat panel within the cabinet. A close-fitting mask is used as a substitute for the mouthpiece of the shutter/transducer assembly. Flow and mouth pressure measurements can be made through the mask connection. Although the subject will not be able to cooperate by performing controlled breathing maneuvers, it is possible to make approximate $V_{TG}$ and $R_{aw}$ determinations with this arrangement.

### Plethysmography for Small Children

Plethysmography can be performed with small children by having the child sit on the lap of an adult who sits within the plethysmograph cabinet. The adult must hold his or her breath during the child's test maneuvers. The child, using a mouthpiece, breathes on the shutter/transducer assembly during test administration.

Generally, non-panting $V_{TG}$ procedures are performed with children. However, some children can be successfully coached to perform panting maneuvers against the closed shutter. When an adult is in the cabinet with the child, the gas displacement corrections for the $V_{TG}$ calculations must include the volumes of both the child and the adult. This is done by using the value of their combined body weights in making the calculations.

## GENERAL CONCERNS FOR LUNG VOLUME DETERMINATIONS

Lung volume determination procedures for infants and young children can be limited by the child's ability to cooperate and follow commands. FRC determinations, on the other hand, are often possible because the procedures generally require little subject cooperation. It may not be possible, however, to gain the cooperation needed for a child to perform a VC maneuver for measurement. As a result, a determination of TLC will not be possible.

There may even be problems with FRC determinations. In the adult subject, FRC is established by the recoil forces of the lungs and the thoracic wall. In infants, additional factors can also affect FRC levels. Glottic (laryngeal) limiting of expiratory flow and the temporary shortening of expiratory time can both contribute to fluctuations in an infant's FRC volume. FRC volumes can actually vary from breath to breath during an infant's breathing. These factors affect the results of FRC determination and also the pulmonary mechanics values that will be described next. If a child is sedated prior to testing, there is a greater chance of having reproducible measurements of values relating to FRC.

# PULMONARY MECHANICS TESTS

## FORCED EXPIRATORY VOLUMES/FLOW RATES

Forced expiratory volumes/flow rates can be measured for children and infants, but the age and ability of the child affects how the procedures are performed.

### Children Six Years of Age and Older

Children six years of age and older are generally able, with patient coaching and practice, to perform FVC maneuvers for testing. However, they must be able to sustain the expiratory effort for at least three seconds. Children generally find it easier to perform FVC maneuvers while standing. The report from a child's pulmonary function study should include the subject's position during the test and the level of cooperation demonstrated. The largest value for VC is the one that should be selected for reporting, regardless of whether it was measured as part of an FVC or an SVC maneuver.

### Children Younger than Six Years of Age

Children younger than six years of age will generally have difficulty performing an FVC maneuver. For these subjects, *a partial forced expiratory volume* (PFEV) maneuver can be accepted. With adults, forced expiratory volumes and flow rates are measured during a maneuver that is begun at the TLC level. For young children, a PFEV maneuver is begun from the tidal volume end-inspiratory level instead of from the TLC level.

The purpose of the maneuver is to generate a partial flow/volume loop without having to have the child cooperate by starting at the TLC level. Although the maneuver is only a partial one, the child's cooperation is still necessary. As with any testing procedure, clear, simple instructions must be given to the child. It may be a good idea to have the child practice the maneuver before beginning breathing on the spirometer for the actual test.

With this maneuver, the subject begins by performing relaxed tidal breathing on the spirometer. Nose clips should be worn by the subject. The tidal breathing flow/volume tracing is recorded in order to identify a stable, end-expiratory baseline volume. Once the baseline volume is established, the child is coached to perform a forced expiratory maneuver for as long as possible at the end of a normal inspiration. Expiration to the RV level is not necessary, but the subject must at least exhale down past the established tidal end-expiratory baseline volume.

A flow/volume tracing like the one in Figure 9–1 is produced by the maneuver. Since the child does not perform a full FVC maneuver, the determinations typically made with an adult subject's forced expiratory test ($FEV_1$, $FEF_{25\%-75\%}$, etc.) cannot be made. Instead, the child's expiratory flow rate at the point of the FRC volume is recorded (see Figure 9–1). This value is referred to as the $\dot{V}_{max}FRC$. The greatest flow value demonstrated from several attempts is the one that is selected for reporting. The value for $\dot{V}_{max}FRC$ can be accepted as representing a maximum flow effort if two or more reproducible curves can be produced and if the subject's effort appears genuine.

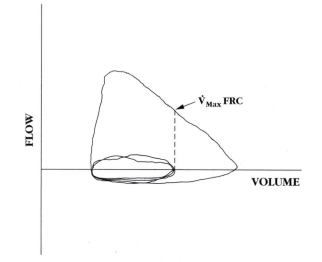

**Figure 9–1** *Tracing for a partial forced expiratory volume maneuver.*

Children with obstructive pulmonary disorders will demonstrate reduced values for $\dot{V}_{max}FRC$. Additionally, the flow/volume loop these children generate will demonstrate the same concave pattern that is shown by adult subjects with obstructive disorders.

## Infants

Tests of this nature can also be performed with infants. A greater degree of technical intervention is required because infants are not capable of even partial cooperation in producing a forced expiratory maneuver. Some form of mechanical assistance is used to produce a "forced expiratory maneuver." The exact procedure that is performed depends on whether or not the infant is **intubated**. As described earlier, a tidal breathing baseline for the subject's FRC value should be obtained before the forced expiratory maneuver is produced.

*Nonintubated Infants.* For a nonintubated infant, external thoracic and abdominal compression is applied to produce a forced expiratory flow. A specially designed inflatable bag that encircles the infant's chest and abdomen is used to generate the compression force. This procedure is usually done after the infant has spontaneously fallen asleep or has been mildly sedated.

Rapid, pressurized inflation of the thoracic/abdominal bag is performed at the end of one of the infant's normal inspirations. In order to be effective, 95% of the bag's peak inflation pressure should be achieved within 100 milliseconds. To ensure that a constant filling pressure is produced during inflation, the bag must be filled from a pressurized reservoir that has a volume at least 10 times that of the bag.

During thoracic/abdominal compression, the infant's expiratory flow rates are measured with a low-deadspace pneumotachometer. A mask with a lubricated face seal is used to direct the infant's expiratory flow through the pneumotachometer.

The purpose of this maneuver is to produce a flow/volume loop tracing. When the test is first performed, the inflating pressure used in the thoracic/abdominal compression bag is at a low level. A flow/volume loop tracing is recorded from the maneuver, and then the test is repeated. With each test, greater bag inflation pressures are used. The procedure is ended at the point where an additional increase in bag pressure no longer produces an increase in expiratory flow rate values.

The goal for the procedure is to create reproducible expiratory flow values that accurately reflect the subject's actual physiology. Unfortunately, it is unclear whether the effects of the externally applied thoracic pressure can be directly related to the effects that intrapleural pressure changes have during a forced expiratory maneuver. The test at least serves as an estimation of actual physiology. Reproducible flow limitations may not always be demonstrated when this method is used to generate expiratory flow rates.

*Intubated Infants.* For infants who are intubated, the forced expiratory flow is produced by a different method. The infant is manually ventilated and is given an inspiration to the TLC level. At end inspiration, a negative pressure is applied to the infant's artificial airway. This results in the "forced expiratory flow." A pneumotachometer is placed in the breathing circuit in such a manner that the expiratory flow created by the negative pressure is drawn through it. The "expiratory flow rate" can then be measured by the pneumotachometer.

This procedure is generally only performed in a critical-care setting on infants who are heavily sedated. If chloral hydrate is used for sedation, caution must be taken with infants who demonstrate clinical signs of wheezing.

*General Information for Infant Forced Expiratory Volume/Flow Rate Testing.* As with the child subjects described earlier, regardless of the procedure used, a tracing is made of the infant's breathing maneuvers and a value for $\dot{V}_{max}FRC$ determined. In normal, healthy infants who are not sedated, factors such as spontaneous inspiratory efforts and glottic closure can produce expiratory flow limitations. These "false" nonpathological flow limitations can actually reduce $\dot{V}_{max}FRC$ values to a greater degree than would many pulmonary disorders. Sedation minimizes the effects of these nonpathological flow limitations. In sedated infants who have an obstructive disorder, the degree of flow limitation identified by the test can be used to reflect the significance of the disorder.

# General Information for Pediatric Forced Expiratory Volume/Flow Rate Testing

Although it cannot completely substitute for the type of information that would be made available from an FVC maneuver, the determination of $\dot{V}_{max}FRC$ can be an effective evaluation tool. In order to provide greater standardization and comparability for the test, the value for $\dot{V}_{max}FRC$ can be standardized by dividing it by a value for FRC determined by indirect spirometry or plethysmography. As a pulmonary assessment tool, $\dot{V}_{max}FRC$ responds to pulmonary disorders in a manner similar to that displayed by other flow measurements made at low lung volumes. The clinical significance of a $\dot{V}_{max}FRC$ value can be related to that of $\dot{V}_{max\ 50}$ or $\dot{V}_{max\ 25}$ values measured in an adult subject.

Unfortunately, the variability in $\dot{V}_{max}FRC$ results can be as much as 30% even among normal subjects. This variability makes $\dot{V}_{max}FRC$ a less sensitive test for differentiating between healthy subjects and asthmatics than $FEV_1$. Regardless, $\dot{V}_{max}FRC$ values do have a role in identifying pediatric pulmonary disorders. $\dot{V}_{max}FRC$ can be used to evaluate infants and young children for normal pulmonary growth and development. Additionally, $\dot{V}_{max}FRC$ can be used in the same way that $FEV_1$ is used in evaluating adults (e.g., bronchoprovocation studies, bronchodilator-benefit studies, etc.). As soon as a child is able to perform an FVC maneuver effectively, however, $FEV_1$ should be used as a measure for these studies.

## AIRWAY RESISTANCE

As with adults, airway resistance ($R_{aw}$) can be measured in children by body plethysmography. Some children, though, are unable to perform the panting maneuver that is required, especially young children who are ill. These children can be tested during tidal breathing if the plethysmograph used will permit it.

Another difficulty in airway resistance testing for small children is the lower air flow rates that may be generated by the child during tidal breathing or panting. $R_{aw}$ determination as described in Chapter 2 is based on a slope measurement being made on the $\dot{V}/P_{Cab}$ tracing between the points of 0.5 l/sec above and below the zero flow point. But some small children may not generate flows as great as 0.5 l/sec. In fact, their flows may even be less than 0.25 l/sec. In this situation, the best method is to calculate $R_{aw}$ based on the tangent of a line that aligns most closely with the straightest portion of the tracing that crosses the zero flow point.

## COMPLIANCE

Lung compliance ($C_L$) measurements can be made on children in the same manner as on adult subjects as long as the child is capable of performing the required breathing maneuvers. For young children and infants, the ability to measure $C_L$ is limited because of their poor cooperation. It is possible, however, to measure a value for total lung/thoracic compliance ($C_{LT}$).

One method for determining a value for $C_{LT}$ involves having the infant or child breathe on a closed-circuit water-sealed spirometer system. Three points are important about this system:

1. Because the subject will be rebreathing on the closed spirometer, it is important for a $CO_2$ absorber to be incorporated into the circuit. If a $CO_2$ absorber is not used, the subject should only breathe on the spirometer for *short* periods of time.
2. The volume of the spirometer's bell must be small—approximately 1 liter.
3. A pressure manometer is connected into the breathing circuit of the spirometer at a point near the subject's mouth.

The test is begun by having the subject breathe on the spirometer while certain baseline measurements are made. These measurements include identifying a stable end-expiratory baseline for the tracing and taking an end-expiratory pressure reading from the manometer in the circuit.

Once these measurements are recorded, a small weight is added to the bell of the spirometer. This weight produces two changes:

1. An increase in the end-expiratory baseline volume level.
2. An increase in the end-expiratory pressure value.

The amount of increase in both of these values should be noted and recorded. A slightly greater weight should then be added to the spirometer bell and the corresponding increases in both volume and pressure again recorded. If desired, this process could be continued in a series of steps, depending on the amount of data needed and the subject's tolerance of breathing under these conditions.

$C_{LT}$ is calculated in the following way:

$$C_{LT} = \frac{\Delta V_{Baseline}}{P_{Mo}}$$

where $\Delta V_{Baseline}$ is the change in volume between the previous end-expiratory volume baseline and the new baseline established by the addition of the weight. $P_{Mo}$ is the pressure measured in the breathing circuit at the new, higher baseline level.

A different method of determining a value for $C_{LT}$ again involves measuring volumes and pressures during breathing. As with the previous procedure, the subject breathes on a spirometer that has a pressure manometer connection placed near the subject's mouth. This time, however, a water-sealed spirometer with a closed circuit is not the only type of spirometer system that can be used. At the end of a normal inspiration, the breathing circuit is occluded to prevent an expiratory air flow. Since the expiratory air flow is blocked, as the subject's inspiratory muscles relax with expiration, the $P_{Mo}$ values will increase to a peak value. This peak value occurs just prior to the $P_{Mo}$ decrease that will result from the next inspiratory effort. With this method, $C_{LT}$ is calculated by

$$C_{LT} = \frac{V_{Insp}}{P_{Mo}}$$

where $V_{Insp}$ is the subject's inspiratory volume and the $P_{Mo}$ is the peak pressure achieved during the subject's inspiratory muscle relaxation. Although this procedure appears relatively simple, acquiring reproducible volume and, especially, pressure readings can be difficult.

Dynamic compliance can be measured in infants and young children in the manner described in Chapter 2. In infants, factors such as their normal rate of breathing and the developmental status in their lung and thoracic structures can make the measurement difficult, specifically because

• Uneven distribution of compliance/resistance characteristics throughout the infant's lung can result in significantly different time constants for alveolar emptying. As a result, true pulmonary pressure equilibrium may not be achieved prior to the start of the next breath.
• The larynx can affect the time constants for alveolar emptying because of its greater contribution to total airflow resistance in infants.

- Due to the greater chest wall compliance that infants have, the distribution of intrapleural pressure can be less even throughout the thorax, and thus the value for esophageal pressure may not be valid.

These troublesome factors cannot be controlled by the technologist, and their effects must be understood and accepted as a limitation of the test procedure.

# DIFFUSING CAPACITY

It is possible to perform diffusing capacity studies on children, but there are procedural difficulties. Smaller children may find it difficult to perform the breath holding needed for the single-breath test. Even if the child can perform the breath holding, some adjustments might have to be made in the procedure. For example, it may be necessary for both the washout volume and the volume of exhaled air collected for analysis to be smaller than usual.

# PREDICTED NORMAL PULMONARY FUNCTION VALUES FOR CHILDREN

Predicted normal pulmonary function values are not as well established for subjects who are newborn to six years old as they are for subjects who are older. Established predictive equations are available for use with children who are at least six years of age.

As stated in Chapter 7, height and gender are the two primary characteristics that affect normal pulmonary function values until a child reaches a height of approximately 60 inches (152 cm). In children, normal values for pulmonary function parameters (FVC, $FEV_1$, etc.) continue to increase until the mid to late teens (18 years for males, 16 years for females) are reached. After this time, there is a relative plateau in normal values until the age of approximately 25 years. Then a decline in pulmonary function begins.

A laboratory can choose to select three separate sets of regression equations for predicting normal values for children, adolescents, and adults. This approach is based on the broad range of subject sizes during childhood through adolescence, the plateau of values in the teens and early twenties, and the decreases in values later in life. Another acceptable and simpler approach is to use a set of children's predictive equations for subjects up to 16 years of age and a second set for older subjects.

Care must be taken when a laboratory selects pediatric predictive equations. Age gaps in the subjects who were studied to establish the equations can be a problem. If the subjects used for the study that produced the children's equations were no older than 16 and the youngest subjects used for the chosen adult equations were 20, then neither set of equations would be appropriate for subjects 17–19 years of age. In making a selection of predictive equations for use in a laboratory, care must be taken to avoid these age gaps.

## Review Questions

Please use the following review questions to evaluate your learning of information from this chapter. It might be helpful to write out your answers on a sheet of paper. If you are unsure of the answers to these questions, review the chapter to reinforce your learning.

1. Relating to the general administration of pediatric pulmonary function testing:
   a. In what ways are pediatric subjects for pulmonary function testing different from adult subjects?
   b. What are the adjustments necessary for testing children?
   c. What functions can be evaluated through pediatric pulmonary function testing?
2. How is indirect spirometry modified for pediatric subjects?
3. Relating to body plethysmography for pediatric subjects:
   a. How is body plethysmography modified for infants?
   b. How is body plethysmography modified for small children?
4. What are some general concerns for pediatric lung volume determinations?
5. Relating to forced expiratory volume/flow rate tests for children:
   a. How are forced expiratory volumes/flow rate tests performed in children older than six years?
   b. How are forced expiratory volumes/flow rate tests performed in children younger than six years old?
   c. How are forced expiratory volumes/flow rate tests performed in infants?
6. How is body plethysmography for airway resistance performed differently for children?
7. Relating to lung/thoracic compliance measurements made on children:
   a. How can lung/thoracic compliance measurements be made on children using a water-sealed spirometer with a closed breathing circuit?
   b. How can lung/thoracic compliance measurements be made with other types of spirometer systems?
8. What are some problems with attempting to measure dynamic compliance in infants?
9. What are possible problems with attempting to perform diffusing capacity tests in children?
10. For which age ranges of children are there more predictive equations available? Fewer predictive equations available?
11. Relating to the normal pulmonary function values in children:
    a. What are the primary factors that affect normal pulmonary function values in children?
    b. What are approaches to selecting pediatric predictive equations for use in a laboratory?
    c. What care must be taken in making a selection of predictive equations?

# CHAPTER TEN

# EQUIPMENT FOR BLOOD GAS ANALYSIS

## RELATED LEARNING

Prior knowledge of the following related information will facilitate understanding and learning of the material in this chapter. The learner will be aided by being able to

1. Relate the information in this chapter to basic concepts of electrochemistry.
2. Describe the mechanisms for the blood transport of oxygen and carbon dioxide.

## LEARNING OBJECTIVES

Upon successful completion of this chapter, the learner should be able to

1. Explain the operating principles of an electrochemical cell.
2. Describe the operation of the following electrochemical blood gas electrodes:
   a. $PO_2$ electrode (Clark electrode)
   b. pH electrode (Sanz electrode)
   c. $PCO_2$ electrode (Severinghaus electrode)
3. Describe the design and operation of a blood gas analysis system.
4. Describe the design and operation of transcutaneous electrodes for measuring $PO_2$ and $PCO_2$.
5. Describe the basic principles of spectrophotometry.
6. Describe the design and operation of CO-oximeters.
7. Describe the design, operation, and use of noninvasive oximetry.

## KEY TERMS

| | |
|---|---|
| ammeter | dermis |
| anode | hygroscopic |
| cathode | pinna |
| contact (salt) bridge | voltmeter |

Blood gas analyzing systems play an important role in assessing pulmonary function. In the last 20 years, they have evolved more than any other type of pulmonary assessment equipment. As a result of this evolution, blood gas assessment now plays a regular and significant role in medical management of pulmonary disorders. Electrochemical and spectrophotometric blood gas analysis systems will both be discussed.

# ELECTROCHEMICAL BLOOD GAS ANALYZERS

Electrochemical blood gas analyzers are used to measure the $PO_2$, pH, and $PCO_2$ in a blood sample. A separate electrode is used for making each measurement. Many blood gas analyzers are also able to measure the $PCO_2$ and $PO_2$ in a nonliquid, gaseous sample. Through the addition of computers, today's blood gas analyzers are capable of a number of sophisticated automatic functions.

## ELECTROCHEMISTRY CONCEPTS

The operation of each electrode in a blood gas analyzer relates in some way to the concept of an *electrochemical cell* (Figure 10–1). This concept also applies, with modifications, to batteries. An electrochemical cell consists of two half-cells, an electrolyte solution that is shared by the half-cells (either directly or by way of a **contact bridge**), and an external electrical connection between the two half-cells. The result of this arrangement, if the related chemical reactions are allowed to occur, is a measurable flow of electrons. This flow is due to an **electrical potential** (EP) difference between the two half-cells. A greater potential produces a greater measurable electron flow. The electron flow can be measured by a meter placed in the external electrical connection of the cell.

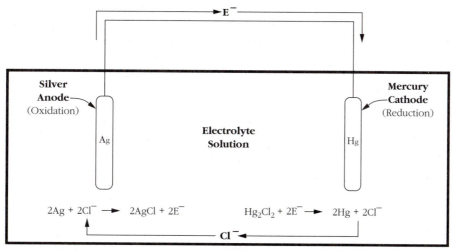

**Figure 10–1** *Concepts of an electrochemical cell.*

Each half-cell is capable of undergoing a chemical reaction that produces an EP; for example:

$$Hg_2Cl_2 + 2e^- \longrightarrow 2Hg + 2Cl^- \ (EP = +0.242 \text{ volts})$$

$$AgCl + e^- \longrightarrow Ag + Cl^- \ (EP = +0.222 \text{ volts})$$

Put together into a single electrochemical cell, the stronger of the two reactions ($Hg_2Cl_2$) will continue in a process of consuming electrons. This half-cell serves as a **cathode** for the cell. The other half-cell (AgCl) will be forced to reverse its reaction and serve as an **anode**. Its smaller value for electrical potential becomes negative. A cell with these two half-cells would have a total potential of +0.020 volts. (Figure 10–1 demonstrates all of the electrochemical events that produce a current flow through the cell.)

Blood gas electrodes make use of the concepts just described. $PO_2$ electrodes measure the electron flow produced by an oxygen-consuming reaction within the cell. Conversely, pH and $PCO_2$ electrodes function on a slightly different electrical principle. They do not measure on the basis of a molecular consumption reaction that produces a flow of electrons. Instead, they both measure how an increase or decrease in pH affects the total electrical potential within a cell.

## PO₂ (CLARK) ELECTRODES

A $PO_2$ blood gas electrode is a polarographic cell that generally consists of a silver anode, platinum cathode, and a potassium chloride electrolyte solution (Figure 10–2). The half-cells are polarized by a voltage of approximately 0.6 volts. The cell is interfaced with the blood sample by a membrane that is selectively permeable to oxygen. This membrane is commonly made of polypropylene.

Oxygen molecules in the blood diffuse across the membrane into the electrode. The number of oxygen molecules that dissolve in the electrode solution is in direct proportion to the $PO_2$ of the sample (**Henry's law**). Once in the cell, the oxygen molecules undergo a reaction at the cathode that produces electrons. *The reaction rate and resulting current flow is in direct proportion to the number of oxygen molecules available and, therefore, the $PO_2$ of the sample.* Greater current flows measured by an **ammeter** in the external electrical connection indicate a larger $PO_2$.

In a blood gas analyzer, the $PO_2$ electrode is carefully designed to contain all of these components in very miniaturized form. One significant point in electrode design is the membrane. It is intended to allow only a slow rate of oxygen diffusion into the electrode. With today's instruments, the blood sample size may only be a fraction of a milliliter. If oxygen were allowed to diffuse from the sample too quickly, it would deplete the sample and eliminate the $PO_2$ diffusion gradient before the electrode responded accurately. Simple calibration can allow this slower rate of diffusion and chemical reaction to accurately reflect the actual $PO_2$ of the blood sample.

The accuracy of $PO_2$ measurements can also be affected by the anesthetic gas *halothane*. This is a factor to be considered in analyzing gas or blood samples from patients who are anesthetized with this agent.

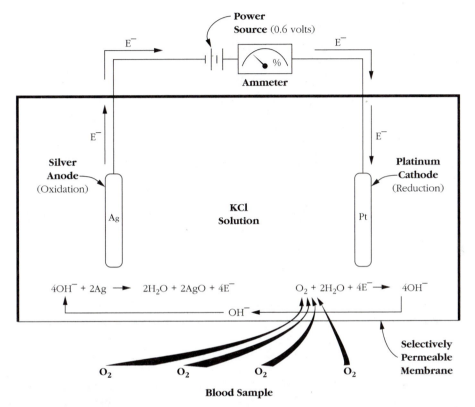

**Figure 10–2** *Basic design of a Clark electrode.*

## THE PH (SANZ) ELECTRODES

The pH electrode uses a more complex electrochemical cell than was earlier described. Along with the two half-cells, it includes an additional component capable of producing its own electrical potential. This component is a special *glass membrane* with **hygroscopic** properties. Protons ($H^+$) in solution attach themselves to the glass by replacing sodium ions ($Na^+$) at the membrane's surface layer (Figure 10–3).

$$Na^+ \; Glass^- + H^+ \longrightarrow H^+ \; Glass^- + Na^+$$
$$\text{(solid) (solution)} \qquad \text{(solid)} \quad \text{(solution)}$$

This process is referred to as *hydration* of the glass. The glass must be fully hydrated in this manner for it to function effectively as a pH sensor.

When a solution is placed in contact with the surface of the hydrated glass, some of the $H^+$ ions leave the glass surface and enter the solution. An equilibrium adjustment occurs between the glass and solution. This adjustment is referred to as an *$H^+$ dissociation* at the glass surface.

$$H^+ \; Glass^- \longrightarrow Glass^- + H^+$$
$$\text{(solid)} \qquad \text{(solid) (solution)}$$

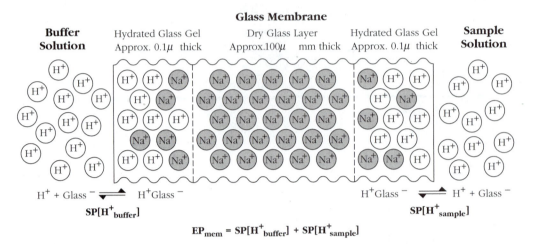

**Figure 10–3** *Concepts of a pH-sensitive glass membrane.*

How far the equilibrium shifts to the right depends on the $H^+$ concentration ($[H^+]$) of the solution. The result of this $H^+$ dissociation is an electrical potential at the glass surface ($SP[H^+]$). Solutions with a greater $[H^+]$ (lesser pH) will cause less of a right shift in the equilibrium. A smaller $SP[H^+]$ results.

The glass membrane in a pH electrode has two surfaces. Each is exposed to a different solution and establishes its own $SP[H^+]$ (see Figure 10–3). When the solutions have different $[H^+]$s, the two surfaces will have different $SP[H^+]$s. The surface having the greater $SP[H^+]$ will be negative with respect to the other surface. This creates an overall potential across the glass membrane ($EP_{mem}$). A greater $[H^+]$ difference between the two solutions causes a greater $EP_{mem}$. Electrical conduction through the dry glass segment in response to the potential is possible but does not easily occur. It involves the infrequent, gradual migration of individual $Na^+$ ions through the glass.

The events creating the glass membrane's $EP_{mem}$ are not electrochemical. As a result, the membrane cannot function as a half-cell in an electrochemical cell. To measure the $EP_{mem}$, the membrane must be added to a complete cell with its own constant, known reference potential ($EP_{ref}$). With the $EP_{ref}$ constant, $H^+$-induced changes in the $EP_{mem}$ would be the only factor that could affect the total system potential ($EP_{sys}$).

$$EP_{sys} = EP_{ref} + EP_{mem}$$

Because blood pH is based on its $[H^+]$, this provides the basis for pH electrode function. The reference cell of a pH electrode uses a Ag/AgCl half-cell and an $Hg/Hg_2Cl_2$ (calomel) half-cell (Figure 10–4A). Both half-cells are saturated to allow the $EP_{anode}$ and $EP_{cathode}$ to remain constant for a constant $EP_{ref}$.

Changes in pH on either side of the glass membrane in a pH electrode can affect the $EP_{sys}$ (Figure 10–4B). The membrane potential due to the blood sample pH ($SP[H^+_{sample}]$), ideally, should be the only factor that changes the EP of the pH-measuring system. To ensure this, a *buffer solution* with a known, constant pH of 6.840 is placed on the reference side of the membrane. It produces a constant membrane potential on the reference side

## A   pH ELECTRODE REFERENCE CELL

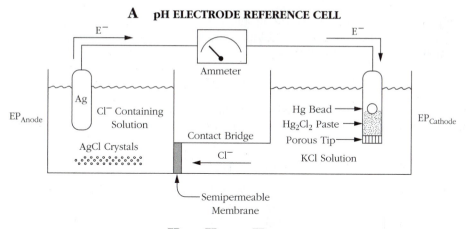

$$EP_{ref} = EP_{Anode} + EP_{Cathode}$$

## B   pH MEASURING ELECTRODE

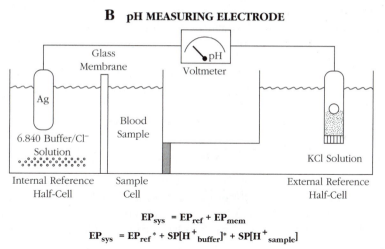

$$EP_{sys} = EP_{ref} + EP_{mem}$$

$$EP_{sys} = EP_{ref}{}^* + SP[H^+{}_{buffer}]^* + SP[H^+{}_{sample}]$$

where "*" indicates a constant (K) electrical potential

$$EP_{sys} = K + SP[H^+{}_{sample}]$$

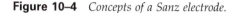

**Figure 10–4**   *Concepts of a Sanz electrode.*

of the glass (SP[H$^+_{buffer}$]). As a result, *all of the factors that may affect the EP$_{sys}$ are constant (K) except for the pH (SP[H$^+_{sample}$]) of the blood sample.*

Glass is an excellent insulator against electrical current flow. Because of the significant electrical resistance caused by the glass membrane, actual current flow through the system is minimal. Current flow, fortunately, is not important to pH measurement. Instead, the ultimate goal of a pH electrode is to measure electrical potential changes within the system. A **voltmeter** in the external electrical connection for the system is used to measure changes in EP$_{sys}$. Its display is calibrated to show units of pH.

The pH electrodes for modern blood gas analyzers have physical configurations that allow for analysis of extremely small blood samples. Sample sizes for some systems may be as small as 25 microliters (.025 ml).

## PCO$_2$ (SEVERINGHAUS) ELECTRODES

The measurement of PCO$_2$ is based on the fact that, in blood, carbon dioxide is transported by an acid/base buffer system. The following equation demonstrates this mechanism.

$$CO_2 + H_2O \longrightarrow H_2CO_3 \longrightarrow H^+ + HCO^-_3$$

Increases in PCO$_2$ result in increased [H$^+$]s in the blood.

PCO$_2$ electrodes are, in essence, modified pH electrodes. The glass membrane in the electrode is separated from the blood sample by a special chamber (Figure 10–5). The chamber has a membrane that is in contact with the blood sample. This membrane is usually made of a silicon-containing material and is selectively permeable to carbon dioxide molecules. A nylon spacer keeps the two membranes physically separated. The space between the membranes is filled with a bicarbonate (NaHCO$_3$) solution. The spacer ensures that the bicarbonate electrolyte solution is in contact with the internal pH-measuring electrode.

Carbon dioxide diffuses readily from the blood sample into the bicarbonate containing chamber. The [H$^+$] in the bicarbonate solution increases directly with a higher PCO$_2$ in the blood sample. The change in bicarbonate solution of [H$^+$] is measured by the pH-sensing component of the electrode and is displayed as PCO$_2$.

## BLOOD GAS ANALYSIS SYSTEMS

Modern blood gas analyzers contain the three types of electrodes just described (Figures 10–6 and 10–7). They are carefully designed, and some systems can measure blood samples as small as 65 microliters (.065 ml). The electrodes are encased within a heated, water-filled jacket. The jacket maintains the electrodes and blood sample at a constant

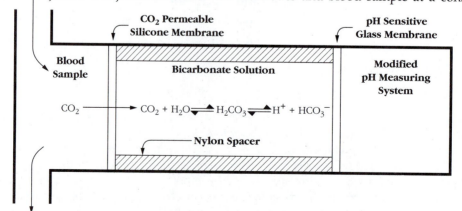

**Figure 10–5** *Basic design of a Severinghaus electrode.*

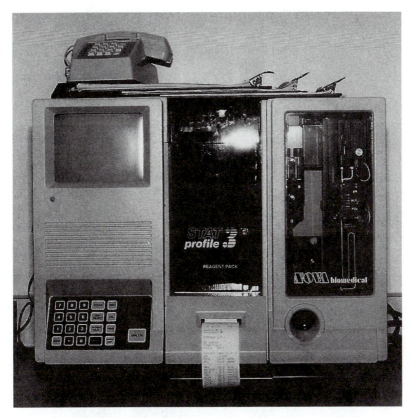

**Figure 10–6** *Blood gas analyzer.*

water-filled jacket. The jacket maintains the electrodes and blood sample at a constant temperature of 37°C so that the measurements are made under physiologic conditions.

Accuracy of electrode function in a blood gas analyzer can be affected by a number of factors. Electrode temperature fluctuations will create measurement errors. Changes in the integrity of the electrode membranes will affect electrode function. Blood protein buildup on the membrane surface can slow down electrode response and create measurement inaccuracies. Tears or holes in the membrane can totally disrupt electrode function. Air bubbles in the blood sample or in the solutions within the electrode can be a source of problems. Finally, physical contact between the outer membrane and the glass inner membrane will cause problems with $PCO_2$ electrodes.

Built-in computers add a number of automated functions to blood gas analyzers:

- Automatic calibration and self-diagnosis of malfunctions.
- Calculation of additional physiologic values such as percent saturation of hemoglobin ($SaO_2$ for arterial blood), plasma bicarbonate, base excess/deficit, and oxygen content of blood. This calculation can be performed with automatic correction for

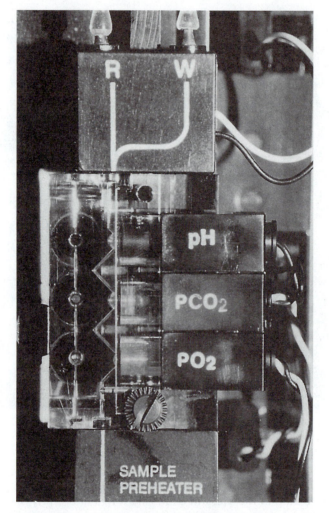

**Figure 10–7**  *Blood gas electrodes within the cuvette of a blood gas analyzer.*

barometric pressure and the patient's actual temperature and hemoglobin values. Generally normal values are assumed for body temperature and $P_{50}$. Some systems allow input of the subject's actual body temperature, however.

- Interpretation and report of blood gas measurement results.
- Electronic storage and retrieval of patient data.

## TRANSCUTANEOUS ELECTRODES

Transcutaneous electrodes are used to measure the gas tensions of oxygen ($PtcO_2$) and/or carbon dioxide ($PtcCO_2$) at the skin's surface. They demonstrate the partial pressure of these gases in the tissues, not in the blood. The skin must be heated to approximately

41°C–45°C to increase local perfusion and tissue gas tensions. Local perfusion must greatly exceed the cellular metabolism rate. This is to ensure that enough oxygen remains in the tissues for measurement by the electrode.

The electrodes are modified versions of the $PO_2$ and $PCO_2$ electrodes described earlier (Figure 10–8). One significant difference is that they have built-in heating systems to raise the temperature at the measuring site. The power source for an electrode heater can supply more or less current as required to maintain a constant temperature. The electrode membrane is placed in direct contact with the skin. It is held in place and sealed against environmental air contamination by an adhesive ring. The site used for electrode placement should, preferably, have no hair and have a relatively thin **dermis** and good local perfusion.

Typically, $PtcO_2$ values are lower than arterial $PO_2$, and $PtcCO_2$ values are higher than arterial $PCO_2$. The difference for a given subject can be established by comparing initial transcutaneous readings with values from an arterial blood sample. Once this difference is established, transcutaneous measurements can be used to indicate the trend of changes in arterial values. Changes in the perfusion at the measurement site and/or loss of electrode integrity can reduce the reliability of transcutaneous measurements.

Transcutaneous systems are useful primarily for infant subjects because of their thinner dermis. Some studies have shown reasonable accuracy with transcutaneous electrodes used on selected adult patients. Because of a lack of consistency, however, use is limited in adults. Transcutaneous electrodes are not frequently used in the pulmonary function laboratory. More often, the noninvasive oximeters (to be described later) are used.

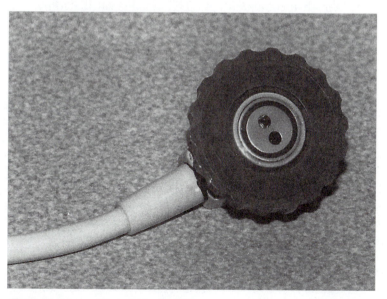

**Figure 10–8**  *Transcutaneous oxygen electrode.*

# SPECTROPHOTOMETRIC BLOOD GAS ANALYSIS

Spectrophotometry is based on the principle that substances absorb or reflect and transmit light in a very characteristic way. As more light is absorbed by a substance, less is reflected and transmitted. The degree of absorption is affected by two factors: the *wavelength of the light* and the *concentration of the substance*. Given these principles, spectrophotometry can be used to determine the concentration of a substance in a test sample. A light with a known, constant wavelength is directed through the sample. The amount of unabsorbed (reflected/transmitted) light passing through the sample can be determined by a photosensitive sensor. Greater amounts of unabsorbed light detected by the sensor indicate low concentrations of the substance.

Spectrophotometric blood analysis systems can differ significantly in their operation and use. Different systems include CO-oximeters and noninvasive oximeters, such as ear oximeters and pulse oximeters.

## CO-OXIMETERS

CO-oximeters provide an accurate assessment of hemoglobin and its variants in a blood sample. They measure total hemoglobin and the amounts of oxyhemoglobin, carboxyhemoglobin, and methemoglobin in the sample. Some microprocessor-operated CO-oximeter systems are capable of making corrections that permit the analysis of specific varieties of hemoglobin, such as fetal or animal hemoglobin. Some CO-oximeter systems can also calculate the volume percent of oxygen in the blood. This calculation is based on the measured values for total hemoglobin and the hemoglobin's percent saturation with oxygen.

Moreover, some CO-oximeter systems can estimate a $P_{50}$ value for the blood sample. This estimated value, when compared with the $P_{50}$ value calculated by a blood gas analyzer, can provide an indication of the amount of left or right shift that exists in the subject's oxyhemoglobin dissociation curve. This procedure works best if the blood sample has a measured $SaO_2$ that is less than 90%.

### Operation of CO-Oximeters

In the measurement system of a CO-oximeter, light from a light source is transmitted by two different pathways within the instrument, and two measuring sensors are used. One pathway is the transmission of the light directly from the source to one of the sensors. The measurements by this sensor provide a reference value for the quantity of light transmission. The second light transmission pathway is from the source, through the blood sample, and then to the second sensor. This pathway is used to analyze the quantity of light that is unabsorbed by the blood sample and passes through the sample to the sensor. Data from the reference and sample light measurements are compared by the system in determining the concentrations of oxyhemoglobin, carboxyhemoglobin, and other hemoglobin variants in the blood.

Hemoglobin and its variants (oxyhemoglobin, reduced hemoglobin, carboxyhemoglobin, etc.) have specific characteristics for light absorption (Figure 10–9). Each has its own

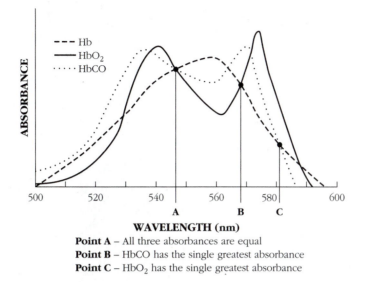

**Point A** – All three absorbances are equal
**Point B** – HbCO has the single greatest absorbance
**Point C** – HbO₂ has the single greatest absorbance

**Figure 10–9** *Concepts of spectrophotometry.*

pattern of absorption over a range of wavelengths. In looking at the patterns, some important facts may be noted.

- At some wavelengths, two or more hemoglobin variants can demonstrate the same degree of absorbance (points A, B, and C in Figure 10–9). The wavelength at which this occurs is called an *isosbestic point*.
- At some isosbestic points in this model, the third variant shows a notably higher level of absorption (points B and C). At points such as these, the concentration of the third variant can be determined by spectrophotometry.
- By means of several carefully chosen wavelengths, each variant can have its concentration determined.
- The wavelength where all variants meet at one isosbestic point (point A) is used to measure changes in total hemoglobin.

A whole-blood sample is aspirated into the sample port of a CO-oximeter, Figure 10–10. Before analysis can be performed, the red blood cells in the sample must be lysed (hemolysis). This is done so that the hemoglobin molecules will be distributed evenly throughout the blood sample instead of being localized within the red blood cells. The hemolysis can be performed by either chemical or physical methods. Sickle cells are not easily lysed. This is especially true when chemical methods are used. Incomplete lysis of sickle cells can result in inaccurate measurements.

Once the hemolysis has been performed, the sample is then moved via a tubing system within the CO-oximeter to the measurement chamber. In the measurement chamber, the blood sample is sandwiched as a thin sheet of blood between two layers of glass. Light

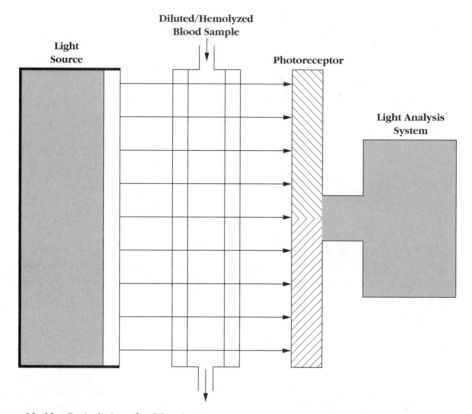

**Figure 10–10** *Basic design of a CO-oximeter.*

of carefully selected wavelengths is transmitted through the sample. Based on the light transmission analysis and related calculations, the quantities of the hemoglobin variants in the sample can be determined. Presence of fetal hemoglobin in the sample can have some effect on the accuracy of the results.

Measurements made by CO-oximeters are the standard against which other forms of spectrophotometry are compared.

## NONINVASIVE OXIMETRY

Spectrophotometry can also be used for noninvasive assessment of oxyhemoglobin saturation values. The basis for noninvasive spectrophotometry is the transmission of light directly through the subject's living tissue (e.g., a finger) to measure the effects of light absorption by blood. Unfortunately, the use of living tissue creates a measurement problem. The tissue not only permits the necessary absorption of the light energy for saturation measurements but also causes the light to be refracted and scattered within the tissue. As a result, the measurements made by noninvasive spectrophotometry are slightly less accurate than those made by CO-oximetry. Two different types of systems available for noninvasive oximetry are described here: ear oximeters and pulse oximeters.

# Ear Oximeters

Ear oximeters were the first noninvasive systems to be used clinically. They are capable of measuring the percent saturation of oxyhemoglobin for blood still within the subject. The system consists of a light source, a fiberoptic cable for light transmission, and an ear sensor. The sensor clips gently onto the **pinna** of the ear and transmits light through this site. It measures the relative absorption of light by blood oxyhemoglobin within the tissue. The ear is heated to cause local vasodilation. The vasodilation and increase in blood flow "arterializes" the site. As a result, the measurements can approach arterial values for oxyhemoglobin saturation.

Ear oximeters have had limited application in general clinical settings. Reasons include the large size of the sensor, the need for heating the site, and the fragile nature of the fiberoptic cable.

# Pulse Oximeters

Pulse oximeters are a more recent development in spectrophotometry. Unlike ear oximeters, pulse oximeters

- Make use of two *light-emitting diodes* (LEDs) that are located within a small sensor at the tissue site. These LEDs are capable of transmitting very bright light. The light from the LEDs is transluminated through the tissue site to a single photodetector in the sensor. The photodetector measures the amount of unabsorbed light that passes through the tissue. This arrangement eliminates the need for a primary light source and a fiberoptic cable to transmit light to the sensor.
- Do not depend on a heated arterialized site for accurate measurements.
- Rely heavily on microprocessor technology.

*Operation of Pulse Oximeters*   Because of the coloration of blood, pulse oximeters operate by considering hemoglobin to be a light filter that permits the passage of light that is primarily in the red and near-infrared wavelength ranges. For this reason, one of the LEDs used in the sensor emits light in the red wavelength range (approximately 660 nm). The other LED emits light in the near-infrared range (approximately 940 nm). At the 660 nm wavelength range, reduced hemoglobin absorbs 10 times the quantity of light that oxyhemoglobin absorbs. At the 940 nm wavelength range, oxyhemoglobin absorbs two to three times more light than reduced hemoglobin.

The ratio (R) of light absorbance at these two wavelengths ($A_{660\,nm}$ and $A_{940\,nm}$) provides a basis for saturation determinations. This is demonstrated by the following equation:

$$R = \frac{A_{660\,nm}}{A_{940\,nm}}$$

A calibration curve for the pulse oximeter is established by first precalculating all of the possible combinations for R between the saturations of 0% and 100%. These calculated values are then compared against actual saturation measurements for blood in the determination of the calibration curve.

The need for heating the tissue measurement site is eliminated on the basis of a theoretical assumption about the tissue at the measurement site. The assumption is that at any given point in time, the light measured by the photodetector through the transluminated tissue can exist in one of only two possible states:

1. A *venous blood and tissue state* (VBT) of light intensity during diastole. This state provides a baseline rate of light absorption.
2. An *arterialized blood state* (AB) of light intensity during systole. This state reflects a changing rate of light absorption that varies with the pulsations of arterial blood. The quantity of light absorption during this state is used to determine an "arterialized" value for oxyhemoglobin saturation.

The oximeter system is able to distinguish between the light-absorbance amounts of these two states. During the VBT state, the quantity of light detected by the sensor provides a stable baseline value. The AB state demonstrates a greater quantity of light absorbance (less light is transmitted on to the photodetector). This is due to the increased quantity of blood in the vasculature. The increased blood quantity represents a momentary "arterialization" of the site during the systolic pulsation of the blood. As a result, the system uses only the light absorbance measurements it makes during the AB state to determine a value for the percent saturation of "arterialized" oxyhemoglobin.

Because the pulse oximeter makes a distinction between the VBT and AB states, the ratio (R) described earlier for calibration of the instrument can be modified in the following way:

$$R = \frac{A - AB_{660\,nm}/A - VBT_{660\,nm}}{A - AB_{940\,nm}/A - VBT_{940\,nm}}$$

This correction in calibration permits the oximeter to eliminate the absorbance variations caused by venous blood, tissue, and skin pigmentation from affecting measurement results.

Adjustment of the brightness of the light emitted by the LEDs allows the oximeter to vary its light-intensity output in response to the nature of the body tissues at the measurement site. When the tissue at the measurement site has greater density, the oximeter can respond by transmitting brighter light from the LEDs. Adjustments in LED brightness are based on baseline measurements made by the oximeter during the VBT state.

The successful performance and accuracy of pulse oximeters rely heavily on microprocessor technology. Microprocessors are responsible for the operation of the LEDs used in the sensor. The microprocessor flashes the LEDs at a rate of 400–500 cycles per second. With each cycle, first one LED alone emits light, then the other alone, then both LEDs are off at the same time. Measurements made by the photodetector during the time that both LEDs are off are used to detect and compensate for the effects of ambient light.

Another function of the oximeter's microprocessor is to perform calibration compensation for the variation in the light output by the LEDs from different sensors that can be used with the unit. The light wavelength output from the LEDs of different sensors can vary by as much as 15 nm. The amount of variation is likely to be greater for the LED that emits light at 660 nm. For the LED operating in this wavelength range, 10 or more different calibration curves are needed. The microprocessor in the oximeter makes it possible for the instrument to make these calibration compensations.

The greater risk for output error for the 660 nm LED is the cause of pulse oximeters having less accuracy at low oxyhemoglobin values (where the amounts of reduced hemoglobin in the blood are greater). As stated earlier, the absorption of 660 nm wavelength light by reduced hemoglobin is significantly greater (10 times) than the absorption of light by oxyhemoglobin. For this reason, greater amounts of wavelength error for the 660 nm LED can have a significant effect on the accuracy of the oximeter measuring reduced hemoglobin.

In addition to the preceding functions, the microprocessor in an oximeter is needed to receive and analyze the complex AB and VBT light signals from the sensor. With the LEDs cycling on and off at rates of 400–500 cycles per second, this is a major task. Additionally, the microprocessor allows the system to perform self-analysis and display error messages.

*Factors Affecting Accuracy of Pulse Oximeters.*   A number of factors can affect the accuracy of pulse oximeter measurements. These factors include the presence of hemoglobin variants and certain dyes in the blood, motion artifact, cardiovascular abnormalities and poor perfusion at the measurement site, and ambient light.

Hemoglobin variants that can affect the accuracy of pulse oximetry measurements include the presence of carboxyhemoglobin, methemoglobin, and/or fetal hemoglobin in the subject's blood. Programmed microprocessor compensation can be used to correct for the presence of fetal hemoglobin when pulse oximeters are used on infants.

Current models of pulse oximeters cannot differentiate between the saturation of hemoglobin with oxygen and saturation with carbon monoxide. Consequently, a subject having abnormally high levels of carbon monoxide in the blood will demonstrate high saturation readings on pulse oximetry. The reading will be nearly that of the combined saturations of oxyhemoglobin and carboxyhemoglobin. This means that a patient's true oxygenation state will be misrepresented if carbon monoxide is present in the blood. Therefore, if the presence of carbon monoxide is suspected, CO-oximetry measurements should be made instead of relying on pulse oximetry measurements.

Medical dyes present in the blood can also affect pulse oximeter measurements. For example, dyes used for vascular flow studies, such as methylene blue and indocyanine green, can cause falsely low readings.

Excessive motion of the digit can produce interference for pulse oximeter sensors and thus erroneous results. This is especially true when the motion is of a prolonged nature, as when the subject is shivering. This motion causes movements in the sensor and fluctuations in the light absorbance readings performed by the sensor. The motion can produce absorbance characteristics that are detected in an approximately equal way by both the red and infrared wavelength sensors. As a result, the value for the VBT reading by the oximeter is falsely elevated and causes an incorrect value for the calibration factor (R). This error in the calibration curve for the instrument will cause the oxyhemoglobin saturation value displayed by the oximeter to be incorrect. Displayed saturation values can decrease to 85% when the subject's actual values are higher.

Cardiovascular abnormalities that reduce peripheral perfusion can also affect the function of pulse oximeters. Such conditions include hypotension, significant hypothermia, and, in infants, a patent ductus arteriosis. Conditions that increase venous pulsations can cause measurement errors as well. These conditions include severe right ventricular failure, tricuspid regurgitation, obstruction of venous return, markedly elevated intrathoracic pressure, and placement of the probe on a dependent limb. Bradycardia experienced by the subject will slow down the response time of a pulse oximeter's measurement.

Most pulse oximeters are only minimally affected by measurement errors caused by ambient light. High-intensity light, such as might be present in the surgical setting, might increase the risk of error, however. The error under these conditions is due to the ambient light affecting the instrument's ability to make absorbance measurements.

*General Information on Pulse Oximeters.*   Pulse oximeters generally provide a display of both the percent saturation of oxyhemoglobin and the pulse rate. The determination of a pulse rate is based on the frequency at which the AB state (systole) occurs. Some pulse oximeters also provide a graphlike display of the quality and/or strength of the arterial pulsations.

Sites that can be used for sensor placement include the finger, toe, earlobe, bridge of the nose, and, on infants, the foot (Figure 10–11). At arterial saturations greater than 80%, the results of pulse oximetry correlate excellently with the results of CO-oximetry. With arterial saturations less than 80%, the accuracy of pulse oximeters declines slightly, but the results are still reasonably reliable. Pulse oximeters may be useful for cardiopulmonary stress testing, sleep studies, transport, assessment of continuous oxygen therapy, and monitoring during surgery.

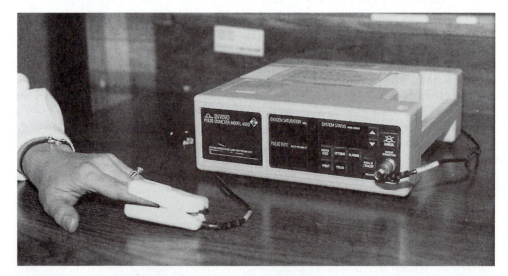

**Figure 10–11**  *Pulse oximeter and sensor.*

## Review Questions

Please use the following review questions to evaluate your learning of information from this chapter. It might be helpful to write out your answers on a sheet of paper. If you are unsure of the answers to these questions, review the chapter to reinforce your learning.

1. Relating to the basic operation of an electrochemical cell:
   a. How is an electron current flow created by an electrochemical cell?
   b. What are electrochemical half-cells?
2. Relating to the design and operation of a $PO_2$ (Clark) electrode:
   a. How are the design and operation of a $PO_2$ (Clark) electrode based on electrochemical principles?
   b. What role does the oxygen molecule play in the electrode's operation?
   c. What other gas molecule can affect the operation of a $PO_2$ (Clark) electrode?
3. Relating to the design and operation of a pH (Sanz) electrode:
   a. What is significant about the glass membrane of a pH (Sanz) electrode having "hygroscopic" properties?
   b. How can a complete electrochemical cell be used to measure the electrical potential that develops through a hygroscopic glass membrane?
   c. How do the preceding factors relate to the operation of a pH (Sanz) electrode?
4. Relating to the design and operation of a $PCO_2$ (Severinghaus) electrode:
   a. What chemical reaction is significant to the operation of a $PCO_2$ (Severinghaus) electrode?
   b. What relation does a $PCO_2$ (Severinghaus) electrode have to a pH-measuring electrode?
   c. How does $PCO_2$ measurement occur when $CO_2$ molecules enter a $PCO_2$ (Severinghaus) electrode?
5. Relating to blood gas analyzer systems,
   a. What is the basic design of a blood gas analysis system?
   b. What factors can affect the accuracy of a blood gas analysis system?
   c. What automated functions are offered by the computer of a blood gas analysis system?
6. Relating to transcutaneous $PO_2$ and $PCO_2$ measuring electrodes,
   a. What is measured by a transcutaneous $PO_2$ and $PCO_2$ electrodes?
   b. What are the basic design and use of a transcutaneous electrode?
   c. How do transcutaneous values for $PO_2$ and $PCO_2$ correspond to arterial values?
7. Relating to the principles of spectrophotometry:
   a. What factors affect the absorbance of light?
   b. How do these factors figure in the operation of a spectrophotometer?
8. Relating to CO-oximetry:
   a. What measurements are performed by a CO-oximeter?
   b. How are CO-oximeters designed to perform spectrophotometry on blood samples?
   c. How are the wavelengths of light evaluated by the CO-oximeter?
   d. What is the process used by a CO-oximeter to perform spectrophotometry on whole blood?

9. Relating to noninvasive spectrophotometry:
   a. What is the principle behind noninvasive spectrophotometry?
   b. How are ear oximeters designed?
   c. What limits the usefulness of spectrophotometry in the clinical setting?
   d. How does the technology of pulse oximeters differ from that of ear oximeters?
   e. What is the basic operation of a pulse oximeter?
   f. In what way does the microprocessor contribute to the operation of a pulse oximeter?
   g. What factors affect the accuracy of the pulse oximeter?
   h. Where are possible placement sites for a pulse oximeter electrode?

# CHAPTER ELEVEN

# TESTS FOR OXYGENATION, VENTILATION, AND ACID/BASE BALANCE

## RELATED LEARNING

Prior knowledge of the following related information will facilitate understanding and learning of the material in this chapter. The learner will be aided by being able to

1. Describe the blood transport mechanisms for oxygen and the factors that affect blood oxygen transport.
2. Describe the significance of the oxyhemoglobin dissociation curve as it relates to factors that affect oxygen transport.
3. Describe the blood transport mechanisms for carbon dioxide.
4. Explain the basic concepts of acid/base balance in the body as they relate primarily to ventilatory and metabolic influences.
5. Describe the operation and use of the following equipment presented in Chapter 10: $CO_2$ analyzers, Clark electrodes, Sanz electrodes, Severinghaus electrodes, blood gas analyzers, and oximeters.

## LEARNING OBJECTIVES

Upon successful completion of this chapter, the learner should be able to

1. Describe the following tests based on the direct assessment of blood gas values:
   a. parameters for the assessment of oxygenation
   b. parameters for the assessment of ventilation
   c. parameters for the assessment of acid/base balance
2. Describe the equipment required for the direct assessment of blood gas values in relation to
   a. blood sampling
   b. blood analysis

3. Describe the test administration required for the direct assessment of blood gas values in relation to
   a. blood sampling
   b. blood analysis
4. Explain the interpretation of tests based on the direct assessment of blood gas values including
   a. parameters for the assessment of oxygenation
   b. parameters for the assessment of ventilation
   c. parameters for the assessment of acid/base balance
5. Describe the use of transcutaneous gas measurement as an indirect indicator of blood gas values.
6. Describe the use of capnography as an indirect indicator of blood gas values.
7. Describe pediatric blood gas assessment in relation to
   a. arterial blood sampling
   b. arterialized blood sampling
   c. alternatives to blood sampling

———————— **KEY TERMS** ————————

| | |
|---|---|
| absorption atelectasis | hyperventilation |
| anemia | hypoventilation |
| ARDS | in vitro |
| arterialized capillary blood | in vivo |
| blood gas | lancet |
| capacity | methemoglobinemia |
| capnogram | mixed venous blood |
| capnography | nonvolatile acid |
| capnometry | polycythemia |
| carboxyhemoglobinemia | shunting |
| cardiac decompensation | Swan-Ganz catheter |
| content | tonometer |
| hypercapnia | volatile acid |
| hypocapnia | |

The primary function of the lungs as an organ system is to provide effective exchange of oxygen and carbon dioxide between inspired air and blood. Additionally, carbon dioxide levels in the blood play an important role in determining the acid/base balance in the body. For these reasons, **blood gas** values and other related values are among the most important basic indicators of how well the pulmonary system is performing its primary function.

The subject of blood gases is large and relates to a number of complex physiologic functions. It includes assessment of pH and other related values that are not technically "blood gases." Excellent books covering the subject in detail are available. The goal for this chapter is to provide a review of key pulmonary function concepts that relate to the assessment of oxygenation, ventilation, and acid/base balance.

Assessment of these functions is based on certain key parameters. Many of these parameters are measured directly from a blood sample. Some are the result of calculations based on measured blood values. Other parameters are used to provide indirect indications of blood gas values. A list of typical direct (and calculated) and indirect blood gas parameters is provided in Table 11–1.

# TESTS BASED ON DIRECT ASSESSMENT OF BLOOD GAS VALUES

## TEST DESCRIPTION

Direct assessment of blood gas values requires the sampling and analysis of blood samples. Arterial blood is used for most of the determinations that are made. Sampling of arterial blood can be performed by needle puncture of an artery or by use of an indwelling arterial catheter. The blood is collected in a syringe.

With infants and small children, arterial puncture may be difficult due to their smaller anatomy. This can present a problem if an indwelling arterial catheter is not available for sampling. Although not a replacement for arterial blood, **arterialized capillary blood** provides information that can, to some degree, be correlated with arterial blood gas values. Sampling of arterialized capillary blood is done by performing a deep skin puncture that produces free-flowing blood. The site must be prepared first by heating it. This increases the local perfusion and "arterializes" the blood in the capillary bed. The blood is collected in a glass capillary tube.

*Mixed venous blood* is used for some blood gas determinations. It is the final mixture of all venous blood from throughout the body just prior to its entry to the lungs for gas exchange. Pulmonary artery catheterization is necessary to allow mixed venous blood sampling. The blood is collected by attaching a syringe to the sampling port of the pulmonary artery catheter. Central venous blood from the inferior vena cava, superior vena cava, or right atrium can, in healthy subjects, provide a reasonable approximation to mixed venous blood. The correlation between these values may not be as close in critically ill patients, however.

*Peripheral venous blood* is of limited use and its values cannot be effectively used as a substitute for mixed venous values. This is because local circulation, perfusion, and metabolism conditions at the sample site can affect the blood gas values. The values may vary from sample site to sample site and be different from mixed venous values in the same subject. Peripheral venous blood can be used to assess extreme pH changes when arterial blood samples are not available.

## Parameters for Assessment of Oxygenation

Oxygenation is important in relation to two key factors:

1. How effectively the arterial blood is oxygenated by the lungs.

## TABLE 11–1  Blood Gas Parameters

### Blood Gas Parameters Commonly Determined Directly from Blood Samples

#### *Measured for Oxygenation Assessment*

$PxO_2$*—partial pressure of oxygen (mm Hg)
Total Hb—total hemoglobin (gm Hb/100 ml of blood or gm%)
$SxO_2$*—percent saturation of hemoglobin with oxygen (%)
%MetHb—percent of methemoglobin (%)
%COHb—percent saturation of hemoglobin with carbon monoxide (%)
$P_{50}$—partial pressure of oxygen that is required to make an $SaO_2$ of 50% (mm Hg)

#### *Measured for Ventilation Assessment*

$PxCO_2$*—partial pressure of carbon dioxide (mm Hg)

#### *Measured for Acid/Base Assessment*

pH—acid/base balance of the blood

#### *Calculated for Oxygenation Assessment*

$CxO_2$*—blood content of oxygen (ml $O_2$/100 ml blood or vol%)
$\dot{T}O_2$—transport rate of oxygen to the tissues (ml $O_2$/min)
$C(a-\bar{v})O_2$—difference between the oxygen content of arterial and mixed venous
   blood (ml $O_2$/100 ml blood or vol%)
$\dot{Q}_{sp}/\dot{Q}_T$—percent of blood that is undergoing physiologic shunting (decimal fraction or %)

#### *Calculated for Acid/Base Assessment*

$HCO_3^-$—plasma bicarbonate ion concentration (mEq/l)
BE—base excess (mEq/l)

### Parameters Used to Indirectly Indicate Blood Gas Values

$PtcO_2$—transcutaneous partial pressure of oxygen (mm Hg)
$PtcCO_2$—transcutaneous partial pressure of carbon dioxide (mm Hg)
$PetCO_2$—partial pressure of carbon dioxide in end-tidal exhaled air (mm Hg)

*x shows the location for the abbreviation that would indicate the source of the blood
   sample. Possible abbreviations are
   a = arterial blood (i.e., $PaO_2$).
atc = arterialized capillary blood (i.e., $PatcO_2$).
   v = venous blood (i.e., $PvO_2$).
   $\bar{v}$ = mixed venous blood (i.e., $P\bar{v}O_2$).

2. How effectively the tissues are oxygenated by the combined functions of arterial blood oxygenation and blood circulation throughout the body.

Given these concerns, oxygenation is assessed by means of a number of parameters: partial pressure of arterial blood oxygen, hemoglobin transport of oxygen, blood oxygen content, intrapulmonary shunting, and tissue oxygenation.

*Partial Pressure of Arterial Blood Oxygen.* The $PaO_2$ indicates how effectively oxygen is being made available to the blood for transport to the tissues. Low $PaO_2$ values can be the result of reduced inspired oxygen pressures. Most often, however, they are due to an abnormality that results in poor intrapulmonary gas exchange or to the presence of intrapulmonary shunting. Low $PaO_2$ values indicate hypoxemia. Hypoxemia will result in tissue hypoxia unless adequate compensation is provided by an increase in cardiovascular function.

*Hemoglobin Transport of Oxygen.* Hemoglobin (Hb) is responsible for transporting 98% of the oxygen carried by blood. Functional hemoglobin that is actively carrying oxygen molecules is referred to as *oxyhemoglobin* ($HbO_2$). Hemoglobin that has released its oxygen is *reduced hemoglobin* (R-Hb).

Dysfunctional hemoglobin can affect the ability of blood to transport oxygen. MetHb is an oxidized form of hemoglobin ($HbFe^{+++}$, as opposed to the normal $HbFe^{++}$) that is in the blood. It is not capable of carrying oxygen. Greater relative quantities of MetHb reduce the capacity of blood to carry oxygen and cause the blood to exhibit a brownish color. Measured values for *%MetHb* indicate the percentage of hemoglobin that consists of MetHb.

The *%HbCO* values indicate the percentage of hemoglobin molecules having gas transport sites that are occupied by carbon monoxide (i.e., the percent of carboxyhemoglobin in the blood). Sites occupied by carbon monoxide are unavailable for oxygen transport. In the case of carbon monoxide poisoning, larger values for %HbCO indicate a greater presence of carboxyhemoglobin and a diminished blood oxygen-carrying capacity. At the same time, however, because this abnormality results from having hemoglobin gas transport sites that are saturated (in this case with carbon monoxide), the blood will still have a "healthy" scarlet appearance. Since carbon monoxide binds with hemoglobin 210 times more easily than does oxygen, relatively low levels of carbon monoxide can begin to cause clinically significant problems with oxygenation.

*Total Hb* is a cumulative total value for all forms of hemoglobin in the blood ($HbO_2$ + R-Hb + MetHb + HbCO). It is useful for indicating the general capacity that blood may have for carrying oxygen. Simply put, more hemoglobin in the blood should be capable of carrying more oxygen. But total Hb alone does not directly indicate how much of the existing hemoglobin is actually participating in oxygen transport.

*SaO_2* values provide a clearer picture of the hemoglobin transport of oxygen. They relate the **content** of actual oxygen carrying hemoglobin in arterial blood to the **capacity** that hemoglobin in the blood has for transporting oxygen. This concept is demonstrated in the following equation, which expresses $SaO_2$ as a percent.

$$SaO_2 = \frac{\text{Content}}{\text{Capacity}} \times 100$$

A value for $SaO_2$ is calculated by some blood gas analyzers based on values for $PaO_2$ and pH. Though convenient, the resulting value can be inaccurate because factors such as patient temperature, %MetHb, and %HbCO are not always taken into account. $SaO_2$ can be measured directly by use of an oximeter. One of two possible methods can be used. The first relates $HbO_2$ content to the total Hb capacity of the blood, or

$$SaO_2 = \frac{HbO_2}{HbO_2 + R\text{-}Hb + MetHb + HbCO} \times 100$$

More sophisticated spectrophotometers, such as CO-oximeters, can determined $SaO_2$ in this way.

$SaO_2$ can also be determined by considering capacity only as the amount of hemoglobin functionally available for gas transport, ignoring quantities of MetHb. This is demonstrated by

$$SaO_2 = \frac{HbO_2}{HbO_2 + R\text{-}Hb + HbCO} \times 100$$

Pulse oximeters generally determine $SaO_2$ in this simpler way. In the same patient, $SaO_2$ determined by the first method will have a slightly smaller value than will the $SaO_2$ determined by the second method.

Blood assumes a more scarlet appearance as $SaO_2$ values increase and a greater percentage of hemoglobin gas transport sites are occupied with oxygen. A smaller $SaO_2$ value indicates that a lesser percentage of the available hemoglobin gas transport sites is being used to carry oxygen. At the same time, the blood assumes a darker, less red appearance.

The overall affinity that hemoglobin has for oxygen is assessed by the value for $P_{50}$. Changes in $P_{50}$ values indicate shifts in the oxyhemoglobin dissociation curve. A smaller than normal value for $P_{50}$ indicates that hemoglobin has a greater affinity for oxygen at a given $PO_2$ value. Thus, a given $PaO_2$ will result in a greater $SaO_2$. This is demonstrated by a left shift in the oxyhemoglobin disassociation curve. The opposite is true for $P_{50}$ values that are greater than normal.

$SaO_2$ values calculated by a blood gas analyzer (described earlier) are generally based on an assumed normal value for $P_{50}$. If factors exist in the blood that create an abnormal value for $P_{50}$, then the calculated values for $SaO_2$ will be inaccurate. If the subject's actual $P_{50}$ is greater than normal, then the calculated value for $SaO_2$ (which assumes a normal $P_{50}$) will be falsely high.

$P_{50}$ is determined by using a **tonometer** to establish a series of low $PbloodO_2$ values in the sample. An oximeter is then used to measure the $SbloodO_2$ at each $PbloodO_2$. The $SbloodO_2$ values can be used to construct a partial $HbO_2$ dissociation curve and the value for $P_{50}$ can be identified on the curve.

*Blood Oxygen Content.* The oxygen content of blood, or **CaO2** for arterial blood, can be calculated based on values for $PaO_2$, Total Hb, and $SaO_2$. $CaO_2$ takes into account all blood transport mechanisms for oxygen. It states directly the quantity of oxygen being carried in the blood. The following equation demonstrates the calculation of $CaO_2$.

$$CaO_2 = (\text{Total Hb} \times 1.34 \times SaO_2) + (.0031 \times PaO_2)$$

The number 1.34 is the binding capacity that hemoglobin has for oxygen. It has the units of ml $O_2$/gm% Hb. Values of 1.36 and 1.39 have also been used by some researchers. For this calculation, $SaO_2$ must be expressed as a fraction (not multiplied by 100) instead of as a percent. The number .0031 is the solubility coefficient for oxygen and has the units ml $O_2$/mm Hg. The oxygen content of mixed venous blood can be calculated by using the appropriate values for $S\bar{v}O_2$ and $P\bar{v}O_2$.

*Transport Rate of Oxygen to the Tissues.* It is possible to make a calculation of the *transport rate of oxygen to the tissues* ($\dot{T}O_2$). This is an important clinical tool, especially in critical care, for two reasons:

1. The calculation of $\dot{T}O_2$ provides a single overall value for tracking a patient's ability to provide oxygen to body tissues.
2. The calculation combines the effects of the two primary factors that affect tissue oxygenation:
   - The amount of oxygen in arterial blood. (This is affected by the lung's ability to oxygenate blood and the blood's ability to carry oxygen.)
   - The cardiovascular system's ability to circulate oxygenated blood.

The calculation of $\dot{T}O_2$ is based on multiplying the oxygen content of arterial blood, just described, times the value for cardiac output. The value for $CaO_2$ takes into account the contribution of the lungs and blood to provide for tissue oxygenation. The value for cardiac output adds the contribution of cardiovascular function to tissue oxygenation.

To calculate $\dot{T}O_2$ for a patient, a value for $CaO_2$ is first determined. However, the units for $CaO_2$ are ml $O_2$/*100 ml* of blood and cardiac output is measured in *liters* of blood per minute. Therefore, the value for $CaO_2$ will need to be multiplied by 10 to covert it from units of ml $O_2$/100 ml of blood to units of ml $O_2$/liter of blood. Now $CaO_2$ can be multiplied times the value for cardiac output.

A value for cardiac output will need to be measured clinically for use in the calculation of $\dot{T}O_2$. Typically, in critical care, a **Swan-Ganz catheter** is used to measure a value for cardiac output.

Once the data needed to calculate $CaO_2$ and a value for cardiac output are available, the final calculation of $\dot{T}O_2$ is based on the following equation:

$$\dot{T}O_2 = (CaO_2 \times 10) \times \text{Cardiac Output}$$

The final units for $\dot{T}O_2$ are ml $O_2$/min delivered to the tissues.

*Intrapulmonary Shunting.* The $\dot{Q}_{sp}/\dot{Q}_T$ is a measure of the physiologic **shunting** ($\dot{Q}_{sp}$) of pulmonary blood as a fraction (or percentage) of cardiac output ($\dot{Q}_T$). It is the amount of the cardiac output that arrives at the left heart without having been totally oxygenated within the lungs. $\dot{Q}_{sp}$ includes the effects of both *true shunting* ($\dot{Q}_s$) and the *shunt effect* occurring within the lungs. True shunting is the result of pulmonary capillary blood flow through alveolar units where there is no ventilation and no gas exchange can take place. The shunt effect occurs in alveolar units where there is blood flow and some amount of ventilation. However, the amount of blood flow is in excess of the amount of ventilation. Gas exchange takes place but it is incomplete.

The classic equation for calculating $\dot{Q}_{sp}/\dot{Q}_T$ is

$$\frac{\dot{Q}_{sp}}{\dot{Q}_T} = \frac{CcO_2 - CaO_2}{CcO_2 - C\bar{v}O_2}$$

The solution of the denominator in this equation indicates how much oxygen would potentially be added to mixed venous blood if no shunting existed. Solution of the numerator indicates the deficit in mixed venous blood oxygenation that occurs as a result of shunting. Division expresses, as a fraction, the amount of arterial blood oxygenation deficit as compared to the total potential for pulmonary blood oxygenation. Since the oxygenation deficit in question is due to a shunting of blood flow, this calculation indicates the fraction of total blood flow that undergoes shunting. *The amount of shunting can be expressed as a percent by multiplying the result of the calculation by 100.*

$CaO_2$ and $C\bar{v}O_2$ are calculated in the manner described earlier. $CcO_2$ is the oxygen content of pulmonary capillary blood. It is calculated as follows:

$$CcO_2 = (\text{Total Hb} \times 1.34 \times ScO_2) + (.0031 \times PcO_2)$$

Since, after gas exchange has taken place, $PcO_2$ can be assumed to be equivalent to the $PAO_2$, the equation can be expressed as

$$CcO_2 = (\text{Total Hb} \times 1.34 \times ScO_2) + (.0031 \times PAO_2)$$

$PAO_2$ can be calculated by using the *alveolar air equation*:

$$PAO_2 = ((P_{Atm} - 47 \text{ mm Hg}) \times FIO_2) - \left[ PaCO_2 \left( FIO_2 + \frac{1 - FIO_2}{R} \right) \right]$$

where R = the respiratory quotient.

The following simplified version of the alveolar air equation can be used clinically to provide an acceptable estimation of $PAO_2$.

$$PAO_2 = [(P_{Atm} - 47 \text{ mm Hg}) \times FIO_2] - \frac{PaCO_2}{0.80}$$

At a $PAO_2$ greater than 150 mm Hg, the capillary hemoglobin can be considered to be completely saturated, and so a value of 1.0 should be used for $ScO_2$. $PAO_2$ of less than 150 mm Hg results in less capillary hemoglobin saturation. For the sake of simplicity, an $ScO_2$ of 1.0 can be assumed and used in all calculations of $CcO_2$. For greater accuracy, however, the following adjustments should be used:

- For $PAO_2$ between 125 and 150 mm Hg, use $ScO_2$ of .99.
- For $PAO_2$ between 100 and 125 mm Hg, use $ScO_2$ of .98.

Another possible adjustment for even greater accuracy is to account for the actual amount of $HbO_2$ in the blood. This is done by subtracting the value for the subject's %HbCO (expressed as a fraction instead of a percent) from the value for $ScO_2$ before calculation of $CcO_2$.

Although ideal for determination of $\dot{Q}_{sp}/\dot{Q}_T$, the calculation just described presents a problem. It requires the sampling of mixed venous blood for analysis so that a value for $CvO_2$ can be calculated. An indwelling pulmonary artery catheter is required for taking the sample. To avoid the need for a mixed venous blood sample, an equation for calculating an *estimated value* for $\dot{Q}_{sp}/\dot{Q}_T$ ($\dot{Q}_{sp}/\dot{Q}_T$ *est*) can be used. By accepting that $(CcO_2 - CaO_2) + (CaO_2 - CvO_2)$ is an equal but different way of representing the oxygen content differences expressed by $CcO_2 - CvO_2$, the denominator for the shunt equation can be changed in the following manner:

$$\frac{\dot{Q}_{sp}}{\dot{Q}_T} \, est = \frac{CcO_2 - CaO_2}{(CcO_2 - CaO_2) + (CaO_2 - C\bar{v}O_2)}$$

Or, by restating $(CaO_2 - C\bar{v}O_2)$ as $C(a-\bar{v})O_2$,

$$\frac{\dot{Q}_{sp}}{\dot{Q}_T} \, est = \frac{CcO_2 - CaO_2}{(CcO_2 - CaO_2) + C(a-\bar{v})O_2}$$

With this change, an estimated value for $C(a-v)O_2$ can be substituted in the denominator and the need for a mixed venous blood sample is eliminated.

A $C(a-\bar{v})O_2$ value of between 4.5 and 5.0 vol% can be used for subjects who have relatively normal cardiovascular function. With critically ill subjects who have poor cardiovascular function, a value of 3.5 vol% should be used. Please note that, because an assumption is being made regarding the function of the subject's cardiovascular system, this is a possible source of error in the determination. The $\dot{Q}_{sp}/\dot{Q}_T$ *est* value can be multiplied by 100 in order to express estimated shunt as a percentage.

It is often assumed that shunt determinations must be made with the subject breathing 100% oxygen ($FIO_2$ of 1.0). Two points should be noted, however.

- Experiments and clinical trials have shown that *clinically useful shunt determinations can be made and compared at any consistently maintained $FIO_2$ level*. There is no absolute need to place a subject on 100% oxygen in order to determine $\dot{Q}_{sp}/\dot{Q}_T$.
- Subjects who have poorly ventilated lung regions (low $\dot{V}/\dot{Q}$ values) and are breathing 100% oxygen will develop **absorption atelectasis**. As a result, there will be an increase in the amount of intrapulmonary shunting and a false elevation of measured shunt.

For these reasons, the use of 100% oxygen is not indicated.

If a standard reference $FIO_2$ is required for comparison of test results, then determinations can be made with the subject breathing 50% oxygen. This value tends to produce beneficial changes in $PaO_2$ without risking the development of additional atelectasis.

For subjects having a $PaO_2$ of 150 mm Hg or greater, a shortcut equation for calculating shunt can be used. With $PaO_2 \geq 150$ mm Hg, the $SaO_2$ can be assumed to be 100%. Additionally, the $ScO_2$ can also be assumed to be 100%. Under these circumstances, the hemoglobin contribution to blood oxygen content can be ignored when determining $\dot{Q}_{sp}/\dot{Q}_T$. Blood oxygen content changes ($CcO_2$ and $CaO_2$) will be reflected by their $PO_2$ ($PAO_2$ and $PaO_2$, respectively) changes alone. Therefore, *for subjects with* *a $PaO_2 \geq 150$ mm Hg, the following shortcut equation for determining $\dot{Q}_{sp}/\dot{Q}_T$ est can be used:*

$$\frac{\dot{Q}_{sp}}{\dot{Q}_T} \, est = \frac{(PAO_2 - PaO_2) \times .0031}{[(PAO_2 - PaO_2) \times .0031] + C(a\text{-}\bar{v})O_2}$$

It is important to note that this method works only if accurate values for $PAO_2$ and $PaO_2$ are used. The greatest likelihood of error is in the determination of $PAO_2$. Using assumptions (such as using 760 mm Hg for the $P_{Atm}$ or 40 mm Hg for the $PaCO_2$) instead of actual values can lead to error in calculating the $PAO_2$.

*Tissue Oxygenation.* $C(a\text{-}\bar{v})O_2$ and $S\bar{v}O_2$ values, in conjunction with $PaO_2$ and hemoglobin values, provide useful tools for assessing how effectively the demands of tissue oxygenation are being met. Normal tissue oxygenation is based on three factors:

- Arterial oxygen content ($CaO_2$).
- Cardiac output ($\dot{Q}_T$).
- Tissue oxygen consumption ($\dot{V}O_2$).

The $CaO_2$ and $\dot{Q}_T$ together determine the amount of oxygen available to the tissues for meeting their needs of $\dot{V}O_2$. This relationship is demonstrated by the following equation:

$$(CaO_2 \times 10) \times \dot{Q}_T = \text{Total Oxygen Availability}$$

The $CaO_2$ is multiplied by 10 to compensate for the difference in units between $CaO_2$ (vol%) and $\dot{Q}_T$ (l/min).

The difference between the $CaO_2$ and the $C\bar{v}O_2$, or $C(a\text{-}\bar{v})O_2$, results from the amount of oxygen extracted from the blood by the tissues. Given normal values for $CaO_2$ (20 vol%) and $C\bar{v}O_2$ (15 vol%), the normal value for $C(a\text{-}\bar{v})O_2$ is 5 vol%. This is the amount of oxygen extracted per unit of blood in order to meet the needs of tissue $\dot{V}O_2$. It amounts to 25% of the oxygen originally available in arterial blood. Seventy-five percent of the oxygen originally available in arterial blood still remains in the mixed venous blood that returns to the lungs for reoxygenation.

A value called *oxygen extraction ratio* ($O_2ER$) can be calculated as follows:

$$O_2ER = \frac{C(a\text{-}\bar{v})O_2}{CaO_2}$$

With normal values for $C(a\text{-}\bar{v})O_2$ and $CaO_2$, the normal value for $O_2ER$ is .25. This corresponds to the 25% of arterial oxygen extraction by the tissues that was described earlier (the 5 vol% of oxygen extracted by the tissues out of the original 20 vol% oxygen in arterial blood). An increased value for $O_2ER$ indicates that the amount of oxygen extracted from the blood by the tissues is greater than normal.

An important relationship exists between $C(a\text{-}\bar{v})O_2$, $\dot{Q}_T$, and $\dot{V}O_2$:

$$\dot{V}O_2 = (C(a\text{-}\bar{v})O_2 \times 10) \times \dot{Q}_T$$

This relationship is significant because *it shows that the only factors affecting the value for $C(a\text{-}\bar{v})O_2$ are changes in either $\dot{Q}_T$ or $\dot{V}O_2$.*

As a generalization, $\dot{V}O_2$ can be assumed to be constant for critically ill patients who are not septic and who have limited muscular activity (no physical agitation, seizures, or shivering). With this assumption, changes in $C(a\text{-}\bar{v})O_2$ can only be due to changes in the level of tissue perfusion ($\dot{Q}_T$). *Therefore, $C(a\text{-}\bar{v})O_2$ values can be used to indicate how effectively a patient's cardiovascular system is working to meet the needs of tissue oxygenation.* An increase in $C(a\text{-}\bar{v})O_2$ values indicates that $\dot{Q}_T$ is reduced, there is less tissue perfusion, and, as a result, a greater amount of oxygen is being extracted from each unit of available blood.

It must be noted that it is possible for a patient's $\dot{V}O_2$ to change. Conditions such as hyperthermia, seizures, shivering, and exercise can increase $\dot{V}O_2$. $\dot{V}O_2$ can be reduced by hypothermia, skeletal muscle relaxation, altered cellular metabolism resulting from cyanide poisoning, and peripheral vascular shunting resulting from sepsis or trauma.

Increases in $\dot{Q}_T$ can, to a limited degree, provide an effective compensatory response to hypoxemia caused by right-to-left shunting. As $\dot{Q}_T$ increases and the $C(a\text{-}\bar{v})O_2$ correspondingly decreases, the result is an increase in $C\bar{v}O_2$ for the blood returning to the lungs for reoxygenation. This elevation of $C\bar{v}O_2$ is significant. It means that the shunted venous admixture is better oxygenated and therefore has less of a reducing effect on the final $CaO_2$.

With exercise, $P\bar{v}O_2$ values decrease and $C(a\text{-}\bar{v})O_2$values increase. This is despite increases in $PaO_2$ and cardiac output. The cause is the increased consumption of oxygen by the working muscles. The resulting increase in blood oxygen extraction has a greater effect than the increased oxygen supply.

Obviously, $C(a\text{-}\bar{v})O_2$ and $O_2ER$ determinations can be made only if a mixed venous blood sample is available. In the absence of regular mixed venous blood sampling, a pulmonary artery catheter that uses a reflectance-type continuous $S\bar{v}O_2$ monitor can be helpful. A decrease in $S\bar{v}O_2$ corresponds to a decrease in $CvO_2$ and indicates that there is a decrease in the oxygen supply to the tissues.

$S\bar{v}O_2$ alone does not indicate whether the problem is related to poor arterial blood oxygenation, poor tissue perfusion, or increased metabolic demands. $S\bar{v}O_2$ values can, however, be correlated with $PaO_2$ and $SaO_2$ values as if $CaO_2$ and $C\bar{v}O_2$ values were being used. This correlation allows for some differentiation according to whether $PaO_2$ changes or $\dot{Q}_T$ changes are responsible for changes in $SvO_2$.

One benefit of continuous $S\bar{v}O_2$ monitoring is that $S\bar{v}O_2$ changes are demonstrated before there are corresponding changes in the subject's arterial blood gas values. *Decreasing $S\bar{v}O_2$ values can be used as an early indicator of impending hypoxemia.*

## Parameters for Assessment of Ventilation

Ventilation is assessed through the evaluation of *$PaCO_2$* values. $PaCO_2$ is not significantly affected by many of the pulmonary factors that affect $PaO_2$ values. This is because carbon dioxide diffuses through the pulmonary tissues between alveolar air and the pulmonary capillary blood approximately 20 times more easily than does oxygen. There is, however, a significant reciprocal relationship between $PaCO_2$ levels and the level of alveolar ventilation ($\dot{V}_A$). As $\dot{V}_A$ increases, $PaCO_2$ values decrease. Likewise, as $\dot{V}_A$ decreases, $PaCO_2$ increases. For this reason, $PaCO_2$ values are used clinically as an indicator of the effectiveness of ventilation.

## Parameters for Assessment of Acid/Base Balance

Assessment of acid/base status requires the measurement of several blood parameters. Arterial blood pH provides a direct statement of the acid/base balance in the body. A pH value greater than normal indicates a condition of *alkalosis*. A pH value less than normal indicates a condition of *acidosis*.

The pH alone, however, does not provide an adequate picture of the events that participated in producing a particular acid/base state. Acidosis can result from either

- More than the normal amount of an acid substance in the blood.
- Less than the normal amount of an alkaline substance in the blood.
- A combination of both of the above factors.

A similar relationship exists for alkalosis. Less than the normal amount of an acid substance, more than the normal amount of an alkaline substance, or a combination of both can produce alkalosis.

Both respiratory and metabolic factors contribute to acid/base balance in the body. The *respiratory* contribution to acid/base balance is evaluated on the basis of $PaCO_2$ levels. This is because carbon dioxide is a *volatile acid*, and it acts as an acid substance in the blood. The primary blood transport mechanism for carbon dioxide is through its conversion to carbonic acid ($H_2CO_3$). $H_2CO_3$ dissociates to form free protons ($H^+$) and bicarbonate ions ($HCO_3^-$). The following equation demonstrates this mechanism.

$$CO_2 + H_2O \longrightarrow H_2CO_3 \longrightarrow H^+ + HCO_3^-$$

$PaCO_2$ levels greater than normal shift this equation to the right and increase the concentration of free $H^+$ in blood.

The concentration of free $H^+$ in the blood determines the pH of the blood. Increases in the concentration of free $H^+$ in the blood cause a decrease in blood pH. Therefore, the increase in the concentration of free blood $H^+$ that results from increased $CO_2$ levels in the blood is directly responsible for causing a decrease in the blood's pH. This produces what is called a *respiratory acidosis*. $PaCO_2$ levels less than normal reverse this action and shift the equation to the left. Fewer free $H^+$ are present in the blood, pH becomes elevated, and a state of *respiratory alkalosis* is the result.

On the basis of these relationships, the level of pulmonary ventilation plays a significant role in maintaining blood pH. Ventilation that maintains a normal $PaCO_2$ level in the blood is sufficient for managing the normal quantities of carbon dioxide produced in the body. The maintenance of appropriate levels of ventilation prevents the development of either respiratory acidosis or respiratory alkalosis.

The *metabolic* contribution to acid/base balance is evaluated on the basis of arterial blood $HCO_3^-$ levels. $HCO_3^-$ is an alkaline substance in the blood and it participates in the carbonic acid/sodium bicarbonate ($NaHCO_3$) reaction. This reaction is significant because it is the primary physiologic acid/base buffering system in the body. As a result, the availability of $HCO_3^-$ plays a central role in blood acid/base balance and pH maintenance.

The kidneys are the body tissues primarily responsible for regulating blood $HCO_3^-$ concentrations. $HCO_3^-$ ions are filtered from the blood into the urine as it is initially produced. The kidneys, however, allow the reabsorption of nearly all of the $HCO_3^-$ back into the blood before the urine is excreted. Changes in $HCO_3^-$ reabsorption are normally responsible for regulating the final $HCO_3^-$ concentration in the blood.

Because of its control of $HCO_3^-$ availability, renal function plays a significant role in maintaining blood pH. Normal levels of renal bicarbonate reabsorption are sufficient for managing the normal quantities of **nonvolatile acids** produced in the body. Maintaining this level of reabsorption prevents the development of either a metabolic acidosis or alkalosis.

Abnormalities that cause a reduction of blood $HCO_3^-$ levels will allow increased levels of unbuffered $H^+$ to remain in the blood. The elevated concentrations of $H^+$ in the blood decrease pH and create a nonrespiratory or *metabolic acidosis.*

The concept of *base excess/deficit* (BE) provides an additional method for quantitating the metabolic contribution to acid/base changes. Use of $HCO_3^-$ values for the alkaline side of acid/base balance only takes the carbonic acid/sodium bicarbonate buffering mechanism into account. Other buffering systems, such as hemoglobin within the red blood cells, have an effect on acid/base balance. Determination of BE includes an accounting of pH and $PaCO_2$ (both are used for $HCO_3^-$ determination) plus the value for Total Hb. The normal value for BE is $\pm 2.0$ mEq/l. Most often, BE is referred to only as *base excess.* With use of this term, a base deficit is referred to, oddly enough, as a negative base excess.

Changes in $HCO_3^-$ and BE follow the same trends. A greater than normal $HCO_3^-$ concentration (greater than 26 mEq/l) and a positive base excess (BE greater than +2 mEq/l) both are caused by the same abnormalities. A base deficit (BE less than −2 mEq/l) corresponds to $HCO_3^-$ values of less than normal (less than 22 mEq/l). *Because an additional buffer factor, hemoglobin, is taken into account, a change in $HCO_3^-$ does not necessarily produce a corresponding numerical change in the BE values.* As a result, a $HCO_3^-$ value of 34 mEq/l (10 mEq/l greater than normal) does not automatically indicate that the corresponding BE value is going to be +10 mEq/l. The value for BE may be slightly greater or less depending on the value for hemoglobin used. For given pH and $PaCO_2$ values, increases in the hemoglobin value used will increase the resulting value for base excess/deficit.

## EQUIPMENT REQUIRED

Direct assessment of blood gas values is a two-step process. First, a blood sample must be obtained. Blood sampling requires certain equipment and procedures. Second, the blood sample must undergo analysis with the appropriate equipment.

### Blood Sampling

Sampling of blood by arterial puncture, regardless of the arterial site used, requires the same basic equipment: an antiseptic agent for the skin, a sampling needle and syringe, and a sterile pad for holding the site after needle removal. The blood gas syringe must contain heparin before the sample is taken. This is to prevent the sample from clotting before analysis can be performed.

In the past, only glass syringes were used for arterial blood gas sampling. This was because of a concern that the diffusion of gases through plastic syringes would affect the gas values in the blood. With the plastic materials used in plastic syringes today, this is no longer a significant concern.

Blood sampling from an arterial, central venous, or pulmonary artery catheter requires two needleless syringes. One is used to withdraw a volume of "waste" specimen from the line prior to the actual blood sample being drawn. The volume of waste specimen withdrawn should be slightly greater than the catheter volume. This waste specimen is withdrawn to prevent the actual blood sample withdrawn next from being contaminated by the solution used to flush out the catheter. With the waste specimen withdrawn, the second syringe is used to withdraw and hold the blood sample. As with arterial puncture, the second "sample" syringe must be preheparinized to prevent clotting of the sample.

Sampling of arterialized capillary blood from a tissue site requires different equipment. A warm wet towel, heat lamp, or some other method is needed to heat the site and increase local perfusion. A skin-antiseptic agent is needed for the skin. A **lancet** for skin puncture and a preheparinized capillary tube for blood collection are also required. As with arterial puncture, a sterile pad is needed for holding the site after the sample has been collected.

## Blood Analysis

Blood analysis is accomplished through use of blood gas analyzers and spectrophotometers. Today's *blood gas analyzers* are very sophisticated instruments. They contain three electrochemical electrodes, one each for determination of $PO_2$, $PCO_2$, and pH.

The electrodes in a blood gas analyzer are held in a heated water bath called a *cuvette* in order to maintain the electrodes at a constant temperature of 37°C (body temperature). This is important because changes in temperature will affect the $PO_2$, $PCO_2$, and pH of blood samples. For example, analysis of a single blood sample first at 37°C and then at a higher temperature will demonstrate higher values for $PO_2$, $PCO_2$, and pH with the second analysis.

Blood samples of 0.2 ml or smaller can be analyzed by some instruments. Samples from both syringes and capillary tubes often can be run on an analyzer. Many analyzers are capable of making $PO_2$ and $PCO_2$ measurements on both liquid (e.g., blood) and gaseous (e.g., collected exhaled air) samples.

Today's analyzers are fully automated to measure and display results for a sample and then to flush out the system when analysis is complete. Periodic calibration checks and warnings of miscalibration can also be automated. Computers within the analyzer can calculate blood gas values that are not directly measured by the instrument (e.g., $HCO_3^-$ and $SaO_2$). Computers can also make corrections for the patient's actual body temperature and hemoglobin levels.

A *CO-oximeter* is used to perform spectrophotometry on **in vitro** blood samples. Spectrophotometry allows determination of $SaO_2$, Total Hb, %MetHb, and %HbCO. *Fiberoptic catheter reflective spectrophotometry* systems allow continuous **in vivo** analysis of $S\bar{v}O_2$ in critical-care settings. The catheter is similar to those commonly referred to as Swan-Ganz catheters but they additionally include two fiberoptic glass bundles within the catheter. One bundle transmits two or three different wavelengths of light into the pulmonary artery blood. The second bundle transmits the reflected light back out of the blood vessel to an external photodetector for determination of $S\overline{v}O_2$. In addition to $S\overline{v}O_2$, the blood pressure measurements normally made with a Swan-Ganz catheter can also be made.

*Pulse oximeters* can be used to perform noninvasive in vivo analysis of $SaO_2$. To differentiate these values for $SaO_2$ determined by pulse oximetry, they are sometimes referred to as $SpO_2$. In the same subject, $SpO_2$ values may differ from $SaO_2$ values for a variety of reasons. The presence of COHb, MetHb, cardiac output dyes in the blood, jaundice, high-intensity ambient light, hypoperfusion at the measurement site (hypothermia and vasopressor drugs), and skin pigmentation can all have at least some effect on the accuracy of $SpO_2$ measurements. Motion artifact caused by shivering can make it difficult for the instrument to correctly detect vascular pulsations and to accurately measure $SpO_2$.

## TEST ADMINISTRATION

As with most pulmonary function tests, the blood sampling and blood analysis techniques used can affect the accuracy of the test results. For the invasive procedures of blood sampling, there is also a significant concern for patient safety.

## Blood Sampling

Several sites can be used for sampling arterial blood by arterial puncture. For adult subjects, the radial and brachial arteries are the sites most often used. Under special circumstances, however, samples can be drawn from the femoral artery and the dorsalis pedis artery along the top of the foot. For infant subjects, arterial puncture can be performed on the radial artery and the temporal artery in the scalp.

Circulation to the hand is generally provided by both the radial and the ulnar arteries. Arterial puncture to the radial artery can potentially damage and cause the loss of circulation through that artery. Before a radial artery is used for arterial puncture, therefore, it is important to evaluate the amount of collateral circulation to that hand. This is done by use of the *modified Allen's test*.

In the modified Allen's test, the technologist uses finger pressure on the subject's wrist to occlude both the ulnar and radial arteries. The subject is instructed to make a fist and then release it. This is to expel blood from the hand and to blanch the skin. Next, the pressure on the ulnar artery is released while pressure on the radial artery is maintained. If coloration returns to the hand within 15 seconds, the test is positive. A positive test means that there is adequate collateral circulation through the ulnar artery to maintain circulation to the hand if the radial artery is damaged. An arterial puncture can be performed on that radial artery. If coloration does not return to the hand within 15 seconds, then the test is negative. In this case, arterial puncture should not be performed on that radial artery.

Because of the invasive nature of blood sampling procedures, strict adherence to aseptic technique for cleaning and palpation of the sample site and handling of the equipment is important. Failure to maintain asepsis can allow transmission of an infection to the subject. Septicemia can be the result.

Once a sample has been taken by arterial puncture, it is imperative that pressure be applied to the wound site. This must be done for *at least* five minutes and must continue until all bleeding has stopped. Care must be taken to examine the wound after pressure application is done to ensure that the bleeding has in fact stopped before the patient is left unattended.

Some patients may require a prolonged time for holding the puncture site after arterial sampling. The prolonged bleeding and need to hold the site are due to the patient having blood coagulation abnormalities. Abnormal blood coagulation can be present in

- Patients receiving treatment with anticoagulant medication.
- Patients with disorders of blood coagulation.

Before arterial puncture is performed, the patient's medical record should be reviewed to identify any problems with blood coagulation.

Once drawn, the blood sample must be handled properly. All air bubbles must be immediately removed from the sample. Bubbles in the sample will alter the gas levels in the blood. $CO_2$ will leave the blood and enter the gas of the bubble because of the minimal $CO_2$ levels in air. This reduces the blood $PCO_2$ and will, as a result, alter pH as well. The $PO_2$ in the air bubble is equal to that of the atmospheric air (approximately 150 mm Hg). Blood $PO_2$ values of more than 150 mm Hg will decrease in the presence of air bubbles. Blood $PO_2$ values of less than 150 mm Hg will increase in the presence of air bubbles. The significance of these changes depends on the size of the bubbles and how long they are present in the sample.

The sample must be placed in a "slush" of ice chips and water as soon as possible after the sample is taken. Failure to do so can result in the blood sample's $PO_2$, pH, and $PCO_2$ values changing. This is the result of continued metabolism by blood cells (primarily white cells) after the sample is drawn. Icing the sample minimizes or suspends blood cell metabolism. An iced sample with a $PO_2$ of less than 150 mm Hg and values for pH and $PCO_2$ that are within a reasonable range can sit for an hour or more without significant changes. Nevertheless, it is still good practice to analyze blood gas samples as soon as possible.

It is possible for blood-borne infections to be transmitted from the subject to the technologist. This is especially true if the subject's blood comes in contact with the technologist's mucus membrane tissue or an open wound. For this reason, it is important that the technologist take adequate safety precautions during blood sampling and with later handling of the sample. Appendix F presents the universal precautions that have been established for the handling of blood.

## Blood Analysis

Analysis equipment must be used and maintained as specified by the manufacturer. Failure to follow the manufacturer's instructions creates a risk of incorrect test results. The key components to a blood gas analyzer are the electrodes. Their proper maintenance is critical. Manufacturer-recommended schedules for electrode membrane and electrolyte replacement must be followed. A frequent problem is blood protein buildup on the electrode membrane. With buildup, electrode response and measurement times will be longer.

As a result, proper calibration may be difficult, and sample analysis can be in error. Routine cleaning or replacement of the membranes will minimize this problem.

Quality assurance procedures must be performed to ensure accurate measurements. Chapter 16 provides specific information on quality assurance for blood gas instruments.

## INTERPRETATION OF TEST RESULTS

Blood gas values provide important information on cardiopulmonary function. Alone, however, they do not provide a complete clinical picture. As with any other clinical data, blood gas values should be interpreted in relation to other indicators of cardiopulmonary function. Normal values for arterial blood gas parameters are provided in Table 11–2.

### Parameters for Assessment of Oxygenation

When assessing oxygenation, it is important to note that there is a difference between hypoxemia and hypoxia. *Hypoxemia* is insufficient arterial blood oxygenation that results from poor function of the pulmonary system. Its presence is indicated by $PaO_2$ values

**TABLE 11–2  Normal Values for Blood Gas Parameters**

#### Oxygenation

$PaO_2$ = 97 mm Hg (80–100 mm Hg)
%MetHb = <1.5% of Total Hb
%COHb = .5%–2% of Total Hb
$SaO_2$ = 97% of Total Hb
$P_{50}$ = 26.7 mm Hg (26–27 mm Hg)
Total Hb = 14–16 gm% (male)
13–15 gm% (female)
$CaO_2$ = approximately 20 vol%
$\dot{T}O_2$ = 900–1200 ml $O_2$/min
$\dot{Q}_{sp}/\dot{Q}_T$ = <5% of cardiac output
$C\bar{v}O_2$ = approximately 15 vol%
$C(a-\bar{v})O_2$ = 5 vol% (4.5–6 vol%)
$P\bar{v}O_2$ = 40 mm Hg (37–43 mm Hg)
$S\bar{v}O_2$ = 75%

#### Ventilation

$PaCO_2$ = 40 mm Hg (35–45 mm Hg)

#### Acid/Base Balance

pH = 7.40 (7.35–7.45)
$HCO_3^-$ = 24 mEq/l (22–26 mEq/l)
BE = ±2 mEq/l

that are less than normal. *Hypoxia* is a condition of insufficient tissue oxygenation. It can exist with or without the presence of hypoxemia. Table 11–3 provides a list of the factors that can cause hypoxemia and hypoxia.

*PaO₂ Values.*   $PaO_2$ values decrease with advancing age. Even in a subject with an $FIO_2$ of .21, they can be increased to as high as 120 mm Hg through the act of hyperventilation alone. For a normal subject breathing 100% oxygen, $PaO_2$ values can be greater than 600 mm Hg. $PaO_2$ values are not affected by changes in total Hb or by changes in factors that affect the binding of oxygen to hemoglobin.

Of the factors that can cause hypoxemia, ventilation/perfusion abnormalities are the most significant problem. Pulmonary units with good matching of ventilation and perfusion create fully oxygenated blood in their capillary beds. Pulmonary units with either poor ventilation or poor perfusion result in poorly oxygenated blood. As a result of the mixing of blood from both types of units, the final $PaO_2$ will be below normal. This reduction in $PaO_2$ is in direct proportion to the number of abnormal pulmonary units contributing blood.

The other factors listed in Table 11–3 as causing hypoxemia have some clinical importance. Their contribution to hypoxemia is generally less significant than that of the ventilation/perfusion disorders, however.

Measurement of $PaO_2$ at rest can be used to indicate the severity of a pulmonary impairment. The nature and degree of severity of a pulmonary disorder can, however, have

## TABLE 11–3   Factors Causing Hypoxemia and Hypoxia

### Factors Causing Hypoxemia

Reduced inspired $PO_2$ ($PIO_2$) (e.g., at high altitudes)
Hypoventilation
Pulmonary diffusion impairments
Right-to-left vascular shunting
Ventilation/perfusion inequalities

### Factors Causing Hypoxia

Hypoxemia
Poor tissue perfusion*
Anemia*
• Absolute—reduced total Hb
• Relative—elevated %MetHb or %HbCO or reduced $P_{50}$
Histotoxicity (e.g., cyanide poisoning)*

*These factors can produce hypoxia even when hypoxemia is not present (i.e., when $PaO_2$ is normal).*

a significant effect on the amount of hypoxemia that results. With pulmonary disorders of only limited severity, $PaO_2$ may remain at normal levels because of compensatory hyperventilation.

Disorders that equally affect both ventilation and perfusion in the same lung regions can also result in relatively normal $PaO_2$ being maintained. This is true even with mild to moderate disorders. Pure emphysema is an example of a pulmonary disorder that does not produce a significant ventilation/perfusion abnormality. Destruction of the pulmonary tissues with emphysema results in the loss of both functional alveolar ventilation and capillary perfusion. Both are reduced by nearly equal amounts. As a result, ventilation/perfusion inequalities do not appear to contribute greatly to hypoxemia. Hypoxemia does develop in emphysema when severity of the disease begins to have a significant effect on the pulmonary diffusing capacity.

Disorders such as chronic bronchitis and acute asthma can rapidly and significantly affect ventilation/perfusion relationships in the lung. Hypoxemia can occur even with only mild disorders. $PaO_2$ as low as 40 mm Hg may be demonstrated by patients with severe disorders. This is true for many restrictive and obstructive disorders.

Use of $PaO_2$ for evaluating pulmonary disorders is best done in conjunction with the use of results from spirometry and other pulmonary function tests. For subjects with obstructive disorders, $PaO_2$ reductions with exercise can be used as an indication of severity. The extent of exercise $PaO_2$ reductions correlates reasonably well with $FEV_1$ and $D_LCO$ reductions. Significantly reduced $D_LCO$ values (less than 50% of predicted) can correspond with hypoxemia at rest as well as during exertion. Unfortunately, it is not possible to directly correlate or predict abnormal $D_LCO$ values with resulting reduced $PaO_2$ values.

A $PaO_2$ of 60 mm Hg correlates with an $SaO_2$ of approximately 90%. For this reason, given a reasonably normal value for Total Hb, the goal of acute oxygen therapy is to maintain a patient's $PaO_2$ at levels that are at least $\geq$ 60 mm Hg.

*Abnormal Non-Oxygen-Carrying Hemoglobin.* Normally the amount of abnormal, non-oxygen-carrying hemoglobin in the blood is small. **Methemoglobinemia** can result from exposure to or ingestion of substances that are strong oxidizing agents (e.g., naphthalene and nitrate compounds). Patients with increasingly severe methemoglobinemia will demonstrate cyanosis. This is because of the greater quantity of non-oxygen-saturated hemoglobin in the blood. Treatment for methemoglobinemia involves the use of a substance called methylene blue. As an "electron carrier," methylene blue participates in a metabolic pathway that converts hemoglobin from the abnormal oxidized form back to the normal, oxygen-accepting reduced form.

Some carboxyhemoglobin is normally produced in small amounts as a by-product of metabolism. **Carboxyhemoglobinemia** results primarily from environmental sources such as smoking, automobile emissions, and other sources of combustion by-products. Smokers often exhibit %COHb levels of 3% to 15%, depending on the amount and frequency of tobacco use. Since $SaO_2$ values decrease by the same amount that %HbCO increases, a 15% increase in carboxyhemoglobin can produce clinically significant hypoxemia (i.e., $SaO_2$ values of less than 85%).

The %HbCO levels can reach 50% in cases of significant CO poisoning. These levels will be maintained or increase as long as a source of CO is present. It should be noted that, because the hemoglobin receptor sites are saturated, cyanosis is not present with carboxyhemoglobinemia. In fact, the patient will exhibit an extraordinarily healthy skin color.

It should be noted that changes in %HbCO levels (and corresponding changes in $SaO_2$) do not relate to the subject's $PaO_2$. A subject can have a normal $PaO_2$ value and yet, because of breathing environmental CO, have an elevated %HbCO and a decreased $SaO_2$. Additionally, pulse oximeters do not yet have the ability to differentiate between oxygen and carbon monoxide hemoglobin saturation. They only register an overall saturation state of hemoglobin. Therefore, $PaO_2$ and $SpO_2$ determinations cannot satisfactorily detect the presence or indicate the significance of CO poisoning. If CO poisoning is suspected in a subject, CO-oximetry is the only means available for providing a proper assessment.

Treatment for carboxyhemoglobinemia is based on two actions:

- Removal of the subject from the source of CO. This allows for the CO gradient within the lungs to be reversed. CO will now diffuse from the blood into the alveolar air and will begin to be eliminated from the body during ventilation. As a result, %HbCO values will begin to decrease.

- Administration of oxygen in high concentrations. The oxygen serves to displace CO molecules from their combination with hemoglobin. Administration of 100% oxygen and possibly hyperbaric oxygen therapy are recommended, especially in cases of significant CO poisoning.

In addition to these actions, an increase in minute ventilation (and therefore alveolar ventilation) will accelerate the elimination of CO from the body.

*Total Hemoglobin.*   Total hemoglobin and related red blood cell abnormalities range from **anemia** to **polycythemia**. With anemia, the reduction of oxygen-carrying hemoglobin in the blood can be a source of hypoxia. Cyanosis is less likely in subjects who are anemic. This is because at least 5.0 gm% of unsaturated hemoglobin must be present before significant cyanosis will be exhibited. As an example, with a 10.0 gm% of total Hb, the $SaO_2$ would have to be nearly 50% before 5.0 gm% of unsaturated hemoglobin—and therefore cyanosis—would be present.

Despite being a compensatory physiologic response to chronic oxygenation problems, polycythemia itself can produce problems. The increased red blood cell/hemoglobin quantities make the blood "thick" and difficult for the heart to circulate. This added cardiovascular work can contribute to the development of heart failure. Cyanosis is more likely to be present in subjects who are polycythemic, even if they are reasonably well oxygenated. The elevation of total Hb makes it possible to have 5.0 gm% or more of unsaturated hemoglobin at higher $SaO_2$ values than would normally produce cyanosis.

*$SaO_2$ Values.*   With $PaO_2$ values greater than 100 mm Hg, changes in $PaO_2$ have little effect on $SaO_2$ values. This is based on the shape of the $O_2$ dissociation curve in this range. $PaO_2$ values as low as 60 mm Hg produce nearly normal (90%) $SaO_2$ values. $PaO_2$ values

of 60 mm Hg down to 40 mm Hg result in $SaO_2$ values of 90%–75%. Clinical signs of hypoxemia and hypoxia (SOB, mental confusion, etc.) become evident as $SaO_2$ values decrease in this range.

$PaO_2$ monitoring provides a more sensitive indicator of changes in pulmonary gas exchange than $SaO_2$ monitoring. This is true until $PaO_2$ values drop down to 60 mm Hg ($SaO_2$ of 90%). Below that, both $PaO_2$ and $SaO_2$ values drop together in a more closely corresponding manner. Either one can be used effectively as an indicator of gas exchange changes. *Assuming reasonably normal total Hb levels,* the therapeutic goal for oxygen therapy is to maintain an $SaO_2$ of at least 90% ($PaO_2$ approximately 60 mm Hg). $SaO_2$ values of less than 90% are used clinically to indicate the need for an increase in oxygen administration. For subjects who have significantly reduced total Hb levels, $SaO_2$ levels of 90% may be too low for adequate blood oxygenation. Consequently, it may be more appropriate to provide amounts of therapeutic oxygen that will maintain $SaO_2$ values at levels greater than 90% in these subjects.

Methemoglobinemia and carboxyhemoglobinemia both reduce the carrying capacity of hemoglobin for oxygen. This effect can create problems with blood gas analyzers that provide a calculated value for $SaO_2$. Calculated values based on $PO_2$ and pH will be inaccurate in these cases. $SaO_2$ values will falsely indicate that hemoglobin is more saturated with oxygen than it actually is. When these disorders are present or suspected, %MetHb and/or %COHb must be measured and taken into account if calculated $SaO_2$ values are being used. Another option is to simply measure $SaO_2$ values directly by oximetry instead of relying on calculated values.

Because of the convenience and frequent use of pulse oximetry, it is easy for the technologist to develop an overconfidence in relating $SpO_2$ values to $SaO_2$ values. $SpO_2$ values may not always accurately reflect the $SaO_2$ values that are actually present. Skin coloration and pigmentation (jaundice, racial differences), presence of abnormal hemoglobin (MetHb, COHb), dyes used for vascular flow studies and hypoperfusion (hypothermia, vasopressor drugs, peripheral vascular disease, hypotension) can all produce inaccuracies in pulse oximetry measurements. Bradycardia in conjunction with drops in arterial saturation can slow down the response time of pulse oximeters.

*$P_{50}$ Values.* Normal values for $P_{50}$ are based on conditions of an arterial blood pH of 7.40, 37°C body temperature, and a $PaCO_2$ of 40 mm Hg. Table 11–4 provides a listing of factors that can cause changes in $P_{50}$ values and shifts in the oxyhemoglobin dissociation curve. Changes in $P_{50}$ affect the ability of hemoglobin to combine with oxygen. A less than normal $P_{50}$ value indicates that hemoglobin will combine with oxygen more easily. A drawback of this, however, is that the hemoglobin will be less willing to release the oxygen to the tissues where it is needed. Elevated $P_{50}$ values indicate the opposite. Oxygen is less attracted to hemoglobin, but at the tissue level, the oxygen is more likely to be released.

Possible abnormalities in $P_{50}$ can be assessed without a direct determination of $P_{50}$ value. This assessment is based on how much the actual measured $SaO_2$ differs from a calculated value for $SaO_2$, given that the same value for $PaO_2$ is used in both cases. The calculated $SaO_2$ is determined from an oxyhemoglobin dissociation curve that is based on

---

**TABLE 11–4  Factors Affecting $P_{50}$ Values**

| Factors That Reduce $P_{50}$ Values | Factors That Increase $P_{50}$ Values |
| --- | --- |
| *(Left shift of the oxyhemoglobin dissociation curve)* | *(Right shift of the oxyhemoglobin dissociation curve)* |
| Increased blood pH | Decreased blood pH |
| Decreased body temperature | Increased body temperature |
| Decreased blood 2,3 DPG levels | Increased blood 2,3 DPG levels |
| Presence of fetal hemoglobin | |
| Presence of carboxyhemoglobin | |

*Note: 2,3 DPG is an organic phosphate related to glucose metabolism.*

---

a normal value for $P_{50}$. If the measured $SaO_2$ has a greater value than the $SaO_2$ calculated for a normal $P_{50}$, then the subject's actual value for $P_{50}$ is decreased.

*$CaO_2$ Values.*  $CaO_2$ values are affected by two key factors:

• The lung's ability to oxygenate blood.
• The ability of blood to carry oxygen.

A disorder that affects either of these factors will cause a reduced arterial blood oxygen content. Pulmonary disorders that cause $PaO_2$ and $SaO_2$ values to decrease will also cause $CaO_2$ values to decrease. Reduction of a patient's hemoglobin values (anemia) will cause $CaO_2$ values to decrease as well. A decrease in $CaO_2$ values indicates that the patient's tissues are at risk for hypoxia. The initial physiologic response to reduced $CaO_2$ values is a compensatory increase in cardiac output. A reduction in cardiac output or localized perfusion can also be a cause of hypoxia. This can be true either with or without normal values for $CaO_2$.

*$\dot{T}O_2$ Values.*  The value for $\dot{T}O_2$ provides a performance measure for the primary factors that affect the transport rate of oxygen to the tissues:

• Arterial oxygen content.
• Cardiac output.

Decreases in $\dot{T}O_2$ values indicate that one or both of these rate factors are not functioning effectively. *The result will be tissue hypoxia.* It is important to note that a deterioration of either of these factors, even if the other factor is unchanged or shows improvement, can still result in a decrease in $\dot{T}O_2$.

  An example of the interaction between the oxygen transport rate factors relates to mechanical ventilation, where *positive end-expiratory pressure* (PEEP) is sometimes used to improve oxygenation. An increase in PEEP can improve a patient's $PaO_2$ and $SaO_2$ and therefore the $CaO_2$. However, the increase in mean intrathoracic pressure that is caused by the increase in PEEP can impair cardiovascular function. The result is a reduction in cardiac output and possibly hypotension. The worsening of cardiac output may be more significant than the improvement of blood oxygenation. If cardiac output is reduced to this extent, resulting decrease in the calculated value for $\dot{T}O_2$ will indicate a worsening of tissue oxygenation.

This concept can be demonstrated with the following example (assuming a normal hemoglobin value of 15 gm %):

- Before PEEP is increased, the patient has a $PaO_2$ of 60 mm Hg, $SaO_2$ of 90% ($CaO_2$ = 18.3 ml $O_2$/100 ml blood), and a cardiac output of 4.8 l/m. The $\dot{T}O_2$ is equal to 878 ml $O_2$/min.
- After PEEP is increased, the patient has a $PaO_2$ of 98 mm Hg, $SaO_2$ of 97% ($CaO_2$ = 19.8 ml $O_2$/100 ml blood). This is an increase in blood oxygen content. However, the increase in PEEP has caused the cardiac output to decrease to 3.5 l/m. As a result, the $\dot{T}O_2$ has now decreased to 693 ml $O_2$/min.

In this situation, it would be better to reduce the PEEP back to the previous level, which will have the following effects:

- A decrease in blood oxygenation (decreased $CaO_2$).
- Better tissue oxygenation because the greater cardiac output provides for the greatest transport rate of oxygen to the tissues (greatest $\dot{T}O_2$).

Calculating a value for $\dot{T}O_2$ provides an opportunity to take all of these factors into account when managing oxygenation.

$\dot{Q}_{sp}/\dot{Q}_T$ **Values.** Increased $\dot{Q}_{sp}/\dot{Q}_T$ values indicate disorders where pulmonary perfusion is in excess of the amount of ventilation (shunt effect), perfusion exists without any corresponding ventilation (true shunt), or both. Most often, pulmonary shunting is the result of disorders that either cause significant atelectasis (**ARDS**) or cause the filling of pulmonary air spaces with foreign substances (aspiration) or infiltrates (infectious pneumonitis).

$\dot{Q}_{sp}/\dot{Q}_T$ determinations can be interpreted on the basis of the following ranges of values:

- A *less than 10% shunt* can be accepted as normal.
- A *10%–20% shunt* indicates a mild disorder. Physiologic compensation of this amount of shunting is not difficult for most patients, however. This level of disorder is not life-threatening.
- A *20%–30% shunt* indicates a clinically significant shunt level. Additional disorders that limit cardiovascular reserves or central nervous system function can add to making this level of shunt a life-threatening disorder.
- A *greater than 30% shunt,* under any circumstances, indicates a potentially life-threatening disorder requiring an aggressive clinical response. Calculated shunts of greater than 60% have been observed in some surviving patients.

$\dot{V}_D/\dot{V}_T$ is often measured in conjunction with $\dot{Q}_{sp}/\dot{Q}_T$ in order to evaluate and compare both as possible sources of hypoxemia.

$FIO_2$ changes must be taken into account when serial shunt determinations are made and compared against $FIO_2$ values of 0.21 to 0.50. $\dot{Q}_{sp}/\dot{Q}_T$ values decrease as a patient's $FIO_2$ increases from 0.21 to 0.50. This is because the shunt-effect (as opposed to true shunting) contribution to $\dot{Q}_{sp}/\dot{Q}_T$ is being therapeutically relieved as $FIO_2$ values are increased up to 0.50. The shunt effect is minimized as a factor that contributes to the overall shunt. With $FIO_2$ values greater than 0.50, the shunt effect is eliminated, and only true shunting remains as a factor affecting $\dot{Q}_{sp}/\dot{Q}_T$. Therefore, $FIO_2$ changes are not a concern in interpreting shunt determinations made at $FIO_2$ values greater than .50.

*C(a-$\overline{v}$)O$_2$ and S$\overline{v}$O$_2$ Values.*   $C(a-\overline{v})O_2$ values made greater than 6 vol% indicate that the cardiovascular system is compromised. In other words, the available $\dot{Q}_T$ is less than adequate for meeting tissue oxygenation needs. As a result, an abnormally large quantity of oxygen is extracted by the tissues from each unit of arterial blood. When this condition occurs in conjunction with arterial blood hypoxemia, then significant tissue hypoxia can result.

$S\overline{v}O_2$ values can be affected either by changes in $PaO_2$ values or by changes in the factors that affect $C(a-\overline{v})O_2$. Changes in $PaO_2$ values must be taken into account in order to make use of $S\overline{v}O_2$ as a substitute for $C(a-\overline{v})O_2$.

Decreases in $PaO_2$ values can cause $S\overline{v}O_2$ values to decrease, even if cardiovascular function remains unchanged. The amount of oxygen in mixed venous blood will be reduced because there was less oxygen in the arterial blood, not because poor perfusion caused more oxygen than normal to be extracted by the tissues.

With normal or unchanged levels of arterial blood oxygenation ($PaO_2$), reduction of $S\overline{v}O_2$ values indicates a worsening of cardiovascular function. Cardiac output is reduced and there is a slower rate of blood movement through the tissue capillary beds. As a result, more than the normal amount of oxygen is being extracted per unit of blood.

The ability of a patient to maintain $S\overline{v}O_2$ values in the 70%–75% range, even in the face of arterial hypoxemia, indicates the availability of good cardiovascular reserves. Cardiac function is demonstrated to be at least marginally adequate as long as $S\overline{v}O_2$ values are $\geq$ 60%. $S\overline{v}O_2$ values less than 60% indicate that **cardiac decompensation** and tissue hypoxia may both be developing. A reduction of $S\overline{v}O_2$ values below 40% indicates significant cardiac decompensation. Clinical problems such as hypoxia, hypotension, arrhythmias, vasoconstriction, respiratory distress, and, possibly, cardiac arrest may soon follow.

It is possible for $S\overline{v}O_2$ values to change even without changes in $PaO_2$, cardiac output, or the general level of tissue oxygen consumption. Blood circulation can be redistributed to provide a greater proportion of the blood supply to organ systems that have a higher rate of oxygen utilization. In this situation, lower $S\overline{v}O_2$ values will result.

## Parameters for Assessment of Ventilation

$PCO_2$ values are inversely proportional to the level of alveolar ventilation. **Hypoventilation** will result in **hypercapnia**; **hyperventilation** will result in **hypocapnia**.

$PaCO_2$ values can be normal or reduced with some pulmonary disorders that cause hypoxemia. This is due to increases in alveolar ventilation. These increases are meant to serve as a compensatory mechanism for the $\dot{V}/\dot{Q}$ disorders that have produced the hypoxemia. Asthma, bronchitis, emphysema, foreign body obstruction, and pneumonia all, at least initially, can produce this pattern of hypoxemia and hypocapnia.

$\dot{V}/\dot{Q}$ disorders cause abnormalities in the alveolar-capillary exchange of both oxygen and carbon dioxide. At least theoretically, both hypoxemia and hypercapnia should result. Despite the fact that hypoxemia does occur, corresponding $PaCO_2$ increases are not often demonstrated. In fact, $PaCO_2$ values can be normal or even possibly reduced. As described above, this is because of the compensatory increases in alveolar ventilation that occur in response to the hypoxemia that is present.

Hypercapnia is often present with advanced pulmonary disorders. Significantly abnormal $\dot{V}/\dot{Q}$ relationships cause poor pulmonary gas exchange in these patients. A failure to adequately increase the compensatory alveolar ventilation level results in a combination of hypoxemia and hypercapnia.

With some pathologies, a poor ventilatory response to $\dot{V}/\dot{Q}$ abnormalities may be due simply to a subject's absolute inability to increase ventilation effectively. This is not always the case, however. In many people, especially those with chronic disorders, the hypercapnia may be due to a physiologic compromise. Some individuals have a low chemoreceptor/ventilatory response to elevated $PaCO_2$ levels. For them, the most comfortable physiologic choice may be to accept the elevated $PaCO_2$ level in order to permit a lower work of breathing (WOB). Other individuals have a greater chemoreceptor/ventilatory response to $PaCO_2$ levels. Their response for comfort will be to elevate ventilation to lower the $PaCO_2$, even if it means having to tolerate a greater WOB.

## Parameters for Assessment of Acid/Base Balance

Abnormalities in acid/base balance relate to the existence of abnormal states of either acidosis or alkalosis. Acidosis is present when arterial blood pH is less than 7.35. Alkalosis is present when arterial blood pH is greater than 7.45.

Abnormal states of acidosis and alkalosis can be caused by respiratory abnormalities alone, metabolic abnormalities alone, or combined metabolic/respiratory abnormalities. Thus, six basic abnormal acid/base states are possible:

---

### Acidosis

---

- Respiratory acidosis
- Metabolic acidosis
- Mixed metabolic/respiratory acidosis

---

### Alkalosis

---

- Respiratory alkalosis
- Metabolic alkalosis
- Mixed metabolic/respiratory alkalosis

Table 11–5 provides an example of normal blood gas values and examples for all of the possible abnormal blood gas values.

*Respiratory acidosis* and *alkalosis* are caused by changes in alveolar ventilation that affect $PaCO_2$ levels. *Metabolic acidosis* and *alkalosis* can result from a great variety of factors. Some of these factors are due to physiologic changes within the body. For example, lactic acidosis from tissue hypoxia will cause metabolic acidosis. Others are due to the ad-

## TABLE 11–5  Acid/Base States

| | pH | PaCO$_2$ (mm Hg) | HCO$_3^-$ (mEq/l) | BE* (mEq/l) |
|---|---|---|---|---|
| **Normal Values** | | | | |
| | 7.40 | 40 | 24 | 0 |
| | 7.35–7.45 | 35–45 | 22–26 | ±2 |
| Normal | 7.38 | 42 | 23.0 | 0.3 |
| **Respiratory (Resp.) Disorders** | | | | |
| **Acidosis** | | **Disorder** | **Compensation** | |
| Uncomp. Resp. Acidosis (Acute) | 7.20 | 63 | 24.0 | 0.0 |
| Part. Comp. Resp. Acidosis | 7.28 | 63 | 28.9 | +0.9 |
| Comp. Resp. Acidosis (Chronic) | 7.38 | 63 | 36.6 | +8.6 |
| **Alkalosis** | | **Disorder** | **Compensation** | |
| Uncomp. Resp. Alkalosis (Acute) | 7.60 | 24 | 24.0 | 0.0 |
| Part. Comp. Resp. Alkalosis | 7.52 | 24 | 19.6 | −1.7 |
| Comp. Resp. Alkalosis (Chronic) | 7.42 | 24 | 15.4 | −7.2 |
| **Metabolic (Met.) Disorders** | | | | |
| **Acidosis** | | **Compensation** | **Disorder** | |
| Uncomp. Met. Acidosis (Acute) | 7.20 | 40 | 15.2 | −13.0 |
| Part. Comp. Met. Acidosis | 7.28 | 33 | 15.2 | −13.0 |
| Comp. Met. Acidosis (Chronic) | 7.38 | 26 | 15.2 | −13.0 |
| **Alkalosis** | | **Compensation** | **Disorder** | |
| Uncomp. Met. Alkalosis (Acute) | 7.60 | 40 | 39.6 | +15.8 |
| Part. Comp. Met. Alkalosis | 7.52 | 49 | 39.6 | +15.8 |
| Comp. Met. Alkalosis (Chronic) | 7.42 | 62 | 39.6 | +15.8 |

**TABLE 11–5** *(Continued)*

### Mixed Respiratory/Metabolic Disorders

| | | Disorder | | Disorder |
|---|---|---|---|---|
| Mixed Resp. Met. Acidosis | 7.20 | 51 | 19.2 | −9.5 |
| Mixed Resp. Met. Alkalosis | 7.60 | 32 | 31.6 | +10.0 |

*Note: A hemoglobin value of 14 gm% and normal body temperature are assumed.*
*Resp. = respiratory.*
*Met. = metabolic.*
*Uncomp. = uncompensated.*
*Part. Comp. = partially compensated.*
*Comp. = compensated.*

ministration/ingestion of chemicals or drugs. For example, methyl alcohol poisoning will cause metabolic acidosis; diuretic therapy can result in metabolic alkalosis.

Some metabolic disorders can be due to therapeutic intervention. For example, metabolic alkalosis can be caused by the use of nasogastric tube suction and multiple blood transfusions. Acidosis or alkalosis resulting from combined respiratory/metabolic origins are caused by the coexistence of multiple factors.

Many clinical factors can cause acid/base abnormalities. For this reason, when an acid/base disorder is identified by blood gases, a thorough clinical evaluation should be made of the possible sources of the disorder.

# INDIRECT INDICATORS OF BLOOD GAS VALUES

In some clinical settings it is helpful to use indirect indicators of blood gas values. Transcutaneous $PO_2$ and $PCO_2$ monitoring and **capnography** both offer the ability to perform indirect assessment of blood gases.

## TRANSCUTANEOUS GAS MEASUREMENT

### Test Description

Transcutaneous measurement of $PO_2$ and $PCO_2$ provides useful trend-monitoring information. $PtcO_2$ and $PtcCO_2$ values can be correlated to $PaO_2$ and $PaCO_2$ values in patients who have a stable cardiovascular system. The measurement of $PtcO_2$ and $PtcCO_2$ is noninvasive and allows for continuous, real-time monitoring and assessment. Transcutaneous gas values cannot completely substitute for the use of arterial blood gas values, however. Correlation between the two sets of values may be good under certain conditions. Under other conditions, though, questionable or poor correlation of results can occur.

The primary reason for inconsistent correlation between the two sets of values is the fact that two different factors determine $PtcO_2$ and $PtcCO_2$ values:

1. The values for $PaO_2$ and $PaCO_2$ that exist. As these values increase or decrease, the values for $PtcO_2$ and $PtcCO_2$ will increase and decrease correspondingly.
2. The rate of local perfusion at the site where the measuring electrode is placed. This rate can be affected either by changes in total systemic circulation or by local changes in perfusion at the site of the electrode. As skin perfusion decreases, values for $PtcO_2$ will decrease, and $PtcCO_2$ values will increase in relation to the actual $PaO_2$ and $PaCO_2$ values. $PtcCO_2$ values are less affected by perfusion changes than are $PtcO_2$ values. As a result, $PtcCO_2$ values may have a greater clinical usefulness in both adults and infants. This is due to the greater diffusibility of $CO_2$ molecules through the body tissues.

The outcome of these two factors is that *a decrease in $PtcO_2$ may be due to hypoxemia, decreased cardiac output (hypotension), or cutaneous vasoconstriction.*

There is a reasonably close correlation between $PaO_2$ and $PtcO_2$ in infants with stable cardiovascular systems. In adults, $PtcO_2$ values generally trend approximately 20% below $PaO_2$ values. These lower values are because of the thicker keratin layer of adult skin. The thickness of this layer creates a greater barrier to oxygen diffusion and reduces the amount of cutaneous oxygen reaching the electrode. For this reason, transcutaneous monitors are more widely used in infant critical care than in adult care.

In neonates, $PtcO_2$ tends to overestimate $PaO_2$ values. In subjects one year old or older, $PtcO_2$ tends to underestimate $PaO_2$ values. The difference in values increases with advancing age.

$PtcCO_2$ values are generally slightly higher than $PaCO_2$ values. These higher values are because of the increased $CO_2$ production that results from the electrode's heating of the skin. The age of the subject has less of an effect on $PtcCO_2$ values than it does on $PtcO_2$ values.

## Equipment Required

Heated electrodes are used to determine transcutaneous gas values. The heat of the electrode has two effects on the skin:

1. Local perfusion increases, and the cutaneous capillary blood becomes "arterialized."
2. The skin lipid structure breaks down, and gas diffusion through the skin occurs more easily.

Both of these factors together allow arterial blood gas values to be approximately measured by electrodes placed on the skin surface. Electrode temperatures of 43.5°C to 45°C are used. With infants, temperatures at the lower end of this range are used.

A heated Clark skin electrode is used for determining $PtcO_2$ values. Monitors are also available for use on the conjunctiva of the eye and on the oropharynx mucus membranes. A heated Severinghaus electrode is used to determine $PtcCO_2$. $PtcCO_2$ electrodes are more difficult to calibrate and have slower response times than $PtcO_2$ electrodes. There are transcutaneous monitors available that combine both a $PO_2$ and a $PCO_2$ electrode in the same sensor unit. As with any gas measurement system, regular calibration must be performed to maintain measurement accuracy.

## Test Administration

A well-perfused skin site with thin subcutaneous layers should be chosen for transcutaneous gas measurements. For infants, sites such as the chest, abdomen, and inner thigh can be used. The forearm, chest, and forehead are good sites for use on adult subjects. Hair at the site must be removed by shaving.

Transcutaneous electrodes must be moved to a different skin site at least every four hours. This practice minimizes the risk of burn injuries that can be caused by the electrode heater. Poor perfusion at the site increases the risk of burn injuries. The electrode must be moved at least every three hours for hypothermic patients or other patients with poor cutaneous perfusion. A reequilibration time of 20–30 minutes will be required each time the electrode site is changed. Until equilibration is complete, the correlation of transcutaneous to arterial values will be less than optimum.

## Interpretation of Test Results

The best correlation between arterial blood and transcutaneous gas values is in patients who maintain a reasonably good level of cardiovascular function. Reduced cardiac output and hypotension can decrease cutaneous perfusion at the location of the electrode. Despite stable $PaO_2$ values, the result is a drop in the measured $PtcO_2$. $PtcCO_2$ values are generally less affected by changes in skin perfusion. This is true as long as the skin is adequately heated by the electrode.

## CAPNOGRAPHY

## Test Description

**Capnography** is the continuous, noninvasive monitoring of $CO_2$ values in the air at the patient's proximal airway. Monitoring is done throughout the breathing cycle. Measurements made during the expiratory phase of breathing provide the most useful information.

Numerical values for $CO_2$ measurements (**capnometry**) and visual representation of $PCO_2$ waveforms during the breathing cycle (capnography) both have clinical significance. With capnography, waveforms demonstrating the changes in $PCO_2$ levels during individual breaths can be displayed, or the trend of end-tidal $CO_2$ levels can be displayed in a series.

The single-breath **capnogram** for a normal subject is shown in Figure 11–1. During inspiration, the measured $PCO_2$ is that of the incoming inspired air and is, for all practical purposes, 0.0 mm Hg. With expiration, the measured $PCO_2$ undergoes considerable change. During Phase I of expiration, unrespired anatomic deadspace gas is being exhaled and measured. The measured $PCO_2$ for this gas is again 0.0 mm Hg.

The measured $PCO_2$ during Phase II rises sharply. This rise represents the mixing and transition from deadspace gas to alveolar gas. Phase III represents the contribution to exhaled air of the millions of emptying alveoli. In a normal lung with well-matched venti-

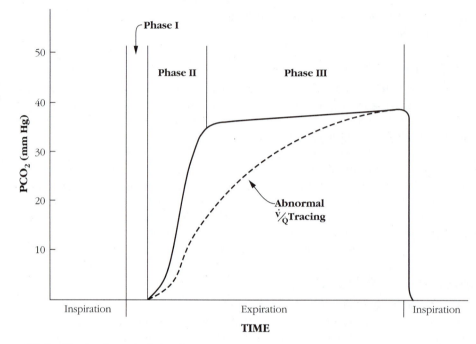

**Figure 11–1** *Tracing for a single-breath capnogram.*

lation and perfusion, the $PCO_2$ values of these alveoli are reasonably uniform. This uniformity results in the Phase III "alveolar plateau" of the normal waveform. The $PCO_2$ value at the end of the Phase III alveolar plateau is called the *end-tidal $PCO_2$* (PetCO_2).

In use, PetCO_2 values are presumed to approximate PACO_2 values. It is necessary to understand the factors that affect PACO_2 in order to understand the significance of PetCO_2 changes. The level of alveolar $PCO_2$ is affected by the following factors:

1. The rate that $CO_2$ is available to diffuse into the alveoli. This is determined by
   • Tissue $CO_2$ *production* and therefore venous blood $CO_2$ levels.
   • The rate of flow for venous blood returning to the lungs (*perfusion*).
2. The level of $CO_2$ that is maintained in the alveoli based on the amount of alveolar ventilation (*ventilation*).

Clinically, PetCO_2 values provide a nonspecific indicator of cardiopulmonary function. Conditions that produce changes in $CO_2$ production, pulmonary perfusion, or pulmonary ventilation can all affect PetCO_2 values.

The significance of this is that PACO_2 and therefore PetCO_2 are both affected by changes in either ventilation or perfusion levels within the lung. Figure 11–2 illustrates the relationship between $\dot{V}/\dot{Q}$ ratio changes and the corresponding changes in PACO_2 that result. For a pulmonary unit with a normal $\dot{V}/\dot{Q}$ relationship, the values for PACO_2 approximate normal PaCO_2 values.

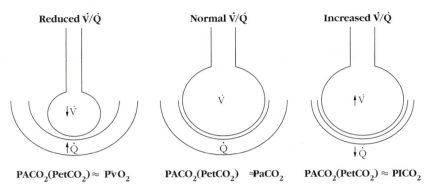

**Figure 11–2** *Relationship between V̇/Q̇ changes and PACO$_2$ changes.*

Abnormalities in V̇/Q̇ relationships affect PACO$_2$ values (see Figure 11–2). If the rate of ventilation to a pulmonary unit is reduced in relation to its perfusion rate (i.e., decreased V̇/Q̇ ratio), the PACO$_2$ values begin to increase and can approximate P̄vCO$_2$ values. This is because alveolar CO$_2$ is not effectively ventilated out in relation to the rate of incoming CO$_2$ from the venous blood. It is not possible for PACO$_2$ values to exceed P̄vCO$_2$ values, however.

When ventilation is increased in proportion to the available perfusion (i.e., increased V̇/Q̇ ratios) there will be less new CO$_2$ entering the alveoli to replace that which is ventilated out. As a result, the PACO$_2$ (and PetCO$_2$ value) will decrease and, in the extreme, can become equal to the PICO$_2$.

As will be discussed later, these relationships provide a basis for using the comparison between PaCO$_2$ and PetCO$_2$ values as an indicator of V̇/Q̇ abnormalities. This comparison is referred to as the *arterial to end-tidal PCO$_2$ difference* [P(a-et)CO$_2$]. P(a-et)CO$_2$ is a more sensitive indicator of increased V̇/Q̇ ratio (deadspace) problems than it is of decreased V̇/Q̇ ratio (shunt) problems. It is more sensitive because there is a greater range of variation between PICO$_2$ and PACO$_2$ values than there is between PACO$_2$ and P̄vCO$_2$ values.

Figure 11–1 also illustrates the effects that nonuniform V̇/Q̇ relationships, and therefore nonuniform PACO$_2$ values, can have on a capnogram tracing. As can be seen, the result is a more gradual increase in exhaled PCO$_2$ values with little or no alveolar plateau.

## Equipment Required

Both infrared and mass spectrometer measurement systems are used for capnometry/ capnography. The infrared systems can use either *mainstream* or *sidestream* sampling methods. Mass spectrometers use sidestream sampling only.

Figure 11–3 illustrates a mainstream sampling system. With mainstream sampling, the sample chamber is located at the patient's airway and the exhaled air passes directly through it. This system permits a precise, nearly instantaneous capnogram with each breath. Unfortunately, mainstream systems are difficult to use in patients who do not have an artificial airway (tracheostomy tube or endotracheal tube) in use. The sensor is likely to be damaged if it is mishandled or dropped. It also adds mechanical deadspace and

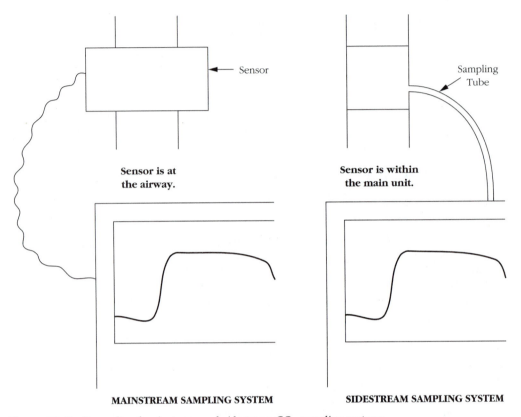

**Figure 11–3**  *Examples of mainstream and sidestream $CO_2$ sampling systems.*

weight to the patient's airway. Fortunately, the newest mainstream sensors minimize these problems.

A sidestream sampling system is also shown in Figure 11–3. With sidestream sampling, the sample gas is continuously aspirated from the patient's airway. The gas is carried to a measurement chamber within the capnometer by way of a small-bore tubing.

Sidestream sampling minimizes most of the problems of mainstream sensor systems. It creates other problems, however. Gas flow through the sample tubing can be obstructed by secretions, condensed moisture, or kinking of the tubing. There is a delay between the initial sampling of gas at the airway and the actual measurement of $CO_2$ concentrations. This delay is affected by both the length and diameter of the sample tubing.

Measurement in sidestream systems is also affected by the flow rate of gas sample aspiration. Aspiration flow rates that are too slow can cause dampening and artifacts of the capnogram waveform. Excessively fast aspiration can result in ambient air being sampled and measured at end-expiration, just prior to the start of the next inspiration. Most units use a sample aspiration flow rate of approximately 150 ml/min.

There are other important factors that can affect the operation of sidestream systems. For example, the sample port must be attached to or near the patient's airway in a manner that prevents ambient air from being aspirated with the sample gas. Ambient air contamination of the gas sample will cause falsely low $PCO_2$ readings. This can be a problem even if the sample aspiration flow rates are reasonable.

The tubing used for sampling should be impermeable to $CO_2$ and free of leaks that might contaminate the sample with ambient air. Secretions and excess moisture are generally removed from the gas sample prior to the gas reaching the measuring chamber. Filters, water traps, and, in some units, reverse gas flow purging of the tubing are used to protect the measuring chamber. It should be noted that reverse flow purging can increase the risk of infection control problems. Table 11–6 lists equipment factors that can affect $PetCO_2$ measurements.

## Test Administration

Both mainstream and sidestream systems can be connected directly to an artificial airway. This connection permits use of capnometry/capnography during mechanical ventilation. Sidestream systems are best for patients who do not have an artificial airway. One method is to incorporate the sample aspiration tube into one of the prongs of a nasal cannula. Gas samples are then aspirated from the gas that is entering and leaving through the nasal cavity.

As stated earlier, sidestream sampling can, inadvertently, permit ambient air to be aspirated during the end-expiratory pause that occurs just prior to the start of the next inspiration. This contamination will cause a drop in the measured $PCO_2$ right at the end of expiration. As a result, a $PetCO_2$ value actually taken at the end of expiration would provide a falsely low reading. An alternative approach can be used to avoid this problem. A peak $PCO_2$ value occurring earlier in the exhaled $PCO_2$ waveform can be used instead of the $PCO_2$ measured at the end of expiration. In this case, terms such as "peak" or "maximal" exhaled $PCO_2$ may be more appropriate than the term "end-tidal $PCO_2$."

---

**TABLE 11–6  Equipment Factors That Can Affect PetCO$_2$ Values**

### Equipment Factors That Can Increase PetCO$_2$ Values

- Leaks in a mechanical ventilation breathing circuit.
- Rebreathing of exhaled air.
- Depletion of the $CO_2$ absorber in a rebreathing type of anesthesia circuit.

### Equipment Factors That Can Decrease PetCO$_2$ Values

- Patient disconnection from a mechanical ventialtor breathing circuit.
- Partial or complete deflation of the cuff of an artificial airway.
- Complete airway obstruction.
- Esophageal intubation.
- Gas-sample contamination with ambient air.

## Interpretation of Test Results

In normal subjects, $PetCO_2$ values generally approximate $PaCO_2$ values. Table 11–7 provides examples of clinical factors that can increase and decrease $PetCO_2$ values. $PetCO_2$ changes can indicate the trend of changing $PaCO_2$ values once the amount of difference between the two has been established.

Capnometers offer only a numerical reading of $PetCO_2$ and do not provide a visual capnogram display. As a result, the clinical usefulness of the information is somewhat limited. Capnogram tracings provide greater clinical information than the use of capnometry alone. Figure 11–4 provides an example of a normal capnogram tracing. Figure 11–4 also provides examples of tracings where $PetCO_2$ values are abnormally elevated and an example of a tracing that can result when $\dot{V}/\dot{Q}$ abnormalities are present in the subject.

The normal value for $P(a\text{-}et)CO_2$ is less than 5 mm Hg. An increase in $P(a\text{-}et)CO_2$ values indicates that the $\dot{V}/\dot{Q}$ ratios within the lungs have increased (increased deadspace ventilation). Poor alveolar emptying can also produce increased $P(a\text{-}et)CO_2$ values. This is because the incomplete emptying results in a falsely low end-tidal $CO_2$ value. Table 11–8 lists specific factors that can cause increases in $P(a\text{-}et)CO_2$ values.

Gross mismatching of $\dot{V}/\dot{Q}$ relationships can occur in subjects with severe obstructive disorders. It is possible, in these individuals, for $PetCO_2$ values to exceed $PaCO_2$ values. The result would be a negative value for $P(a\text{-}et)CO_2$.

# PEDIATRIC BLOOD GAS ASSESSMENT

The determination of blood gas values in infants and children differs from that in adult subjects. The differences include the sampling sites, the size of the blood sample, and the choice of methods (i.e., arterial samples, arterialized samples, transcutaneous monitoring, and pulse oximetry).

## ARTERIAL SAMPLING

The sampling procedures for arterial blood gas determinations present special problems in pediatric patients, especially for newborns, infants, and very young children. The choice of arterial sampling sites, the sample size, and the alternative arterial sampling methods used are all different in pediatric cases.

## Arterial Puncture

Sampling sites for arterial puncture are more limited with infants than with adults. For children, sampling from brachial and femoral sites presents a greater risk of nerve palsy, osteomyelitis, and bleeding problems. These sites should not be used at all in infants and young children. Rather, the temporal arteries in the scalp and the radial arteries are preferred sites for these subjects. A heparin-washed, 25-gauge scalp vein needle can be used on a blood gas syringe for performing arterial puncture at the temporal artery site. As

TABLE 11–7  **Clinical Factors Affecting PetCO$_2$ Values**

### Clinical Factors That Can Increase PetCO$_2$ Values

*As related to an increased diffusion rate of CO$_2$ into the alveoli:*

- Increased CO$_2$ Production
   Bicarbonate administration
   Hyperthermia (fever)
   Increased metabolic rates
   Sepsis
   Seizures
   Use of nutritional support that produces a higher respiratory quotient

*As related to decreased alveolar ventilation:*

- Central nervous system depression
- Central nervous system disorders (direct trauma, bacterial or viral infection, cancers/tumors, primary idiopathic alveolar hypoventilation)
- Musculoskeletal disorders
- Neuromuscular disorders
- Obstructive pulmonary disorders

### Clinical Factors That Can Decrease PetCO$_2$ Values

*As related to a decreased diffusion rate of CO$_2$ into the alveoli:*

- Decreased CO$_2$ Production
   Hypothermia
   Use of nutritional support that produces a lower respiratory quotient

- Decreased CO$_2$ Delivery to the Lungs
   Cardiac arrest
   Hemorrhage
   Hypotension
   Pulmonary embolism
   Pulmonary hypoperfusion

*As related to increases in alveolar ventilation:*

- Cerebrovascular disorders
- Certain drugs (salicylates, progesterone, aminophylline)
- Head trauma
- Hypoxemia
- Response to metabolic acidosis
- Psychogenic hyperventilation
- Vagally mediated stimulation of pulmonary receptors due to interstitial disorders

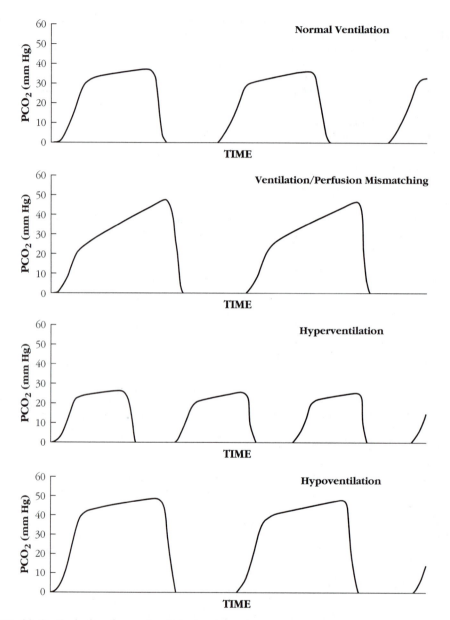

**Figure 11–4** *Examples of normal and abnormal capnograms.*

with adult subjects, the modified Allen's test must be performed before a radial artery puncture is performed.

The majority of pediatric patients will cry during an arterial puncture procedure. Generally children will hyperventilate during the procedure even if they are not crying. Small infants with pulmonary disorders can easily have their $PaO_2$ values affected by such factors as breath holding and crying during the procedure.

---

**TABLE 11–8  Factors Increasing P(a-et)CO$_2$ Values**

---

### Conditions Resulting in Increased Deadspace Ventilation

---

#### *Pulmonary Conditions/Ventilatory State*

---

- Emphysema and, to some degree, asthma and chronic bronchitis
- High rate, low tidal volume ventilatory patterns
- Positive pressure ventilation (especially with PEEP)

---

#### *Cardiovascular/Vascular Conditions*

---

- Cardiac arrest
- Hypotension with pulmonary hypoperfusion
- Pulmonary embolism
- Lateral decubitus body position

---

### Conditions Resulting in Incomplete Alveolar Emptying

---

- Tachypnea in subjects with airway obstruction:
    Asthma, chronic bronchitis, emphysema
    Upper airway obstruction
    Partial obstruction of an artificial airway

---

### Poor Gas Sampling Technique

---

- A large leak around the artificial airway that results in loss of a portion of the tidal volume.
- The airway adapter is placed too close to a flow source of fresh gas.
- A monitor with a slow sensor response time is being used on a tachypneic subject.
- A sidestream monitor with a high gas sample aspiration flow rate is being used on a subject with small tidal volumes.

---

## Arterial Catheterization

It is possible to perform arterial catheterization on children. There are significant potential hazards related to catheterization, however, primarily because of the child's smaller size. As for any subject, hemorrhage and infection are a risk. With children, the risks of thromboembolism and ischemia in the tissues distal to the catheter site are probably greater, again because of the child's smaller size.

In infants, the umbilical artery can be catheterized if the procedure is performed within the first 48 hours following birth. Having an umbilical artery catheter can certainly make infant arterial blood sampling more convenient. But use of an umbilical artery catheter can lead to a significant problem with anemia.

In an infant, the total blood volume is approximately 85 ml/kg of body weight. For the typical term infant, this amounts to approximately 300 ml of total blood volume. Given the same weight/blood-volume relationship, a preterm infant can have a total blood volume of 150 ml. It can even be as little as 60 ml in extremely small preterm infants. Because of these small blood volumes, the blood sample size taken from the infant and the frequency of sampling become important. A sick preterm infant can rapidly become anemic as a result of frequent blood sampling.

Three clinical practices can be used to offset the negative effects of arterial blood sampling in infants:

- Keeping the frequency of blood sampling and sample size to a minimum. Most blood gas analyzers can operate effectively on less than 1 ml of blood.
- Using replacement blood products to offset the development of anemia.
- Using noninvasive methods for monitoring blood gas values (e.g., transcutaneous monitoring and pulse oximetry) in order to minimize the need for blood sampling.

## ARTERIALIZED BLOOD SAMPLING

Arterialized blood sampling is an alternative to using arterial blood to assess infants and small children. Although not an equivalent replacement for arterial blood gas values, arterialized blood pH, $PO_2$, and $PCO_2$ values can be used as an *estimate* of arterial blood values.

Arterialized blood samples provide adequate estimation of arterial pH and $PCO_2$ values. Arterial ($PaO_2$) and arterialized ($PacO_2$) $PO_2$ values demonstrate a lesser degree of correlation. The correlation is poorest when

1. Samples are taken during the first few days of a newborn's life, especially if the actual arterial $PO_2$ is greater than 60 mm Hg.
2. Subjects have either local (at the site of sampling) or systemic reductions in circulation.

Additionally, the procedure used to procure the blood sample can greatly affect measurement. Squeezing or milking of the sample site, for instance, will produce falsely low $PacO_2$ values as compared with actual $PaO_2$ values.

## ALTERNATIVES TO BLOOD SAMPLING

The applications of transcutaneous $PO_2$ and $PCO_2$ monitoring and pulse oximetry for $SpO_2$ values are very effective in infants. These methods of assessment can have a significant impact on decreasing the number of blood samples that must be drawn from a subject. Additionally, they permit for *continuous* monitoring of values.

## Review Questions

Please use the following review questions to evaluate your learning of information from this chapter. It might be helpful to write out your answers on a sheet of paper. If you are unsure of the answers to these questions, review the chapter to reinforce your learning.

1. Relating to the blood samples that might be used for blood gas assessment:
   a. What are different types of blood samples that might be used for assessment of blood gas values?
   b. How are each of the different types of samples useful?
2. Relating to parameters measured for the assessment of oxygenation:
   a. What is the clinical significance of measurements for the partial pressure of oxygen?
   b. What is the clinical significance of measurements such as %MetHb, %HbCO, Total Hb, $SaO_2$, and $P_{50}$ for evaluating the hemoglobin transport of oxygen?
   c. What is the clinical significance of the blood oxygen content determination?
   d. What are the different methods for determining the amount of intrapulmonary shunting?
   e. Is it necessary for a patient to be on 100% oxygen when a value for shunt is determined?
   f. What shortcut equation can be used for determining a value for shunt?
   g. What is the clinical significance of values such as $C(a-\bar{v})O_2$, $O_2ER$, and $S\bar{v}O_2$ for assessing tissue oxygenation?
3. What is the clinical significance of $PaCO_2$ for the assessment of ventilation?
4. Relating to assessment of acid/base balance:
   a. How is pH significant to the assessment of acid/base balance?
   b. How is the $PaCO_2$ significant? How is $HCO_3^-$ significant?
5. Relating to equipment needed for blood sampling:
   a. What equipment is required for arterial blood sampling?
   b. What equipment is required for arterialized blood sampling?
6. Relating to blood analysis:
   a. How is a blood gas analyzer used to perform blood analysis?
   b. How is a CO-oximeter used to perform blood analysis?
   c. How is a pulse oximeter used to perform blood analysis?
7. Relating to performing arterial blood sampling for blood gas analysis:
   a. How is arterial blood sampling performed when it is to be used for blood gas analysis?
   b. How is the modified Allen's test performed?
   c. What is the significance of the modified Allen's test?
   d. How should the blood sample be handled once it has been drawn?
   e. What precautions should be taken by the technologist to avoid the risk of blood-borne infection?
8. What are concerns for use and maintenance of blood gas analyzers?
9. Relating to normal blood gas values:
   a. What are normal values for blood gas assessment of oxygenation?

    b. What are normal values for blood gas assessment of ventilation?

    c. What are normal values for blood gas assessment of acid/base balance?

10. What is the difference between hypoxemia and hypoxia?

11. Relating to circumstances that may change $PaO_2$ values:

    a. What happens to $PaO_2$ values with advancing subject age?

    b. What happens to $PaO_2$ values when 100% oxygen is breathed?

12. Relating to abnormalities of oxygenation:

    a. What are the factors that can cause hypoxemia?

    b. Which one of these factors is most significant for causing hypoxemia?

    c. How are $PaO_2$ values that are measured at rest clinically useful?

    d. What is the effect on $PaO_2$ values of disorders that have an equal impact on both ventilation and perfusion?

    e. How do significant ventilation/perfusion abnormalities affect $PaO_2$ values?

    f. How do $PaO_2$ values relate to spirometry values when pulmonary disorders are present?

    g. What is the clinical significance of methemoglobinemia?

    h. How is methemoglobinemia treated?

    i. What is the clinical significance of carboxyhemoglobinemia?

    j. How is it carboxyhemoglobinemia treated?

    k. What is the clinical significance of anemia?

    l. What is the clinical significance of polycythemia?

    m. How can $SaO_2$ values be used to evaluate arterial blood oxygenation?

    n. What is the clinical significance of $P_{50}$ values?

    o. What is the clinical significance of $CaO_2$ values?

    p. What is the clinical significance of shunt determination?

    q. What is the relationship between the percent of shunt and the severity of pulmonary disorder?

    r. What is the clinical significance of $C(a\text{-}\bar{v})O_2$ and $S\bar{v}O_2$ determinations?

13. Relating to abnormalities of ventilation:

    a. What is the relationship between hypoventilation, hyperventilation, hypercapnia, and hypocapnia?

    b. What is the relationship between hypoxemia and hypocapnia?

    c. What is the relationship between ventilation/perfusion abnormalities and $PaCO_2$ values?

14. Relating to acid/base abnormalities:

    a. What are the six possible abnormal acid/base states?

    b. What are the causes of these states?

15. Relating to transcutaneous gas measurements:

    a. How are transcutaneous gas measurements clinically useful?

    b. Why is there inconsistent correlation between transcutaneous gas values and arterial blood gas values?

    c. How is this inconsistent correlation clinically significant?

    d. What equipment is required for transcutaneous gas measurement?

    e. How is transcutaneous gas measurement administered?

    f. What conditions produce the best correlation between transcutaneous gas and arterial blood gas measurements?

16. Relating to capnography:
    a. How is capnography performed?
    b. What is the appearance of a capnogram produced during a single tidal breath?
    c. How do PetCO$_2$ values relate to pulmonary perfusion and ventilation?
    d. What equipment is required for capnography?
    e. What is the difference between a mainstream and a sidestream sampling system?
    f. What are some clinical concerns when capnography is administered?
    g. What clinical factors can increase PetCO$_2$ values?
    h. What clinical factors can decrease PetCO$_2$ values?
    i. What clinical factors can alter the shape of a capnogram?

17. Relating to blood gases for pediatric patients:
    a. How can arterial blood sampling be performed for pediatric patients?
    b. How close is the correlation between arterialized blood gas values and arterial values?
    c. What are some alternatives to the sampling of blood for pediatric blood gas assessment?

# CHAPTER TWELVE

# EXERCISE PHYSIOLOGY

───────── **LEARNING OBJECTIVES** ─────────

Upon successful completion of this chapter, the learner should be able to

1. Describe the physiologic needs to be met during both rest and exercise in relation to
   a. physiologic energy requirements
   b. pulmonary ventilation
   c. external respiration
   d. cardiovascular function
   e. internal respiration
   f. metabolism
2. Describe the general physiologic adaptions that take place during exercise in relation to
   a. metabolism
   b. the systemic capillary bed
   c. the heart and vascular system
   d. the pulmonary capillary bed
   e. ventilation
3. Describe significant physiologic adaptations and parameters during exercise, including
   a. metabolism parameters
   b. pulmonary parameters
   c. cardiovascular parameters

## KEY TERMS

acid
acidotic
arteriolar constriction
buffing system
bulk flow
cytoplasm
diffusion
enzyme
homeostasis
interstitial fluid

interstitial space
mitochondria
mole
organelle
oxygen content
proprioceptors
sedentary
skeletal muscle
smooth muscle

A basic understanding of exercise physiology is helpful to understanding the concepts of exercise testing. If studied in depth, exercise physiology is a very complex subject. The goal for this chapter, however, is to provide a simple but complete overview of exercise physiology.

# PHYSIOLOGIC NEEDS DURING REST AND EXERCISE

Whether at rest or performing exercise, the human body has a need for energy. Nutrients are taken into the body, but in their ingested form, they cannot serve directly as an energy source. The nutrients must first be converted into a chemical form that is physiologically usable.

## PHYSIOLOGIC ENERGY REQUIREMENTS

All physiologic work performed within the body and physical work performed by the body require some degree of work at the cellular level. The broad range of different intracellular chemical processes that are used in order meet these needs is collectively called *metabolism*. A physiologic source of energy must be available to the cells in order for the chemical processes of metabolism to take place.

Physiologically, the chemical energy source used by all living organisms is the compound *adenosine triphosphate* (ATP). The chemical breakdown of ATP to form *adenosine diphosphate* (ADP) releases the energy that is stored in ATP. This is demonstrated by the following equation:

$$\text{ATP} \xrightarrow{\text{enzyme}} \text{ADP} + \text{P} + \text{energy}$$

where an **enzyme** is used to facilitate the chemical reaction, and P represents the phosphate radical released during the reaction.

Each cell in an organism must be capable of manufacturing ATP for its own use. ATP production is itself a form of metabolism. For this reason, it requires the use of at least some ATP in order to initiate and move the process of ATP production along. ATP production is based on reversing the earlier equation.

$$ADP + P + energy \xrightarrow{\text{enzyme}} ATP$$

Muscular work in humans requires the use of tremendous amounts of ATP as an energy source. In order for ATP to be produced and used effectively, two physiologic requirements must be met:

1. The fuel needed for ATP production must be supplied.
2. Waste products that result from ATP production must be removed.

Unless these requirements are met, the amount of muscular work that an individual is capable of performing will be limited.

## OVERVIEW OF PHYSIOLOGIC MECHANISMS

The majority of ATP-producing metabolism takes place within the **mitochondria** of a cell. In single-cell organisms, the processes of fuel supply and waste removal for ATP production are easily met by movement of the substances across the cell's membrane or wall. Since humans are large, multicellular organisms, we require more complex mechanisms to support cellular function. The three basic mechanisms used to meet the needs of cellular work for muscle cells in humans are transport, exchange, and metabolism.

*Transport* is the **bulk flow** or movement of the substances needed to support muscle cell work. Transport is demonstrated through

- Pulmonary *ventilation*, which accomplishes the movement of oxygen (fuel) into and carbon dioxide (waste) out of the body.
- Cardiovascular *circulation*, which carries oxygen from the lungs and to the muscle tissue for use and carries carbon dioxide from the muscle tissue and to the lungs for removal.

*Exchange* takes place by means of the **diffusion** of substances. Exchange is demonstrated through

- *External respiration* within the lungs. External respiration is the movement of oxygen from the alveolar gas and into the pulmonary capillary blood and the movement of carbon dioxide from the pulmonary capillary blood and into the alveolar gas. The *respiratory exchange ratio* (R) is the ratio of this exchange within the lungs between oxygen ($\dot{V}_L O_2$) and carbon dioxide ($\dot{V}_L CO_2$). The ratio is expressed in the following way:

$$R = \frac{\dot{V}_L CO_2}{\dot{V}_L O_2} = \frac{200 \text{ ml/min}}{250 \text{ ml/min}} = 0.80$$

where, using normal resting values for $\dot{V}_L O_2$ and $\dot{V}_L CO_2$, the normal value for R is 0.80.

- *Internal respiration* within the muscles. Internal respiration is the movement of oxygen from the muscle tissue capillary blood into the muscle tissue cells and the movement of carbon dioxide from the muscle tissue cells into the muscle tissue capillary blood. The exchange of nutrients (carbohydrates, for example) between the blood and the muscle tissue cells also occurs at this level.

*Metabolism* normally requires that oxygen is consumed in the production of ATP and that carbon dioxide is produced as a waste. This ratio of $O_2$ consumption ($\dot{V}O_2$) to $CO_2$ production ($\dot{V}CO_2$) is called the *respiratory quotient* (RQ). The ratio is expressed in the following way:

$$RQ = \frac{\dot{V}CO_2}{\dot{V}O_2} = \frac{200 \text{ ml/min}}{250 \text{ ml/min}} = 0.80$$

where, using normal resting values for $\dot{V}O_2$ and $\dot{V}CO_2$, the normal value for RQ is 0.80.

As can be seen, the normal value for both R and RQ is 0.80. What this represents is that the rate of oxygen supply and carbon dioxide removal in the lungs is equal to the rate of oxygen consumption and carbon dioxide production in the tissues. These equal rates of exchange are necessary for maintaining physiologic **homeostasis**.

Figure 12–1 demonstrates the relationships between all of these physiologic mechanisms. In the diagram, an effort has been made to show the interconnections between the mechanisms. This is done by using a gearlike linkage of the rotational directions taken by the mechanisms. A reduction or loss of function in any one mechanism will result in the others also being made less functional in supporting the needs of the body.

The processes used in transport, exchange, and metabolism will now be discussed in greater detail.

## PULMONARY VENTILATION

The purpose of pulmonary ventilation is the exchange of gases between the atmosphere and the alveolar-capillary interface. This exchange serves to

- Supply oxygen from the atmosphere into the lungs for use in the external respiration exchange process.
- Remove carbon dioxide in the lung that results from the external respiration exchange process and eliminate it into the atmosphere.

The overall ventilation of the lung ($\dot{V}_E$) is affected by a combination of the *respiratory rate* (f) and *tidal volume* ($V_T$) used in breathing. This can be represented in the following way:

$$\dot{V}_E = f \times V_T$$

Increases in f, $V_T$, or both will increase ventilation.

Not all lung ventilation effectively reaches the alveolar gas/blood exchange interface. *Physiologic deadspace volume* ($V_D$) is the total volume of the areas in the lung where gas exchange with alveolar capillary blood is not possible. $V_D$ includes both the volume of the conducting airways in the lungs (*anatomic deadspace volume*, $V_Dan$) and the alveolar re-

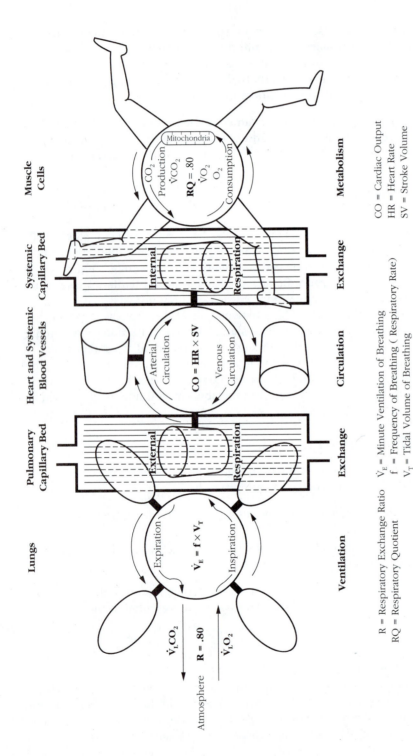

**Figure 12–1** *Relationships between the physiologic mechanisms that support muscular work.*

gions where pulmonary capillary blood flow for gas exchange has been significantly reduced or has been lost (*alveolar deadspace volume*, $V_D$alv). The portion of the $V_T$ that does ventilate alveoli with the capillary blood flow needed for gas exchange is called the *effective alveolar volume* ($V_A$eff).

In normal individuals, there is no loss or reduction of the alveolar capillary blood flow needed for gas exchange, and $V_D$alv does not exist. Therefore, in the normal lung, the $V_D$ is comprised solely of and is equal to the $V_D$an.

Normally, between 20% and 40% of each breath's $V_T$ is $V_D$. The $V_D$an and thus the $V_D$ are relatively fixed in their values (approximately 1 ml/lb of lean body weight). This is significant because *in situations where an increase in $V_T$ occurs, the $V_D$ accounts for a lesser percentage of each breath's volume*. In other words, as breathing volumes increase, a greater proportion of each breath is $V_A$eff and a lesser proportion is $V_D$. Stated still another way, for a constant level of lung ventilation, changes in breathing rate and volume will affect the proportion of lung ventilation that is deadspace.

- Small breaths and fast breathing rates used to maintain a constant level of ventilation will increase the proportion of ventilation that is deadspace.
- Large breaths and slow breathing rates used to maintain the same constant level of ventilation will decrease the proportion of ventilation that is deadspace.

In a normal individual, $V_T$ is approximately 500 ml and $V_D$ is approximately 150 ml. This means that the $V_A$eff for each breath is approximately 350 ml.

The purpose of ventilation is to increase the quantity of $O_2$ and decrease the quantity of $CO_2$ in the blood that passes through the alveolar capillary bed. Increases in ventilation will only slightly increase the quantity of $O_2$ per unit volume of blood. However, it will significantly decrease the quantity of $CO_2$ in the blood.

## EXTERNAL RESPIRATION

The purpose of external respiration is the exchange of $O_2$ and $CO_2$ between alveolar air and the blood in the pulmonary capillary bed. The physiologic mechanism for this exchange is diffusion. Factors affecting the rate of diffusion with external respiration are

- Diffusibility of the gas. This diffusibility primarily affects oxygen, because carbon dioxide has the ability to diffuse through liquids, and therefore tissues, at a rate 20 times faster than the rate for oxygen.
- Surface area of the alveolar/capillary interface (normally approximately 70 $m^2$).
- Thickness of the alveolar/capillary interface (normally 0.4–2.0 microns).
- Gas gradient driving diffusion across the alveolar/capillary interface (normally 60–65 mm Hg for $O_2$ and 5 mm Hg for $CO_2$). $CO_2$ requires less of a diffusion gradient because of its previously described faster rate of diffusion.

The rate of gas exchange across the alveolar/capillary interface is normally quite rapid. The amount of time that a volume of blood spends passing through the alveolar capillary bed is approximately 0.75 second. Gas exchange for oxygen (the slower diffusing gas) is completed within the first one third (approximately 0.25 second) of the blood's transit time. The rate of exchange for carbon dioxide is accomplished even more quickly because of its faster rate of diffusion. The pressures for oxygen and carbon dioxide in the blood exiting the pulmonary capillaries become approximately equal to their alveolar air values (105 mm Hg for $O_2$ and 40 mm Hg for $CO_2$).

Two factors can affect the process of external respiration:

- The ability of the gases (primarily oxygen) to undergo diffusion. Diffusion is limited by abnormalities in the factors that were described earlier as affecting diffusion.
- The pulmonary capillary blood transit time. Transit time is affected by the rate of blood flow through the pulmonary capillaries.

The normal difference between the alveolar air and systemic arterial blood oxygen partial pressures [$P(A-a)O_2$] is about 10 mm Hg. This is despite the fact that the pulmonary capillary blood leaving the alveoli has a $PO_2$ equal to that of the alveolar air value. What this means is that the blood $PO_2$ somehow becomes reduced between the time that the blood leaves the alveolar capillary beds and the time that it is pumped out by the heart.

Anatomic shunting is responsible for the $P(A-a)O_2$ difference. The shunting is largely due to poorly oxygenated blood from the bronchial venous circulation being added into the newly oxygenated blood leaving the pulmonary capillary beds. This results in a normal arterial $PO_2$ ($PaO_2$) of approximately 95 mm Hg. The arterial partial pressure of carbon dioxide is not affected by the shunting of blood. The $PaCO_2$ value remains unchanged and is still approximately equal to the alveolar values.

Oxygen and carbon dioxide are transported in the blood by different mechanisms. The quantities of $CO_2$ in the blood have a significance beyond just transport of the gas. $CO_2$ levels in the blood also affect the blood's pH. This is because at least 60% and, more often, up to 90% of the $CO_2$ in blood is transported in a manner that causes it to be hydrated to form carbonic acid ($H_2CO_3$). The process is demonstrated by the following equation:

$$CO_2 + H_2O \longrightarrow H_2CO_3$$

The carbonic acid produced in the reaction then dissociates to form a free proton ($H^+$) and a bicarbonate ion ($HCO_3^-$):

$$H_2CO_3 \longrightarrow H^+ + HCO_3^-$$

The next equation shows the process in its entirety:

$$CO_2 + H_2O \longrightarrow H_2CO_3 \longrightarrow H^+ + HCO_3^-$$

The quantity of carbon dioxide transported in this manner serves as a significant acid/base **buffering system** in the body. Increased amounts of an **acid** in the body causes an increase in the concentration of free protons ($H^+$) in the blood. The increase in free protons makes the blood more acid (reduced pH values). These free protons ($H^+$) are buffered, and hence the acidity of the blood is reduced, by having the free protons chemically bind with bicarbonate ions that are available in the blood. The result is that the equation stated previously is driven in the opposite direction:

$$H^+ + HCO_3^- \longrightarrow H_2CO_3 \longrightarrow CO_2 + H_2O$$

Greater quantities of chemically unbound carbon dioxide are the result, increasing the levels of $CO_2$ in the blood. The final step in this buffering process is an increase in the levels of lung ventilation. The lung ventilation serves to eliminate the additional carbon dioxide that has accumulated in the blood from the chemical buffering process. The end result of this mechanism is that blood pH is maintained at a stable level.

The reverse of this process can result in an increase in the acidity of the blood. Poor lung ventilation will cause an accumulation of $CO_2$, and therefore $H_2CO_3$, in the blood. The dissociation of the carbonic acid results in greater concentrations of $H^+$ and $HCO_3^-$. The greater concentrations of $H^+$ cause greater blood acidity (reduced pH) when ventilation is poor.

## CARDIOVASCULAR FUNCTION

The cardiovascular system transports oxygen from the lungs to the sites of muscular activity and then transports carbon dioxide from these sites to the lungs. Cardiac function provides the driving force for circulation of the blood. *Cardiac output* (CO) is a function of the *heart rate* (HR) and the *stroke volume* (SV) of cardiac contraction. This relationship can be expressed in a manner similar to that of the relationship between $\dot{V}_E$, f, and $V_T$:

$$CO = HR \times SV$$

The amount of *blood pressure* (BP) in the vascular system is a combined function of the cardiac output and resistance to blood flow through the systemic vasculature (peripheral vascular resistance). Increases in either cardiac output, the peripheral vascular resistance, or both can result in increased blood pressure.

All of the blood leaving the heart to be distributed throughout the body has the same amount of driving pressure. Therefore, a factor other than pressure is needed in order to control the varying amounts of blood distribution to different body sites.

Control of the distribution of circulation is performed by controlling the degree of **arteriolar constriction** (local vascular resistance) at each of the different body sites. This mechanism is used to control and regulate the distribution of blood circulation to specific organs and body regions. An area of the body with a greater temporary need for blood flow (e.g., muscles during exercise) can increase its blood supply by reducing the degree of constriction of the arterioles serving the site.

## INTERNAL RESPIRATION

The purpose of internal respiration is the exchange of gases between the tissue capillary blood and the tissues. As with external respiration, gas exchange (diffusion) is completed early in the transit time of the tissue capillary blood.

**Interstitial fluid** $PO_2$ values are approximately 40 mm Hg. This results in an arterial-tissue $PO_2$ diffusion gradient of approximately 55 mm Hg. Intracellular $PO_2$ is lower than that of the interstitial fluid because oxygen is constantly being consumed in the cell by metabolism. Intracellular $PO_2$ ranges from 0 to 40 mm Hg, with a mean value of 6 mm Hg. An intracellular $PO_2$ of at least 1–5 mm Hg is required for metabolic processes to continue. The extraction of oxygen by the muscle tissues results in a venous $PO_2$ ($PvO_2$) of approximately 40 mm Hg as the venous blood leaves the tissue capillary beds.

Intracellular $PCO_2$ values are 46 mm Hg. $PCO_2$ values in the interstitial fluid are 45 mm Hg. These values are as compared with the arterial values of 40 mm Hg. Diffusion of carbon dioxide from the cells into the interstitial fluid and into the systemic capillary blood occurs quickly and easily because of carbon dioxide's ease of diffusibility. Venous $PO_2$ ($PvO_2$) values of approximately 45 mm Hg result as the venous blood leaves the tissue capillary beds.

## METABOLISM

Metabolism produces ATP and provides the energy required for muscle function. The aerobic metabolism of carbohydrates (glucose) provides a very simple picture of the chemistry of metabolism:

$$C_6H_{12}O_6 + 6\ O_2 \longrightarrow 6\ CO_2 + 6\ H_2O + energy\ (ATP)$$

Aerobic metabolism of glucose is not the only means by which ATP can be produced. Lipids and proteins can also undergo aerobic metabolism to produce ATP. In addition to aerobic metabolism, glucose can also undergo anaerobic metabolism. Both aerobic and anaerobic metabolism of carbohydrates will be discussed.

## Aerobic Metabolism of Carbohydrates

Glycogen is the primary form of stored carbohydrate in the body. It is a large polymer form of glucose. Glycogen is produced in the body from ingested carbohydrates and is stored by the body for later use as a source for carbohydrate metabolism. It is available in all cells but is primarily stored in the liver and in skeletal muscle cells. Epinephrine, physiologically released into the blood stream, can stimulate the conversion of glycogen to glucose for metabolism.

Carbohydrate metabolism is accomplished in four metabolic stages:

- Substrate phosphorylation (or glycolysis).
- Conversion of pyruvic acid to acetyl coenzyme A.
- The Krebs (or citric acid) cycle.
- Oxidative phosphorylation (or the electron transfer chain).

*Substrate Phosphorylation (or Glycolysis).* *Substrate phosphorylation* is a series of 10 chemical reactions that occurs in the **cytoplasm** of muscle cells (Figure 12–2). As can be seen, substrate phosphorylation produces a net gain of 2 **moles** of ATP for each mole of glucose that is metabolized. The chemical result of the process is pyruvic acid.

The conversion of *nicotinamide adenine dinucleotide* (NAD) to NAD-$H_2$ serves as an important enzyme reaction in the process of substrate phosphorylation. In order for the process to continue, the NAD-$H_2$ that results must be converted back to NAD for later reuse. If the supply of NAD is not renewed, substrate phosphorylation will not continue. As will be described later, the fourth stage of aerobic metabolism—oxidative phosphorylation—is responsible for this conversion.

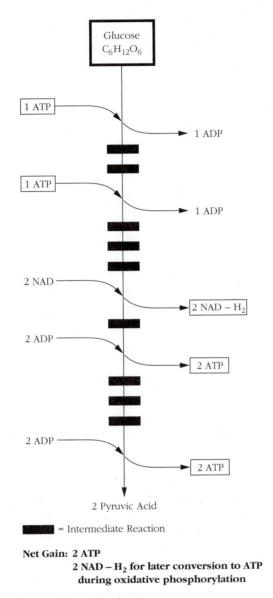

Net Gain: **2 ATP**
**2 NAD – H₂ for later conversion to ATP
during oxidative phosphorylation**

**Figure 12–2** *Substrate phosphorylation (glycolysis).*

*Conversion of Pyruvic Acid to Acetyl Coenzyme A.* As can be seen in Figure 12–3, the *conversion of pyruvic acid to acetyl coenzyme A* (acetyl CoA) is a single-stage reaction. As with substrate phosphorylation, this conversion occurs in the cytoplasm of the muscle cells. No ATP is produced at this stage. It should be noted, however, that additional NAD-H₂ is produced. Also, the acetyl CoA that results from this reaction is needed as the initial ingredient to trigger the next stage of metabolism.

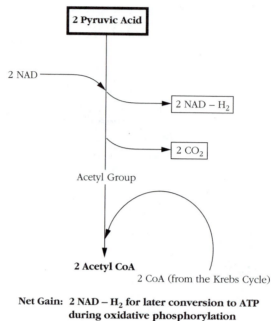

**Net Gain:  2 NAD – H$_2$ for later conversion to ATP
during oxidative phosphorylation**

**Net Waste:  2 CO$_2$**

**Figure 12–3**  *Conversion of pyruvic acid to acetyl CoA.*

As with substrate phosphorylation, in order for this reaction to continue, NAD must continue to be made available by the reconversion of NAD-H$_2$. *Carbon dioxide is produced as a waste product in this reaction.*

*The Krebs (or Citric Acid) Cycle.*  This cycle is a series of eight chemical reactions/conversions (Figure 12–4). It begins with the release of the acetyl group from acetyl CoA at the membrane of muscle cell mitochondria. This acetyl group is then used within a mitochondrion to convert oxaloacetic acid to citric acid, thereby triggering the Krebs cycle.

As with the conversion of pyruvic acid to acetyl CoA, the Krebs cycle does not directly produce any ATP. Again however, quantities of NAD-H$_2$ are produced. Additionally, quantities of a similar *carrier*-H$_2$ substance, involving *flavin adenine dinucleotide* (FAD), are produced (FAD-H$_2$). *Carbon dioxide is a waste product of this stage of metabolism.*

*Oxidative Phosphorylation (or the Electron Transfer Chain).*  *Oxidative phosphorylation* is the key stage in the aerobic metabolism of carbohydrates (Figure 12–5) for three reasons:

- The majority of ATP is produced in this stage.
- The stage cannot function unless oxygen is present. *It is the need for oxygen in this stage of carbohydrate metabolism that makes the process aerobic.*
- Large quantities of NAD-H$_2$ and FAD-H$_2$ are converted back to NAD and FAD for reuse in continuing the previous stages of metabolism.

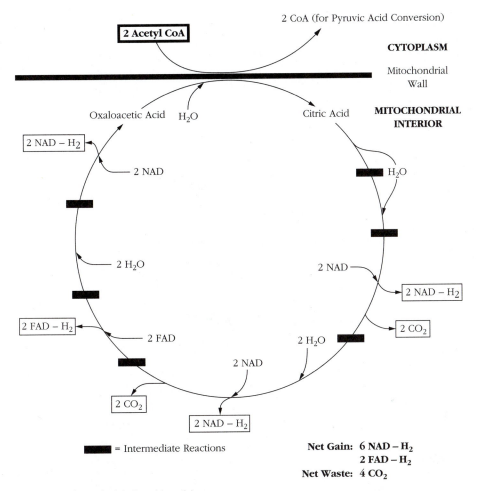

**Figure 12–4** *Krebs cycle (citric acid cycle).*

Without oxygen and the resulting products of oxidative phosphorylation, the process of aerobic carbohydrate metabolism would quickly diminish and end. *Water is produced as a waste product of this stage.*

*Summary of Aerobic Metabolism of Carbohydrates.* Figure 12–6 provides an overview of the stages of aerobic carbohydrate metabolism. For each mole of glucose that undergoes aerobic metabolism, *38 moles of ATP are produced.* This is based on the following contributions:

- Substrate phosphorylation = 2 moles of ATP.
- Oxidative phosphorylation = 36 moles of ATP.

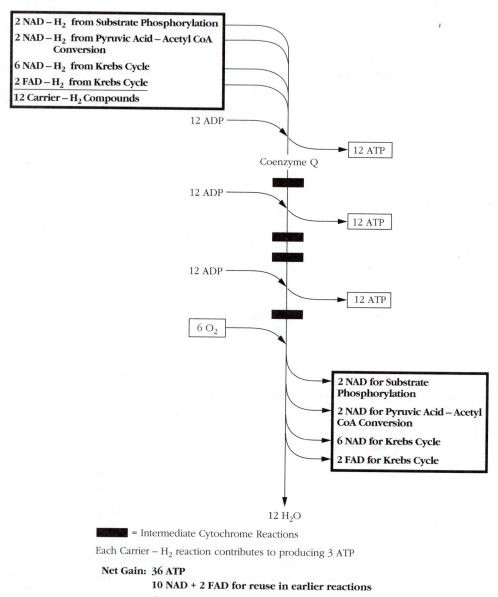

2 NAD – H$_2$ from Substrate Phosphorylation
2 NAD – H$_2$ from Pyruvic Acid – Acetyl CoA Conversion
6 NAD – H$_2$ from Krebs Cycle
2 FAD – H$_2$ from Krebs Cycle
12 Carrier – H$_2$ Compounds

12 ADP

12 ATP

Coenzyme Q

12 ADP

12 ATP

12 ADP

12 ATP

6 O$_2$

2 NAD for Substrate Phosphorylation
2 NAD for Pyruvic Acid – Acetyl CoA Conversion
6 NAD for Krebs Cycle
2 FAD for Krebs Cycle

12 H$_2$O

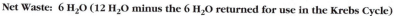 = Intermediate Cytochrome Reactions

Each Carrier – H$_2$ reaction contributes to producing 3 ATP

**Net Gain: 36 ATP**
**10 NAD + 2 FAD for reuse in earlier reactions**
**Net Waste: 6 H$_2$O (12 H$_2$O minus the 6 H$_2$O returned for use in the Krebs Cycle)**

**Figure 12–5** *Oxidative phosphorylation.*

Aerobic metabolism is a comparatively slow process for producing energy because of its many steps. However, because later stages of the process recycle and provide components for earlier stages, aerobic metabolism is very efficient. As long as oxygen continues to be available, the metabolic process can be continued for extended periods of time.

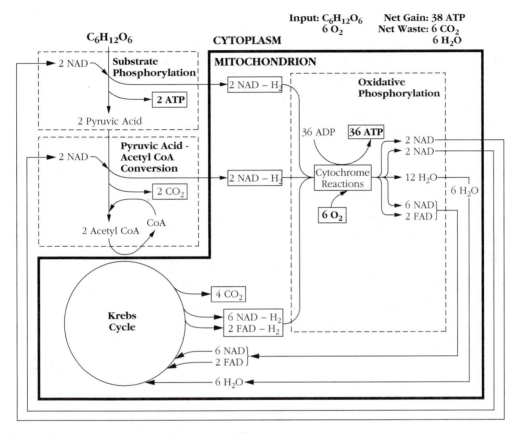

**Figure 12–6** *Summary of carbohydrate metabolism.*

The waste products of aerobic metabolism are carbon dioxide and water. The carbon dioxide is easily eliminated by the normal ventilation of the lungs. The water waste generated is also easily compensated for by normal physiologic mechanisms.

Of the 686,000 calories of energy available in one mole of glucose, 304,000 calories are converted for storage and later use in the form of ATP. This represents a 44% efficiency in energy conversion. The rest of the calories of energy from metabolism are released as heat and are used to maintain body temperature.

The series of reactions in the metabolism of carbohydrates results in a respiratory quotient of 1.0. Given a normal oxygen consumption of 250 ml/min, then, there would be a corresponding carbon dioxide production of 250 ml/min:

$$RQ = \frac{\dot{V}CO_2}{\dot{V}O_2} = \frac{250 \text{ ml/min}}{250 \text{ ml/min}} = 1.0$$

## Anaerobic Metabolism of Carbohydrates

Normally, the metabolism of carbohydrates is performed through aerobic metabolism. However, *anaerobic metabolism* of carbohydrates is possible. As with aerobic carbohydrate metabolism, the anaerobic metabolism of carbohydrates begins with substrate phosphorylation. But this is where the similarity ends (Figure 12–7). Without oxygen, oxidative phosphorylation is not possible. Consequently,

- The stage of metabolism most responsible for ATP production (oxidative phosphorylation) does not occur.
- The method normally used to convert NAD-$H_2$ back to NAD (and FAD-$H_2$ to FAD) (again, oxidative phosphorylation) does not occur.
- An alternative method for converting NAD-$H_2$ to NAD must be used.

Without a supply of oxygen, there is only one way that muscle cells can convert NAD-$H_2$ back to NAD. This is done through a process that converts pyruvic acid (from sub-

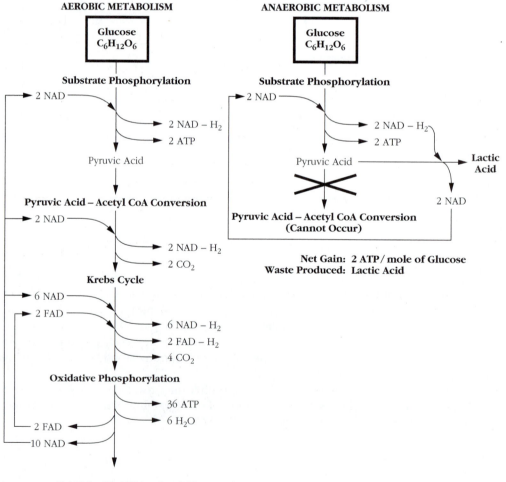

**Figure 12–7** *Comparison between aerobic and anaerobic carbohydrate metabolism.*

strate phosphorylation) to lactic acid. The needed conversion is accomplished, but with the following drawbacks:

- Only limited quantities of NAD-$H_2$ are converted to NAD.
- The pyruvic acid normally available from substrate phosphorylation is consumed in the conversion to produce lactic acid. Consequently, pyruvic acid is not available for conversion to acetyl CoA, and the Krebs cycle cannot function.
- *Lactic acid*, instead of carbon dioxide and water, is produced as a waste product of metabolism.

Given this situation, *the outcome of anaerobic metabolism is that, for every mole of glucose metabolized, only 2 moles of ATP are produced.* This is significantly less than the 38 moles of ATP per mole of glucose produced by aerobic metabolism. Only 14,000 calories of energy stored as ATP are produced per mole of glucose. Efficiency is only 2%.

Fortunately, the process of substrate phosphorylation alone is much faster than ATP production that passes through all four stages of aerobic metabolism. Although only 2 moles of ATP are produced per mole of glucose, the rapid pace of the production means that significant amounts of ATP can nevertheless be produced. Unfortunately, this also means that, as a result, the body's supply of glucose (glycogen) will be more rapidly depleted. Anaerobic metabolism is a rapid process for producing energy, but it can only be continued for short periods of time before glucose stores are consumed.

Moreover, the lactic acid waste from anaerobic metabolism creates physiologic problems that must be managed:

- The only way that lactic acid can be eliminated is by its conversion back to pyruvic acid. This process requires oxygen and cannot begin until oxygen is again available and aerobic metabolism replaces anaerobic metabolism.
- The lactic acid accumulating in the tissues and therefore in the blood is a problem for acid/base balance. It must be buffered in order to prevent it from increasing the acidity (decreasing the pH) of the blood.

The acidity of lactic acid ($H_6C_3O_3$) is buffered by the bicarbonate/carbonic acid/carbon dioxide buffering mechanism described earlier. This can be demonstrated by the following equation:

$$H_6C_3O_3 \longrightarrow H^+ + H_5C_3O_3^- \xrightarrow{NaHCO_3} H^+ + HCO_3^- \xrightarrow{NaH_5C_3O_3} H_2CO_3 \longrightarrow CO_2 + H_2O$$

As can be seen, the process of buffering lactic acid results in the production of carbon dioxide and water. Because so much lactic acid is being produced in an attempt to maintain ATP production, much more $CO_2$ is produced than would normally be produced by aerobic metabolism. Thus, an extra burden is placed on the lungs to increase ventilation and eliminate the greater amounts of $CO_2$ from the body.

## LIPID METABOLISM

Lipids can participate in aerobic metabolism. The process of lipid metabolism begins with the breakdown of neutral fat demonstrated in the following equation:

Neutral Fat → Glycerol + 3 Fatty Acids

As can be seen in Figure 12–8, glycerol can undergo substrate phosphorylation and be converted to pyruvic acid and then acetyl CoA. From there, the Krebs cycle and oxidative phosphorylation can proceed. The fatty acids are converted directly to acetyl CoA, which again leads to participation of the Krebs cycle and oxidative phosphorylation.

Lipids are much more effective sources of ATP than are carbohydrates. One mole of neutral fat produces 463 moles of ATP. *This is 12 times more ATP than can be produced by one mole of glucose.* The respiratory quotient that results from lipid metabolism is approximately 0.71 (approximately 178 ml/min of $CO_2$ produced for each 250 ml/min of $O_2$ consumed).

## PROTEIN METABOLISM

Proteins also can participate in aerobic metabolism. Usually, however, proteins are metabolized only after sources of carbohydrates and lipids have been exhausted. In order to be metabolized, a protein must first be broken down into its amino acid building blocks. There are 20 different amino acids that, in various numbers and combinations, can be used in the makeup of a protein.

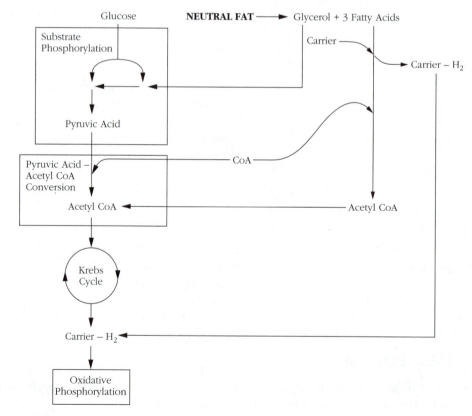

**Figure 12–8** *Lipid metabolism.*

It is the amino acids derived from the breakdown of proteins that participate in aerobic metabolism. As can be seen in Figure 12–9, the amino acids can enter the stages of aerobic metabolism at a variety of points. Only glycolysis is missed as a stage of amino acid participation.

Because of the great difference in the composition of proteins, the amount of ATP produced through protein metabolism varies widely. Generally, however, the respiratory quotient for protein metabolism is approximately 0.80–0.85 (approximately 200–213 ml/min of $CO_2$ produced for every 250 ml/min of $O_2$ consumed).

## METABOLISM SUMMARY

Normal metabolism at rest is performed through a combined metabolism of carbohydrates and lipids. These nutrients are generally used at the rate that they are ingested into the body. Under these normal conditions, 250 ml/min of oxygen is consumed by metabolism, and 200 ml/min of carbon dioxide is produced as waste. This results in a respiratory quotient of 0.80.

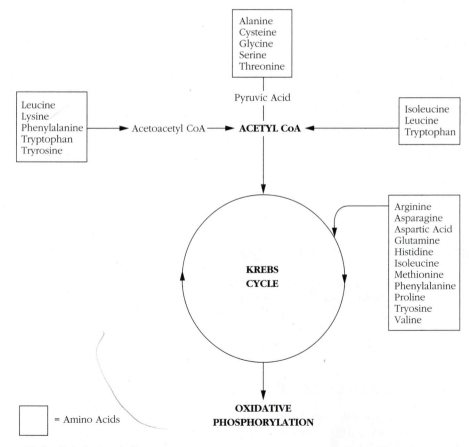

**Figure 12–9** *Protein metabolism.*

# GENERAL PHYSIOLOGIC ADAPTATIONS DURING EXERCISE

At rest, the muscular work performed by the body is largely limited to the diaphragm and intercostal muscles (both **skeletal muscles**) for breathing, the gastrointestinal **smooth muscles** for the digestive process, and the heart for blood circulation. With exercise, the muscles of the limbs and torso (all skeletal muscles) significantly add to the level of muscular work.

During exercise, there are adaptations by all of the previously described mechanisms that are used to support cellular function. Figure 12–10 demonstrates the general physiologic adaptations that occur during exercise. A brief description of each adaptation follows.

## METABOLISM

In order to have the energy needed to perform increased muscular work, an increase in the amount of ATP available in the muscle cells is necessary. This requires an increase in the metabolism used to produce ATP. Correspondingly, the rates of cellular oxygen consumption and carbon dioxide production must also increase.

During heavy exercise of a short duration, carbohydrates in the form of stored glycogen are the primary nutrient source used for muscle cell ATP production. With moderate exercise of a long duration, one half of carbohydrates (mostly from stored glycogen) and one half of lipids (mostly from adipose stores) are used. There is a greater reliance on the metabolism of lipids for ATP production as the duration of exercise becomes more prolonged.

## SYSTEMIC CAPILLARY BED

During exercise, the arterioles controlling perfusion to the muscle tissue capillary bed undergo dilation. This increases the rate of blood flow to the muscle tissue. As a result, greater amounts of oxygen can be supplied to the muscle tissue, and greater amounts of carbon dioxide can be carried away.

## HEART AND VASCULAR SYSTEM

Both the stroke volume and contraction rate of the heart increase when exercise is performed. As a result, both arterial blood pressure and cardiac output increase. These adaptations are needed to compensate for the increases in blood volume that must be circulated per minute through the working muscles. *These increases in heart action and corresponding increases in perfusion to the muscles have the greatest effect on increasing the availability of oxygen to the tissues.*

## PULMONARY CAPILLARY BED

With exercise, there are increases in the amount of perfusion in the pulmonary capillary bed. This occurs as a result of recruitment of capillary beds in the upper portions of the lung where both ventilation and perfusion are usually reduced. The vascular recruitment

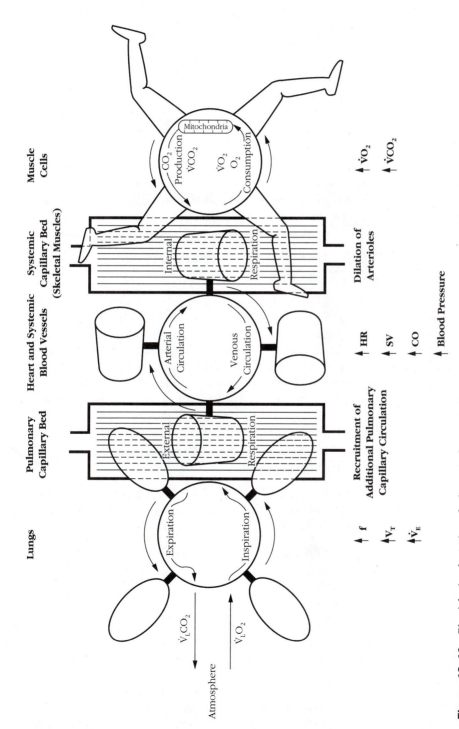

**Figure 12–10** *Physiologic adaptations during exercise.*

and increases in pulmonary perfusion make the lung an even more effective organ of gas exchange.

## VENTILATION

Exercise produces increases in both the rate and volumes used in breathing. To some degree, these changes increase the availability of oxygen for entering the blood. However, they have a much more significant effect on increasing the lung's ability to eliminate carbon dioxide from the blood.

# SIGNIFICANT PHYSIOLOGIC ADAPTATIONS AND PARAMETERS DURING EXERCISE

## OVERVIEW OF THE PROGRESSION OF PHYSIOLOGIC ADAPTATIONS DURING EXERCISE

An exercise model must be created in order to provide a framework for describing the progression of physiologic adaptations that occur during exercise. A good example is that of a normal, **sedentary** individual riding a bicycle up a hill that gradually becomes more steep. As a result of this gradual increase in hill steepness, more and more work must be performed over time by the cyclist. At some point, the cyclist will become exhausted by the level of work that is being performed and will have to stop the activity.

At the start of exercise, at the bottom of the hill, the cyclist's muscles make use of aerobic metabolism for producing the ATP needed for muscle function. As the level of exercise increases, the rate of ATP producing metabolism also increases. This means more consumption of oxygen and more production of carbon dioxide. Increases in ventilation and circulation occur correspondingly with these increases in muscular work and metabolism.

Aerobic metabolism increases and continues alone as the source of ATP until a work level is reached that is approximately 55%–65% of the maximum work level of which that individual is capable. At this time, two factors become significant:

1. The amount of ATP needed to perform muscular work is greater than can be provided by aerobic metabolism alone.
2. Anaerobic metabolism begins and shares the responsibility of ATP production along with aerobic metabolic mechanisms.

The point at which anaerobic metabolism joins aerobic metabolism in producing ATP is called the *anaerobic threshold* (AT). The *anaerobic threshold is the greatest work level (or oxygen consumption level) that can be achieved without the production of lactic acid as a metabolic by-product.*

As described earlier, the lactic acid produced by anaerobic metabolism must be buffered in order to prevent the development of a blood acidosis. Because of this buffering, there is a rapid increase in the amount of $CO_2$ to be eliminated by the body.

To the cyclist, this is experienced as a new, urgent need to increase breathing significantly.

As exercise continues and the work level increases, there continue to be increases in metabolism, ventilation, and cardiovascular function. At some point, the cyclist experiences exhaustion. This exhaustion is due to a combination of three factors:

- The level of work required to perform carbon dioxide eliminating ventilation has become excessive.
- The cardiovascular system has reached a limit of its ability to supply greater amounts of oxygen to the tissues.
- The body's stores of glycogen have become depleted, largely because of the accelerated rate of carbohydrate metabolism that occurs with anaerobic metabolism.

With exhaustion, the cyclist ends muscular work. However, *for a period of time, muscle tissue oxygen consumption continues to be maintained at greater than resting level.* This consumption is performed by the body in order to compensate for what is referred to as the *oxygen debt.* The continued increased oxygen consumption of oxygen debt serves three functions.

1. Replenishing stores of oxygen within the muscle tissue cells.
2. Performing the aerobic conversion of lactic acid back into pyruvic acid.
3. Replenishing the energy stores of glycogen within the body.

Muscle tissue oxygen consumption continues at an elevated level until these needs have been met.

## CHANGES IN SIGNIFICANT PHYSIOLOGIC PARAMETERS DURING EXERCISE

A great deal of research has been done on how the human body responds to exercise. As a result, a series of parameters has been identified for defining and evaluating exercise tolerance. These parameters relate specifically to the metabolism, cardiovascular function, and pulmonary function that contribute to exercise performance.

### Metabolism Parameters

Figure 12–11 demonstrates the changes that occur in key metabolic parameters during exercise. Note that the horizontal axis of this graph is meant to indicate work level, not a time frame of reference. This is important because, in terms of time, exhaustion generally occurs soon after the onset of the anaerobic threshold.

*Oxygen Consumption.* The *normal oxygen consumption at rest* ($\dot{V}O_2$rest) averages 250 ml/min (3.5–4.0 ml/min/kg). With exercise, oxygen consumption ($\dot{V}O_2$) increases directly with the level of muscular work being performed. $\dot{V}O_2$ increases continue until exhaustion occurs and a *maximum level of oxygen consumption* ($\dot{V}O_2$max) is reached. Once exhaustion occurs and $\dot{V}O_2$max is reached, no further increases in oxygen consumption are possible.

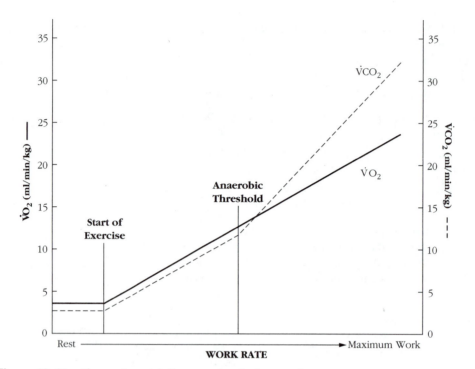

**Figure 12–11** *Changes in metabolic parameters during exercise.*

For each individual, $\dot{V}O_2$max is a reproducible, well-defined physiologic end-point. The $\dot{V}O_2$max a person can achieve indicates to a large degree the capacity that individual has for performing muscular work. For this reason, *$\dot{V}O_2$max is used as a definitive indicator of an individual's muscular work capacity.* Training can increase a person's $\dot{V}O_2$max level.

$\dot{V}O_2$max, for the normal sedentary adult, is approximately 1700 ml/min (approximately seven times the normal resting value). For a trained athlete, $\dot{V}O_2$max may be as great as 5800 ml/min (approximately 23 times the normal resting value). One way of relating resting to maximum $\dot{V}O_2$ values is by means of units called *METS.* One MET is equal to the amount of oxygen consumed by the body at rest. This is generally about 250 ml $O_2$/min or, more specifically, approximately 3.5 ml/min/kg of body weight. Therefore, for a person weighing 80 kg, one MET is calculated by the following equation:

$$80 \text{ kg} \times 3.5 \text{ ml } O_2/\text{min/kg} = 280 \text{ ml } O_2/\text{min}$$

METS are multiples of resting oxygen consumption. If the subject of the preceding equation were to increase oxygen consumption to 2240 ml $O_2$/min (eight times the 280 ml $O_2$/min consumed at rest) this eight-fold increase in oxygen consumption would represent a metabolic increase of 7 METS above resting oxygen consumption.

Calculation of METS is based on dividing the $\dot{V}O_2max$ value demonstrated by an individual by the normal value for $\dot{V}O_2rest$. A value for METS can be calculated by the following equation:

$$\text{METS} = \frac{\dot{V}O_2max}{3.5 \text{ ml } O_2/\text{min}/\text{kg} \times \text{kg of Body Weight}}$$

Given this, a normal sedentary subject can increase his or her $\dot{V}O_2$ by approximately 7 METS with maximum exercise. Trained athletes can produce metabolic increases of as much as 23 METS.

*Carbon Dioxide Production.* During the initial phase of progressively increasing exercise workloads, carbon dioxide production ($\dot{V}CO_2$) increases at approximately the same rate as $\dot{V}O_2$. Once the anaerobic threshold has been reached, $\dot{V}CO_2$ increases at a faster rate than $\dot{V}O_2$. This faster rate is the result of additional $CO_2$ production from the $HCO_3^-/CO_2$ buffering mechanism described earlier. Normal $\dot{V}CO_2$ is approximately 200 ml/min (2.8 ml/min/kg). $\dot{V}CO_2$ can increase to 20 times the normal resting value during extremes of maximum exercise.

*Anaerobic Threshold.* In normal individuals who have sedentary lifestyles, the onset of the anaerobic threshold occurs at approximately 60% ($\pm10\%$) of the maximum work level for that person (60% of the person's $\dot{V}O_2max$). In people with athletic training, the onset of the AT may not occur until a work level of 90% of maximum is reached (90% of that person's $\dot{V}O_2max$).

As described previously, with the onset of the AT, there is a marked increase in $CO_2$ production because of lactic acid buffering and a corresponding compensatory increase in ventilation. Shortly after the onset of the AT, a breathlessness develops and a burning sensation begins in the working muscles. Muscle fatigue also soon begins to take place.

*Respiratory Quotient.* As a result of increases in $CO_2$ production during exercise, especially after the AT has been achieved, the respiratory quotient increases from resting levels of 0.80 to levels beyond 1.0. Once the RQ reaches 1.0, the subject will be able to continue exercising for only a short period of time. RQs of as much as 1.5 are possible at the end of intense, short-duration exercise.

*Blood pH.* Blood pH remains relatively unchanged, with values of approximately 7.40 until after the onset of the anaerobic threshold. This pH value stability is based on the body's ability to buffer changes in proton ($H^+$) concentration. With workloads beyond the AT, the blood gradually becomes more **acidotic** as the body is less able to buffer the excessive acid ($H^+$) produced by anaerobic metabolism. The pH may become as low as 7.0 with maximum exercise work levels.

## Pulmonary Parameters

Figure 12–12 demonstrates the changes that occur in key pulmonary parameters during exercise. (As with Figure 12–11, it is important to note that the horizontal axis of this graph is meant to indicate *work level*, not *time* as a frame of reference.)

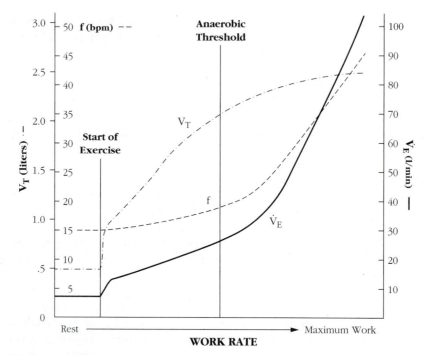

**Figure 12–12** *Changes in pulmonary parameters during exercise.*

*Minute Ventilation.* Ventilation increases begin at the very start of an exercise effort. The immediate increase in minute ventilation is the result of two physiologic factors:

- The brain motor cortex causes stimulation of the respiratory centers in the brain stem. This occurs at the same time that the motor cortex sends nerve stimulation to the working skeletal muscles. The result is that there are immediate increases in $V_T$ and $\dot{V}_E$ even before there are significant increases in $\dot{V}O_2$ and $\dot{V}CO_2$.
- Body movement causes excitation of the joint **proprioceptors** in the limbs of the body. This excitation causes the proprioceptors to send stimulating transmissions to the respiratory centers in the brain.

Humeral factors (normal chemoreceptor mechanisms for controlling ventilation) do the fine-tuning of ventilation once the initial increases have occurred.

The level of ventilation performed by an individual increases correspondingly with increases in workload. This pattern changes with the onset of the anaerobic threshold. At that point, ventilation increases occur at a rate that is greater than the rate of workload increase. The ventilation increases are meant to compensate for the additional $CO_2$ produced during anaerobic metabolism. Minute ventilation increases in response to lactic acid buffering generally begin during the range of 60%–90% of an individual's maximum exercise work level (60%–90% of $\dot{V}O_2$max).

Normal minute ventilation values of 5–6 l/min can increase to as much as 100 l/min during maximal exercise work performed by normal sedentary individuals. $\dot{V}_E$ can increase to as much as 200 l/min in conditioned athletes. Despite significant increases in ventilation, there is little change in arterial $PCO_2$ during exercise. That is because the rates of increase for both $\dot{V}CO_2$ and $\dot{V}_E$ are equal.

*Tidal Volume.* Tidal volumes increase early in exercise and are initially responsible for the increases in ventilation. An individual's tidal volume can increase from a normal value of 0.5 liter (10% of vital capacity) to 2.3–3.0 liters (50% of vital capacity) during exercise.

*Breathing Rate.* Increases in breathing rate are more responsible for the increases in minute ventilation that occur late in maximal exercise. This is especially true after the anaerobic threshold is reached. Normal breathing rates of 12–16 bpm can increase to as much as 40–50 bpm. Increases in respiratory rate occur even earlier and are more significant to increasing ventilation in subjects who have limited $V_T$ capabilities resulting from disorders that reduce lung compliance.

*Deadspace/Tidal Volume Ratio.* Deadspace/tidal volume ratios ($V_D/V_T$) decrease significantly during exercise. Normal values of 0.20–0.40 ($V_D$ is 20%–40% of $V_T$) can decrease to values between 0.04 and 0.20. These ratio reductions are based on a combination of two factors:

- The tidal volume increases just described.
- The fact that during exercise the volume of deadspace in the lungs does not change.

As a result, as $V_T$ values increase, the values for $V_D/V_T$ decrease.

Because of the reductions in $V_D/V_T$ during exercise, there is a narrowing of the difference between the $PCO_2$ of exhaled gas ($PECO_2$) and the $PCO_2$ of gas in the alveoli ($PACO_2$).

*Pulmonary Capillary Blood Transit Time.* Increases in cardiac output during exercise significantly reduce the pulmonary capillary blood transit time. The normal transit time of 0.75 second can be reduced to be as little as 0.38 second. In normal individuals, this is still an adequate amount of time for oxygen diffusion; only approximately 0.25 second is needed. In an individual with a pulmonary diffusion defect, however, a greater time for oxygen diffusion may be required than is available. The result will be less than sufficient oxygenation of the pulmonary capillary blood.

*Alveolar-Arterial Oxygen Difference.* The normal difference between alveolar and arterial $PO_2$ [$P(A - a)O_2$] of 10 mm Hg changes little until a heavy workload is achieved. This is because of the increased pulmonary efficiency that results during exercise. With maximum exercise, however, $P(A - a)O_2$ values can increase to 20–30 mm Hg.

*Oxygen Transport.* Oxygen transport by hemoglobin and the release of oxygen by hemoglobin at the tissue level respond to changes in the needs of the perfused tissues. Local conditions of increased temperature, increased $PCO_2$, and a relative acidosis in the muscle tissues participating in exercise make hemoglobin less able to hold onto oxygen. This results in a greater release of oxygen by the blood for use by the tissues for metabolism.

## Cardiovascular Parameters

Figure 12–13 demonstrates the changes that occur in key cardiovascular parameters during exercise. (As with the previous two graphs, the horizontal axis of this graph should not be confused as indicating time as a frame of reference.)

*Cardiac Output.* Cardiac output increases linearly with increases in the workload during exercise. This linear increase continues until a point of exhaustion is reached. At work levels of up to approximately 50% of an individual's exercise capacity, the increases in cardiac output are due to increases in heart rate and stroke volume together. After this point, the continued increases in cardiac output are due only to increases in heart rate.

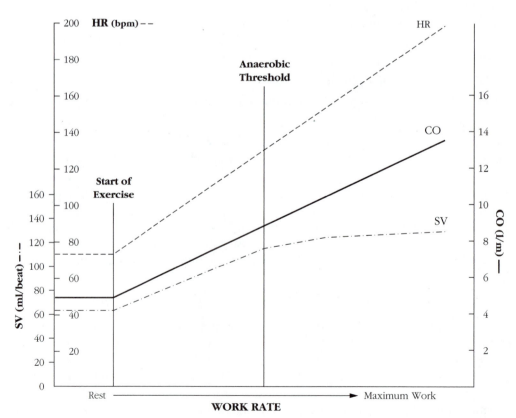

**Figure 12–13** *Changes in cardiovascular parameters during exercise.*

Given normal resting cardiac output values of 4–6 l/min, the maximum cardiac output for a normal sedentary adult is approximately 20 l/min. The maximum cardiac output for a conditioned athlete can be as great as 40 l/min.

*Arterial-Venous Oxygen Content Difference.*    During maximal exercise, the arterial-venous **oxygen content** difference increases to become 2.5–3 times the resting value. Given a normal arterial-venous oxygen content difference of 5 vol%, the difference during maximal exercise can increase to as much as 15 vol%. This increase is due to the greater amounts of oxygen that are extracted by the working muscle tissue during exercise.

*Stroke Volume.*    The stroke volume of the heart increases linearly with increases in workload until a maximum value is achieved. Normal stroke volume values of 50–80 ml can nearly double during exercise. Generally, a maximum stroke volume value is achieved at approximately 50% of an individual's capacity for exercise. After a heart rate of about 120 bpm is reached, there is little additional increase in cardiac stroke volume. Increases in cardiac output after this time are based primarily on increases in heart rate.

*Heart Rate.*    Resting values for HR can be as high as 100 bpm in normal sedentary adults and as low as 30 bpm in the conditioned athlete. During exercise, heart rates increase in a direct, roughly linear manner with increases in the work level that is being performed. The HR increases can be as much as 2.5–4 times that of the individual's resting HR.

With maximum exercise, a *maximum heart rate* (HRmax) is achieved just prior to the point of total exhaustion. HRmax is important because it is a definable and reproducible physiologic end-point for each individual. Normal values for HRmax decrease with the increasing age of an individual. The following two equations provide a mean value for HRmax:

$$\text{HRmax} (\pm 10 \text{ bpm}) = 210 - (0.65 \times \text{age})$$

$$\text{HRmax} (\pm 10 \text{ bpm}) = 220 - \text{age}$$

The first equation produces higher predicted values in older adult subjects. The second equation gives slightly higher values for younger adult subjects.

*Oxygen Pulse.*    In order to meet the demands of increasing muscle work during exercise, each heart contraction must deliver a greater quantity of oxygen out to the body. *Oxygen pulse* ($O_2$pulse) relates the rate of oxygen consumption by the body during exercise to the exercise heart rate. It is the portion of the oxygen consumption rate that is met by the blood pumped out with each heart beat. $O_2$pulse is calculated by the following equation:

$$O_2\text{pulse} = \frac{\dot{V}O_2}{HR}$$

In normal sedentary adults, the $O_2$pulse at rest is approximately 2.5–4.0 ml $O_2$/heart beat. $O_2$pulse values can increase to become as much as 10–15 ml $O_2$/heart beat during extremely heavy exercise.

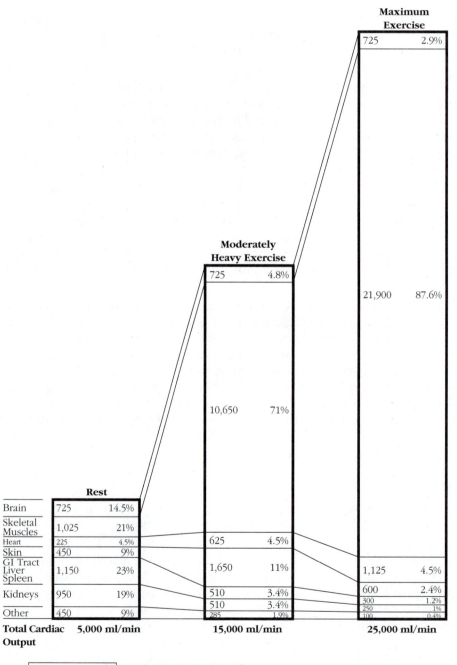

Note: | 725          14.5% |  indicates that the blood flow to this tissue is 725 ml/min and that this value
represents 14.5% of the total blood flow.

**Figure 12–14** *Changes in the distribution of circulation during exercise.*

*Blood Pressure.* During exercise, systolic blood pressure increases significantly while diastolic blood pressure remains relatively stable. Given a normal value of approximately 120 mm Hg, systolic blood pressure can increase to 200 mm Hg or higher during exercise. There is little change in diastolic pressure from a normal value of 80 mm Hg. Diastolic blood pressure can increase to 90 mm Hg with maximum work efforts during exercise.

The difference between the systolic blood pressure and the diastolic blood pressure values is referred to as the *pulse pressure*. The changes in blood pressure just described result in a significant increase in the pulse pressure of each cardiac contraction during exercise.

*Distribution of Circulation.* Figure 12–14 demonstrates the effects of exercise on the distribution of blood flow throughout the body. Circulation to the skeletal muscles increases significantly and is primarily responsible for the increases in cardiac output during exercise. Circulation to the heart also increases. Skin perfusion increases as a cooling mechanism for the body but can decrease at extreme exercise levels. This decrease is in response to the muscles' significant need for blood flow. Cerebral (brain) circulation undergoes almost no change during exercise, regardless of the work level being performed. Circulation to tissues other than those of the skin and muscles decreases during exercise.

At rest, the perfusion of skeletal muscle capillary beds is approximately 10% of the muscles' blood flow capacity. With exercise, there can be up to a 100% capillary recruitment in the muscles.

## Review Questions

Please use the following review questions to evaluate your learning of information from this chapter. It might be helpful to write out your answers on a sheet of paper. If you are unsure of the answers to these questions, review the chapter to reinforce your learning.

1. How are the basic energy requirements of the body met?
2. Relating to physiologic mechanisms for transport and exchange within the body:
   a. What basic physiologic mechanism is used for transport within the body?
   b. What are two examples of where this mechanism is used?
   c. What basic physiologic mechanism is used for exchange?
   d. What are two examples of where this mechanism is used?
3. Relating to pulmonary ventilation:
   a. What is the purpose of pulmonary ventilation?
   b. What are the relationships between minute ventilation, tidal volume, respiratory rate, and deadspace volume?
4. Relating to external respiration:
   a. What is the purpose of external respiration?
   b. What factors affect the process of external respiration?
   c. What factors affect the rate of diffusion with external respiration?
   d. How does the quantity of carbon dioxide in the blood affect acid/base balance?

5. Relating to cardiovascular function:
   a. What role does the cardiovascular function play in gas transport?
   b. What is the relationship between cardiac output, heart rate, and stroke volume?
   c. What is the role of arteriolar constriction?
6. Relating to internal respiration:
   a. What is the purpose of internal respiration?
   b. What are gas pressure relationships for oxygen and carbon dioxide at the tissue level?
7. Relating to carbohydrate metabolism:
   a. What is the primary form of stored carbohydrate in the body?
   b. What is the contribution of substrate phosphorylation to the aerobic metabolism of carbohydrates?
   c. What is the contribution of the conversion of pyruvic acid to acetyl coenzyme A to the aerobic metabolism of carbohydrates?
   d. What is the contribution of the Krebs cycle to the aerobic metabolism of carbo-hydrates?
   e. What is the contribution of oxidative phosphorylation to the aerobic metabolism of carbohydrates?
   f. How does anaerobic carbohydrate metabolism differ from the aerobic metabo-lism of carbohydrates?
   g. What is the effect of lactic acidosis?
8. Relating to lipid and protein metabolism:
   a. How does lipid metabolism differ from the carbohydrate metabolism?
   b. How does protein metabolism differ from carbohydrate metabolism?
9. Relating to physiologic changes that occur during exercise:
   a. How does metabolism change with exercise?
   b. How do systemic capillary beds change with exercise?
   c. How do the heart and vascular system change with exercise?
   d. How does the pulmonary capillary bed change with exercise?
   e. How does ventilation change with exercise?
10. Relating to metabolic parameters and exercise:
    a. What is the significance of oxygen consumption?
    b. What is the significance of METS?
    c. What is the significance of carbon dioxide production?
    d. What is the significance of aerobic threshold?
    e. What is the significance of respiratory quotient?
    f. What is the significance of blood pH?
11. Relating to pulmonary parameters and exercise:
    a. What is the significance of minute ventilation?
    b. What is the significance of tidal volume?
    c. What is the significance of breathing rate?
    d. What is the significance of pulmonary capillary blood transit time?
    e. What is the significance of alveolar-arterial oxygen difference?
    f. What is the significance of oxygen transport?

12. Relating to cardiovascular parameters and exercise:
    a. What is the significance of cardiac output?
    b. What is the significance of the arterial-venous oxygen content difference?
    c. What is the significance of stroke volume?
    d. What is the significance of heart rate?
    e. What is the significance of oxygen pulse?
    f. What is the significance of blood pressure?
    g. What is the significance of the distribution of circulation?

# CHAPTER THIRTEEN

# EQUIPMENT USED FOR CARDIOVASCULAR STRESS TESTING

## RELATED LEARNING

Prior knowledge of the following related information will facilitate understanding and learning of the material in this chapter. The learner will be aided by being able to

1. Recall equipment concepts from Chapter 1, specifically relating to spirometers, directional breathing valves, and directional control valves.
2. Recall equipment concepts from Chapters 3 and 10, specifically relating to gas analyzers and oximeters.
3. Describe the basic equipment and application of ECG monitoring systems.
4. Describe, in basic terms, the equipment and procedures required for measuring blood pressure with both a cuff-based system and arterial catheterization.
5. Describe, in basic terms, the design and application of a Swan-Ganz type of pulmonary artery catheter.
6. Describe the operation and use of the basic equipment needed to administer low-flow oxygen by nasal cannula.

## LEARNING OBJECTIVES

Upon successful completion of this chapter, the learner should be able to

1. Describe the equipment used to create a measurable physical activity during exercise testing, including
   a. treadmills
   b. cycle ergometers
   c. arm ergometers
   d. rowing/paddling exercises
   e. swimming ergometry
2. Describe the equipment used for measuring breathing volumes during exercise testing.

3. Describe breathing valves used during exercise testing.
4. Describe gas collection/mixing systems used during exercise testing.
5. Describe gas analysis and blood gas evaluation instrumentation used during exercise testing.
6. Describe cardiovascular monitoring systems used during exercise testing.
7. Describe oxygen therapy equipment used during exercise testing.
8. Describe cardiopulmonary stress testing systems used during exercise testing.

## ─── KEY TERMS ───

ergometer
flywheel
homogenous
Korotkoff sounds
metronome

ramp study
thermodilution cardiac output determination
watt
workload

There are two major factors that relate to the effective administration of cardiopulmonary stress testing:

- The subject must perform a physical activity that is measurable in some way. Preferably, this activity should make use of large skeletal muscles groups.
- Pertinent physiologic measurements must be made either during the time the subject is performing the physical activity or immediately after the exercise is ended.

Depending on the complexity of the testing performed by a laboratory, the equipment required can vary considerably. It can be as simple as a watch with a second hand and a walking circuit with a known distance to be walked by the subject. Conversely, very complex, expensive systems for both creating a physical activity and performing multiple, simultaneous physiologic measurements are available.

## EQUIPMENT FOR CREATING A MEASURABLE PHYSICAL ACTIVITY

Being able to quantify the amount of physical work performed by a subject during cardiopulmonary stress testing is very important. Doing so permits a fuller interpretation of the types of physiologic responses the subject demonstrates during a test. Ideally, the muscular work during the testing can be performed in one of two ways:

- While an exercise that requires progressively higher levels of muscle power output is being performed, up to the point the subject is exhausted by some maximum work level.

- While an exercise that requires a constant, submaximal level of muscle power output is performed for a fixed period of time.

Whichever method is selected, the equipment used for creating a measurable physical activity for cardiopulmonary stress testing should

- Require the use of large muscle groups, preferably those of the legs and buttocks, in performing the work.
- Permit the technologist to quantify and control the **workload** (muscle power output per minute—**watts**) that the subject must exert in performing the exercise.
- Require a physical activity that is already known or is easily adapted to by the subject.
- Minimize the risk of injury to the subject while the exercise is being performed.
- Reasonably permit the desired physiologic monitoring to be performed during use of the equipment.

## TREADMILL

### Description of Operation

Figure 13–1 shows a treadmill set up for cardiopulmonary stress testing. It consists of a continuous belt on which the subject can walk. The belt is mounted between two rollers and is motor driven. The belt's speed is controlled by the technologist operating the sys-

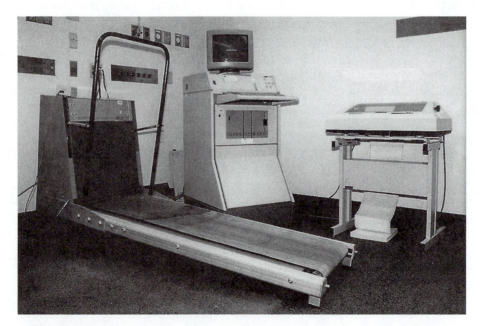

**Figure 13–1** *Treadmill.*

tem. The forward end of the treadmill can be raised to cause the walking surface to be at an incline. Increases in the treadmill belt speed and in the amount of incline can both be used to increase the workload for the subject. The treadmill should have handrails to help the subject maintain balance.

The speed of the treadmill should be adjustable, 1.5–10 mph. It should have incline capabilities ranging from a 0% to a 30% grade. Percent grade is calculated in the following way:

$$\% \text{ Grade} = \frac{\text{Length of Treadmill}}{\text{Vertical Height of Elevation}}$$

The workload (in units of watts) generated by having a subject perform exercise on a treadmill is calculated in the following way:

$$\text{Workload} = \text{Wt} \times \text{v} \times \text{sine} \angle$$

where Wt is the subject's actual weight, v is the speed of the treadmill belt, and sine $\angle$ is the sine of the angle of incline (in degrees) of treadmill elevation. The diagram in Figure 13–2 demonstrates the source of each of these values in relation to the construction of a treadmill. The subject's workload in units of watts can be determined by dividing the workload in KPM/min by 6.12.

## Benefits of Treadmill Use

The treadmill provides an exercise that is familiar to most subjects and that is most appropriate to daily living. A treadmill is the device preferred by many laboratories for this reason.

## Drawbacks to Treadmill Use

Treadmills create some difficulty in being able to set a specific desired workload for a subject. This is because the actual workload depends on a variety of factors. As described earlier, the subject's weight and the speed and incline of the treadmill are the primary factors affecting workload. However, the subject's stride length and walking pattern can

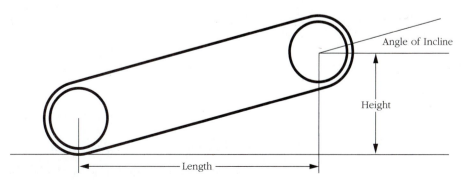

**Figure 13–2**  *Basis for determination of treadmill workload.*

also affect the workload. Additionally, body lift from the subject's use of the handrails is variable and unmeasurable in terms of its effect on workload.

Other problems associated with use of a treadmill for stress testing include

- Difficulty in making some physiologic measurements (e.g., blood pressure, arterial blood sampling).
- Danger of falling for subjects who become tired and cannot meet the workload of the device. This is made more of a problem by the fact that the treadmill's belt cannot be stopped rapidly.
- Some subjects find treadmill walking uncomfortable while they are attached to the mouthpiece and breathing valve assembly needed for more complex physiologic monitoring.

Finally, treadmills are rather large, noisy, and expensive devices.

## Use of Treadmill Devices for Testing

Subjects should be given a brief orientation and training session on the treadmill before the actual test is performed. Signaling between the subject and the technologist may be difficult when the subject is nearing exhaustion and needs to stop the exercise. For this reason, a signal system must be prearranged with the subject in order to avoid the risk of miscommunication and injury during the test.

The belt should not be stopped rapidly at the end of the procedure. Instead, it should be slowed steadily but gradually until it is stopped. A more gradual slowing of the belt will give the subject a better opportunity to adjust her or his exercise pace as the belt is slowing down.

## CYCLE ERGOMETER

## Description of Operation

Figure 13–3 provides a picture of a cycle **ergometer**. The cycle ergometer is a type of stationary bicycle where the muscular work used to spin the pedals causes a **flywheel** on the cycle to spin. Changes in pedaling rate and changes in the amount of resistance to flywheel rotation both can affect the workload created by this device. Generally, pedaling frequency is limited to a certain range, and adjustments to a flywheel braking mechanism are used to change workload. Flywheel braking is often accomplished by tension adjustments to a strap around the flywheel.

Workload (in watts) for a cycle ergometer is based on the following equation:

$$\text{Workload} = \text{FwR} \times d \times f \times \pi$$

where FwR is the flywheel braking force, d is the diameter of the flywheel, f is the pedaling frequency, and $\pi$ is the symbol for pi (pi = 3.14).

Two basic types of cycle ergometers are available for use in the laboratory.

- *Mechanical cycle ergometers.* These devices are purely mechanical in operation and do not permit any control interactions with computers or other electronic control systems. Figure 13–4 shows a mechanical cycle ergometer.

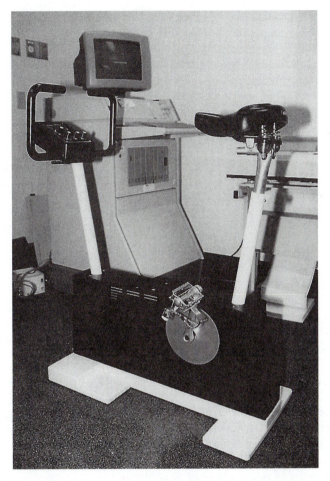

**Figure 13–3** *Cycle ergometer.*

- *Electromechanical cycle ergometers*. These devices use a combination of electronic and mechanical mechanisms and do permit control interactions with computers and other electronic control systems.

*Mechanical Cycle Ergometers.* Mechanical cycle ergometers generally use a flywheel braking mechanism that consists of an adjustable resistance strap around the flywheel. Figure 13–4 demonstrates this arrangement. The flywheel braking force is based on the braking strap tension, $T_1 - T_2$ (see Figure 13–4).

The braking strap is generally attached to a weighted balance that has a readout scale for workload. As tension adjustments are made to the resistance strap, the resulting workload changes are reflected on the readout scale of the balance mechanism. This arrangement allows for manual adjustment of workload levels by the technologist.

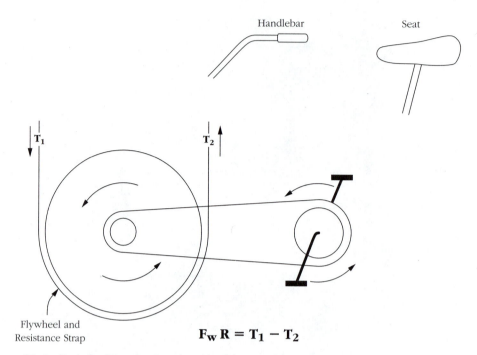

**Figure 13–4** *Basis for determination of workload for a mechanical cycle ergometer.*

Mechanical cycle ergometers permit only a narrow range of pedaling rates to be used by the subject (generally, 50–60 cycles per minute). Pedaling rates faster or slower than this range will result in the workload scale on the ergometer being incorrect. A **metronome** or similar device is often used to indicate the proper pedaling rate to the subject. This type of cycle ergometer is relatively easy to calibrate.

*Electromechanical Cycle Ergometers.* Electromechanical cycle ergometers make use of electronically controlled flywheel braking mechanisms. The braking is generally based on a magnetic field that produces resistance to flywheel rotation. Changes in the level of braking are based on electronic control of the strength of the magnetic field.

As stated earlier, this arrangement allows workload (flywheel resistance) changes to be made automatically by a computer-controlled testing system. Additionally, workload changes can be made in smaller steps or increments. These qualities make it possible to conveniently perform **ramp studies** for cardiopulmonary stress tolerance.

The electronic control mechanisms of electromechanical cycle ergometers permit use of a wider range of pedaling rates (40–80 cycles per minute) by the subject. This can be a benefit with some subjects who have difficulty in maintaining pedaling rates over a limited range. Because of their greater complexity, though, calibration of electromechanical cycle ergometers is more difficult than for mechanical ergometers.

## Benefits of Cycle Ergometer Use

Cycle ergometers are less expensive, smaller, and quieter in operation than many treadmill systems. Also, unlike with treadmills, the workload generated by a cycle ergometer is not affected by the subject's body weight. Cycle ergometers permit rapid, simple adjustments in subject workload. Additionally, a subject who becomes distressed during a test can immediately stop pedaling and reduce the workload level to zero.

Cycle ergometers are safer than treadmills for use because the subject sits on the device during testing. As a result, there is little chance of the subject falling during a test. Also, because of the relative stability of the subject, some physiologic measurements (blood pressure, etc.) are more easily made during testing.

## Drawbacks to Cycle Ergometer Use

For some (especially older) subjects, cycle ergometers present a less familiar exercise. The type of exercise performed also relates less to normal daily activities. Subjects tend to experience more muscle discomfort at high workloads than with treadmill exercises. This is noticed primarily as a mild burning sensation in the anterior thigh muscles.

When the same subject is tested on both a treadmill and a cycle ergometer, there are some differences in the test results. For the same maximum workload level (in watts) and $HR_{max}$ attained, the results of testing on the cycle ergometer, in comparison to the treadmill values, will demonstrate

- Oxygen consumption value that is less (by 5%–10%).
- Minute ventilation level that is greater.
- Lactic acid production that is greater.

These differences are thought to be due to the difference in the muscle groups used. Because the differences are relatively minor, they are not considered clinically significant. Either device is considered to be acceptable for use in testing.

## Use of Cycle Ergometer Devices for Testing

It is important that the physical configuration of the cycle ergometer be made appropriate for the subject being tested. Such positional factors as the seat height, handlebar height and reach, and possibly pedal crank length can be adjusted to make the subject more comfortable.

The seat should be adjusted so that, for a pedal turned to its lowest position, the subject's leg is almost fully extended. In this position, the knee of the subject's extended leg should be almost but not quite straight. Foot straps may or may not be used, depending on the comfort of the subject.

# OTHER MECHANICAL DEVICES FOR CREATING A MEASURABLE PHYSICAL ACTIVITY

## Arm Ergometer

There are occasions when a subject has only limited or no use of his or her lower extremities. In this situation, an *arm ergometer* (Figure 13–5), can be used to create a measurable physical activity. The arm ergometer is similar in design to a cycle ergometer ex-

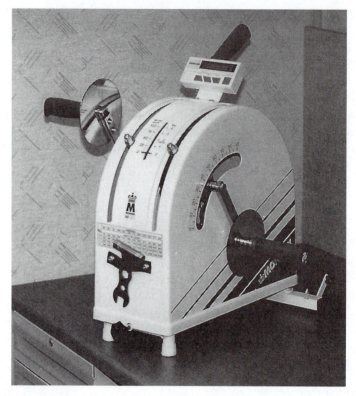

**Figure 13–5** *Arm ergometer.*

cept that the pedal cranks are elevated to the shoulder level. The subject is positioned so that the arms are fully extended on the outward "pedal" stroke. Generally, a "pedaling" frequency of approximately 50 cycles/minute is used.

With this device, both the $\dot{V}O_2$max achieved and the $\dot{V}_E$max are 50%–70% less than with a cycle ergometer. Interestingly enough, $HR_{max}$ values are only 2%–12% less.

A variation of the arm ergometer is to have the wheels of a wheelchair coupled to the flywheel of a cycle ergometer system.

## Rowing/Paddling Exercises

*Rowing machines* and water-based setups for rowing or paddling can be used as a basis for exercise testing. Although they are not typically used for most subjects, paraplegics or racing oarsmen (and other similar athletes) can be tested in this manner.

## Swimming Ergometry

Special systems have been developed to study the physiologic effects of swimming as an exercise. A *swimming ergometry* system consists of a small "swimming pool" where the subject swims against a current of moving water within the "pool." Because of the moving water, the swimmer remains stationary within the pool. With the swimmer being stationary, it is possible to make physiologic measurements on the subject during this type of exercise.

# EQUIPMENT USED FOR MEASURING BREATHING VOLUMES

Measurement of breathing volumes is an important part of major cardiopulmonary stress testing. A variety of spirometer systems have been used for this purpose. As previously described in the chapters on pulmonary function testing, the volume measurements made by a spirometer are under conditions of ATPS. The measurement results generally need to be converted to BTPS conditions in order to be physiologically meaningful. Some applications of the volume measurements require the ATPS conditions to be converted to STPD.

Two devices that were used in the past to measure breathing volumes during exercise are the dry gas meter and the Tissot spirometer. Although neither device is commonly used today, they still are available as effective methods for measuring exercise breathing volumes. The pneumotachometer is used more often today as the method for volume measurement during exercise testing. Each of these devices will be discussed here.

## DRY GAS METER

The *dry gas meter* used for measuring breathing volumes is similar in construction to the common mechanical gas meter used for measuring the amount of natural gas used in a home. The main difference is that, for breathing volumes, it has a readout dial calibrated in liters.

Dry gas meters are best used for measuring gas volumes as they are *inhaled* by the subject. Moisture in exhaled air will condense within the instrument and affect its operation. During use, the volume of each inspiration is measured. A value for the total accumulated volume during the time of the exercise is then displayed by the device. The measured volume must be converted to a physiologic value by use of the following equation:

$$\dot{V}_I = \frac{\dot{V}_{Meas} \times 60}{T_{Meas}} \times BTPS\ Conversion\ Factor$$

where $\dot{V}_I$ is the inspired minute ventilation that was performed by the subject during the test, $\dot{V}_{Meas}$ is the measured volume displayed on the spirometer, $T_{Meas}$ is the amount of time (in seconds) that volume measurement was performed (60 is used to convert the final value to l/min), and the *BTPS conversion factor* is to convert the ATPS measured value to BTPS conditions.

Some newer versions of dry gas meters include a potentiometer that allows the volume measurements to be converted to an analog electrical signal. The signal can then be linked to a digital readout or even integrated to a computer system through an analog-to-digital signal converter.

## TISSOT SPIROMETER

As described in Chapter 1, the *Tissot spirometer* is a large water-sealed primary volume measuring (PVM) spirometer. Because of its large capacity (up to 600 liters), a Tissot spirometer is generally able to manage the volumes of air exhaled by an exercising subject.

If exhaled air is to be withdrawn from the Tissot spirometer for gas analysis, it is important for the subject to breathe for a while into the spirometer system before the test is begun. This procedure will wash out any room air that was originally within the spirometer. The amount of time needed to wash out room air from the spirometer will vary depending on how much air volume remains within the spirometer when it is completely "emptied." Once the spirometer is washed out, the bell must be returned to the zero volume position before volume measurements are made during exercise.

As with the dry gas meter, Tissot spirometers can have either a scale to display the measured volume or a potentiometer incorporated into the system. A value for expired minute ventilation ($\dot{V}_E$) can be calculated in the same manner as $\dot{V}_I$ was calculated for the dry gas meter.

## PNEUMOTACHOMETER

As stated earlier, the *pneumotachometer* is the device most commonly used today for making volume measurements during exercise testing. Chapter 1 provides a description of how a pneumotachometer works. With cardiopulmonary stress testing systems, the pneumotachometer is linked to a computer that integrates the flow signal from the spirometer into a readout of volume. The computer can also make all ATPS-to-BTPS and ATPS-to-STPD conversions that are needed for calculation of the test results.

# BREATHING VALVES

A *directional breathing valve* is needed as part of any testing system that is used to make measurements of oxygen consumption ($\dot{V}O_2$) and carbon dioxide production ($\dot{V}CO_2$). The design of directional breathing valves was discussed in Chapter 1.

The purpose of the valve is to have the subject inspire ambient room air and to make the subject's exhaled air available for measurement by gas meters and a spirometer system. The design of the breathing circuits used in these systems will be discussed later in this chapter.

# GAS COLLECTION/MIXING SYSTEMS

Exhaled air samples that are used for making $\dot{V}O_2$ and $\dot{V}CO_2$ measurements must represent a **homogenous** mixed expired sample. As will be described later, breath-by-breath systems perform this by continuously analyzing the subject's exhaled air and by integrating this data with spirometric volume measurements.

Less sophisticated systems must provide a means of properly preparing the subject's exhaled air for analysis. This can be done through use of either exhaled gas collection devices or mixing chamber devices.

## GAS COLLECTION DEVICES

With some testing systems, a portion of the subject's exhaled air is collected and a gas sample is drawn for analysis from the volume of collected air. The fact that a quantity of the exhaled air is collected before any of the air is sampled results in a well-mixed, representative physiologic sample.

Both *Douglas bags* (see Chapter 4, "Key Terms") and *neoprene meteorological balloons* have been used as exhaled gas collection devices. It is important that these devices be thoroughly washed out with the subject's exhaled air before any samples are taken for analysis. As with the Tissot spirometer, it is necessary to wash out any room air from the device this way before use.

## GAS MIXING DEVICES

*Gas mixing chambers* are sometimes used instead of volume collection devices (Figure 13–6). These chambers are generally made of a clear Plexiglas material. They must be designed to not produce a resistance to the gas flowing through them. Baffles within the chamber produce a mixing of the exhaled air that passes through it. This mixing is important because it makes the gas leaving the chamber more homogenous. Gas sampling for analysis is done after the subject's exhaled air exits the mixing chamber.

Mixing chambers generally have an internal volume of 5–6 liters. Chambers of this size work most effectively under conditions where changes in the subject's $\dot{V}_E$, $FEO_2$, and $FECO_2$ values occur relatively slowly during the test. If there are rapid changes in the

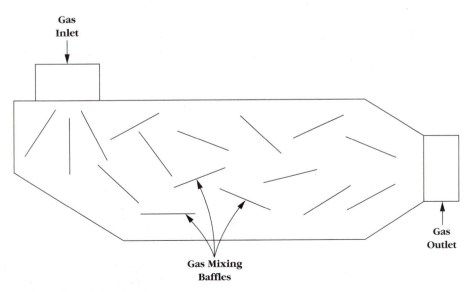

**Figure 13–6** *Gas mixing chamber.*

subject's level of ventilation during the test, time must be allowed for gas equilibrium to occur within the chamber before sampling is done.

# GAS ANALYSIS AND BLOOD GAS EVALUATION INSTRUMENTATION

Depending on the complexity of the cardiopulmonary stress testing being done, exhaled gas analysis and/or evaluation of blood gas values may be included as part of the procedure.

## GAS ANALYZERS

Analysis of exhaled $O_2$ and $CO_2$ concentrations must be performed when values for $\dot{V}O_2$ and $\dot{V}CO_2$ are being determined. One way of doing this is to make use of two separate analyzer systems—a dedicated oxygen analyzer and a separate dedicated carbon dioxide analyzer.

Another alternative is to make use of a mass spectrometer for analysis of exhaled gas samples. This way just one device performs the analysis of both $O_2$ and $CO_2$ concentrations. Because of their complexity and expense, however, mass spectrometers are less frequently used than dedicated oxygen and carbon dioxide analyzers.

## BLOOD GAS EVALUATION

Blood gas measurements made during exercise can provide a more complete picture of a subject's response to exercise. The particular method used depends on the nature of the testing to be done. Either invasive or noninvasive methods can be used for blood gas evaluation.

### Invasive Methods

Direct sampling of arterial blood is done by either arterial puncture or arterial catheterization. The blood sample can also be used to measure lactate (lactic acid) levels in the blood.

*Arterial Puncture.*   It is possible to perform *arterial puncture* on an exercising subject, but it can be extremely difficult. This is especially true for a subject nearing exhaustion. The chances of injury to the subject are also greatly increased. Use of a cycle ergometer does, to some degree, make arterial puncture during exercise less difficult.

A sample drawn even shortly after exercise has been stopped will demonstrate a change from the subject's blood gas values during exercise. Unless the sample is drawn *immediately* at the moment exercise is ended, the results will be different than if the sample had been drawn just prior to exercise being ended. Values for $PaO_2$ and $P(A-a)O_2$ are most affected by a delay in sampling.

Because of the difficulty in performing arterial puncture during exercise testing, repeat or serial testing of blood gas values is not generally attempted.

*Indwelling Arterial Catheterization.* Use of an *arterial catheter* with a sampling stopcock can improve the capability of sampling arterial blood during exercise. Either the radial artery or the brachial artery can be catheterized prior to the start of exercise. The catheter should be well secured to prevent problems with arterial injury or the loss of catheter patency during exercise.

Arterial catheterization permits blood sampling to be performed under a broader range of exercise methods than arterial puncture and allows serial samples to be drawn. Continuous measurement of systemic arterial blood pressure is also made possible through use of an indwelling arterial catheter. This is done by means of a pressure transducer connected in-line with the catheter.

Care should be taken when indwelling arterial catheters are used for testing subjects who have known peripheral vascular disease. There is a greater risk of injury in these subjects.

## Noninvasive Systems

Oximetry can be used to monitor arterial blood oxyhemoglobin saturation ($SaO_2$) levels. Ear oximetry has been employed, but today pulse oximetry is usually the chosen method, and values for $SpO_2$ are monitored. Pulse oximeters also provide a display of the subject's heart rate. Although a convenient indicator of heart rate, the pulse oximeter's display should not be depended on as the primary source of heart rate data.

Oximetry monitoring permits *continuous* measurement of arterial oxyhemoglobin saturation values. This feature is useful for evaluation of subjects who are suspected of having pulmonary disorders. In these subjects, decreases in $PaO_2$ and therefore in $SpO_2$ can occur rapidly with exercise.

It should be noted that $SaO_2$ (and $SpO_2$) values do not usually decrease significantly until a subject's $PaO_2$ values drop below 60 mm Hg. This results in a clear correlation between $SaO_2$ changes and $PaO_2$ changes for $PaO_2$ values less than 60 mm Hg. Conversely, there is a less distinct correlation between $SaO_2$ and $PaO_2$ changes with $PaO_2$ values greater than 60 mm Hg. Although this limitation does not significantly affect the usefulness of the device, it should be kept in mind.

# CARDIOVASCULAR MONITORING SYSTEMS

Cardiovascular monitoring is often performed during cardiopulmonary stress testing. Heart rate and rhythm and blood pressure are all parameters that are commonly monitored. In some situations, pulmonary artery catheterization may also be performed.

## ELECTROCARDIOGRAM (ECG) MONITORS

If heart rate and rhythm are monitored during stress testing, they should be monitored continuously throughout the test. Monitoring should be accompanied by a hard-copy tracing of the ECG results during the test. Various options are available for ECG monitoring.

## General Requirements

In order to work effectively, any ECG system used in exercise testing must include electronic filters that are capable of minimizing or eliminating the tracing artifact that can result from the subject's movement during exercise. Without the motion artifact filtering, it is difficult to assess changes in the ST segments of the subject's tracing adequately. When treadmill or cycle ergometer testing is done, the limb leads must be moved to the torso of the subject. This is to minimize problems with artifacts in the ECG record.

The quality of the tracing produced by the ECG system should permit assessment of heart rhythm intervals and segments. This tracing quality should continue for heart rates up to the subject's $HR_{max}$. Additionally, significant changes in the subject's ST segment should be identifiable up to the subject's $HR_{max}$.

## Monitor Types

Various ECG monitor types can be applied to exercise testing. Systems can have as few as one or as many as 12 leads.

A *single-lead ECG system* can be used for basic applications. This provides monitoring only for heart rate determination and for the identification of gross arrhythmias. Monitoring of ECG at this minimum level may not be adequate for subjects having suspected or known cardiovascular disease, however. The addition of $V_1$–$V_6$ *chest leads* and full *12-lead ECG monitoring* permits a greater capability for evaluation of the cardiovascular response to exercise.

Many sophisticated ECG monitoring systems offer certain special features. They may provide the capacity to "freeze-frame" a section of ECG tracing that is displayed on screen. This permits careful evaluation of that tracing section while the testing and ECG recording continues.

With computerized systems, the tracing data can be digitalized and displayed in unique ways. One is for "median" ECG complexes, averaged from a series of heart beat complexes, to be synthesized and displayed by the system. This type of tracing image manipulation can create problems in evaluating the degree of S-T segment depression the subject demonstrates during exercise.

## Application

Motion artifact is the main source of ECG recording problems during exercise testing. Proper skin preparation, application of the electrode pads, and connection of the lead wires all contribute to effective ECG monitoring with a minimum of motion artifact.

An exercise trial practice with the subject connected to the ECG system should be done before the exercise test is actually begun. This will allow for the system's operation to be checked out and for problems to be corrected before stressful conditions are created for the subject.

With 12-lead systems, the subject should have a pre-test resting ECG done while wearing the lead arrangement that will be used during the test. This will help to ensure that proper comparisons can be made between the exercise testing ECG results and previous resting ECGs that were done with normal lead arrangements.

Care must be taken in evaluating the subject's heart rate based on ECG data. Relying on the heart rate readout provided by an automated system can be a source of error. These systems generally determine heart rate based on averaging the interval from R-wave to R-wave over several heart beats. This can work effectively if the ECG complexes are relatively normal. Under some conditions, however, inaccurate heart rates can be displayed. Heart rhythms that have variable patterns, such as nodal or ventricular arrhythmias, can cause inaccurate counting of heart rates by the system. Elevated T-waves falsely identified as R-waves and motion artifact are also possible sources of heart rate display error.

## BLOOD PRESSURE MONITORING

As with ECGs, there are different options available for blood pressure monitoring. Either noninvasive or invasive methods can be used.

### Noninvasive Blood Pressure Monitoring

The most basic approach for measuring systolic and diastolic blood pressure values is manual use of a *blood pressure cuff* and a *stethoscope*. This measurement must be performed by the technologist who is administering the stress test. Although possible, it can be a very difficult procedure to perform on an exercising subject. It is especially difficult if treadmill exercising is used.

Automated cuff-type blood pressure monitors are easier to use on an exercising subject. Once the monitor's cuff and sensor are in place on the subject's arm, blood pressure checks can be done without the technologist having to make physical contact with the subject. With any cuff-based system, however, it is going to be difficult to measure blood pressure values accurately during maximum exercise. The **Korotkoff sounds** normally used to indicate the blood pressure are difficult to detect during maximum exercise. This is especially true with the subject arm movements that occur when treadmill exercising is used during the test.

### Invasive Blood Pressure Monitoring

As described earlier, blood pressure can be monitored through use of an *indwelling arterial catheter* attached to a pressure transducer and monitor. A well-secured catheter, inserted into either the radial or brachial artery, can be used.

In addition to values for systolic and diastolic pressure, values for mean blood pressure and a continuous tracing of blood pressure values can be obtained. Unfortunately, even with use of an indwelling arterial catheter it may be impossible to obtain accurate readings of blood pressure values during peak exercise.

## PULMONARY ARTERY CATHETERIZATION

*Pulmonary artery catheterization* can be employed in conjunction with cardiovascular stress testing. Generally, a balloon-tipped Swan-Ganz catheter is used. The catheter must be inserted, secured, and tested for proper operation prior to the start of any actual stress testing.

Having a pulmonary artery catheter in place permits monitoring of pulmonary artery pressure, pulmonary capillary wedge pressure, and mixed venous blood gases. It also makes **thermodilution cardiac output determinations** possible.

Because placement of a pulmonary artery catheter is a significant invasive procedure, it is used only in special circumstances. For example, it may be helpful when studying the effects of exercise on a subject who has significant pulmonary hypertension.

# OXYGEN THERAPY EQUIPMENT

Although not a regular part of every stress test administration, testing is often done to evaluate the benefits of oxygen therapy during exercise. Only basic oxygen therapy equipment is required. The oxygen can be supplied through a flowmeter from either a cylinder or a wall outlet. A nasal cannula is the appliance most often used to supply oxygen to the subject during exercise testing. This is reasonable because if oxygen is later prescribed for the subject, it is most likely to be by nasal cannula administration.

Generally, the oxygen should be humidified prior to its administration. This is true even if lower oxygen flow rates are administered. The increased rates of ventilation during exercise alone can have a drying effect on the subject's airway mucosa. The addition of even low flows of dry oxygen can increase subject discomfort.

# CARDIOPULMONARY STRESS TESTING SYSTEMS

## "MINIMAL" EQUIPMENT SYSTEMS

It is possible to perform stress testing with only a minimum of equipment. Some simple, measurable form of physical activity must be performed by the subject as a source of exercise. Activities such as walking a measured hallway or circular course (e.g., around a gymnasium) are suitable. Having the subject climb a stairway or make repeated steps up and down using a single or double stationary step setup can also be used as a source of exercise.

Only basic data collection is performed with tests of this nature. Prior to the test, a physical examination of the subject should be completed. During the test, the subject should be observed closely for symptoms of distress, and the nature of those symptoms should be identified.

Immediately following the end of the exercise, certain physiologic measurements can be made. These postexercise measurements include respiratory and heart rates and blood pressure. A small portable pulse oximeter may also be used to assess desaturation of arterial oxyhemoglobin during the exercise.

## BASIC SYSTEMS (WITHOUT EXPIRED GAS ANALYSIS)

Cardiopulmonary stress testing can be performed under more controlled circumstances if some additional basic equipment is used. A significant improvement is use of a treadmill or cycle ergometer as a source of exercise. These devices permit the technologist to have a greater control over the workload being performed by the subject.

Because the treadmill and cycle ergometer both provide a more stationary form of exercise, they permit serial measurements of heart rate and blood pressure to be made *during* the exercise. Additionally, one-, three-, or twelve-lead ECG monitoring can be included as a part of the testing. Oxygen administration for evaluating its effects on the subject during exercise is also made easier.

## SYSTEMS WITH EXPIRED GAS ANALYSIS AND EXHALED VOLUME MEASUREMENT

Stress testing systems that permit analysis of expired gases and measurement of exhaled volume during exercise significantly increase the physiologic data obtained. With all of these systems, the subject breathes on a one-way breathing valve assembly, inspiring room air and exhaling into or through one device to permit gas analysis and another for volume measurement. The same basic measurements are made with all systems of this type.

- Analysis of end-tidal $O_2$ (FetO$_2$) and $CO_2$ (FetCO$_2$) concentration values. These are then converted to PetO$_2$ and PetCO$_2$ values through use of the following equation, where FetX can represent either FetO$_2$ or FetCO$_2$ and PetX either PetO$_2$ or PetCO$_2$.

  PetX = ($P_{Atm}$ − 47 mm Hg) × FetX

- Analysis of expired $O_2$ (FEO$_2$) and $CO_2$ (FECO$_2$) concentration values. These values are used in determining values for the subject's $\dot{V}O_2$ and $\dot{V}CO_2$ during exercise.
- Measurement of exhaled minute ventilation ($\dot{V}_E$). Values for $\dot{V}_E$ are used directly for evaluating the subject's response to exercise. They are also a part of calculating values for the subject's $\dot{V}O_2$ and $\dot{V}CO_2$.

Additionally, two other types of data are recorded during use of these systems. Respiratory rate is recorded as a part of evaluating the subject's response to exercise. The temperature of the expired gases at the point at which inhaled volumes are measured is recorded for use in certain calculations.

Although they all include the analysis of expired gases and measurement of exhaled volumes, the systems that will be presented here differ in the following ways.

- How the expired gas is managed before analysis.
- Whether expired gas measurements are performed individually at periodic intervals or can be performed continuously throughout the test.
- The type of exhaled volume measurement that is done.
- The degree of automation that exists for data management and the types of test results that can be generated for reporting.

The inclusion of a computer into the test system permits a greater ability to manage the gas analysis and volume measurement test data. This has two significant effects on stress test administration and data reporting:

1. The calculations needed for generating test results can be made almost instantaneously, with an immediate display of their values.

2. The test results can easily be displayed and reported showing relationships between two or more variables during exercise. For example, the simultaneous changes in $\dot{V}O_2$ and $\dot{V}CO_2$ can be displayed against the exercise workload at which they occur.

More sophisticated testing systems include computers that accept direct input from cardiovascular measurement systems, such as for ECG and blood pressure monitors. It is also possible, by using a digital-to-analog converter, for the computer system to automatically make workload changes on the device used to create exercise for the subject.

There are three possible system configurations that permit expired gas analysis during exercise testing:

- A *gas collection device* to collect a sample of mixed expired gas. This sample will undergo analysis separate from the main flow of gas moving through the breathing circuit for the system.
- A *mixing chamber* to create a continuously flowing mixed expired gas sample that can easily be analyzed within the breathing circuit.
- *Continuous breath-by-breath sampling* of expired gases where a computer is used to integrate the analysis data to determine a mixed expired value.

In addition to the differences in how the expired gases are analyzed, these systems can also differ in how exhaled volume measurements are made during exercise. Each of these systems will be discussed.

## Systems Making Use of Gas Collection Devices

Figure 13–7 provides an example of a cardiopulmonary stress testing system that includes a gas collection device for use in expired gas analysis. This arrangement allows for timed collections of mixed expired gases to be made at periodic intervals during the test.

The gas sampling port at the subject's breathing valve permits analysis of $PetO_2$ and $PetCO_2$ values. The gas sampling port at the gas collection device is used for analysis of the mixed expired gases within the device. A gas sample control valve must be included to selectively control whether the analyzers are used to analyze end-tidal samples or mixed expired samples. The gas analysis test results can be recorded manually from the gas analyzers. Inclusion of a multichannel recorder allows for more convenient recording of gas analysis value changes during the test.

In the system shown in Figure 13–7, a Tissot spirometer is used for the measurement of exhaled gas volumes. As with any spirometer of this type, the gas temperature within the spirometer must be measured in order to make conversions from ATPS to BTPS and STPD.

Testing systems of this type allow for periodic, noncontinuous sampling of expired gases. Two sets of measurements are taken at each planned workload level:

1. Analysis of mixed expired gas samples collected from volumes of the subject's exhaled air.
2. Measurement of the subject's exhaled volumes.

Both of these measurements are performed during a measured period of time. Analysis of $FetO_2$ and $FetCO_2$, for calculation of the subject's $PetO_2$ and $PetCO_2$, can also be per-

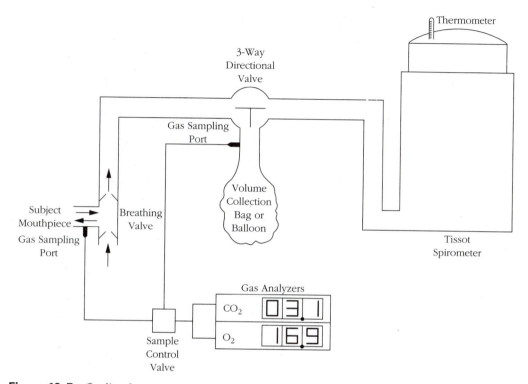

**Figure 13–7** *Cardiopulmonary stress testing system using a gas collection device.*

formed during the measurement time period. Respiratory rate can be measured by use of a sensor at the subject's breathing valve. All of these measurements may be repeated at different exercise workloads during the test.

There are two ways in which the gas analysis and exhaled volume measurements for each timed period can be made. One is for all of the subject's exhaled air during the measurement time period to be collected in the gas collection device. The gas concentration of this mixed gas sample is then analyzed. After analysis is completed, the gas in the device is expelled into the spirometer in order to measure the volume of collected gas.

Another method is for the subject, during the measurement time period, to exhale most of his or her air volume into the Tissot spirometer for volume measurement. Meanwhile, at some point during the time period a smaller exhaled air sample is collected in a gas collection device for mixed expired gas analysis. As before, after analysis, the gas volume collected for analysis will also have to be measured and added to the subject's total exhaled gas volume during the measurement time period.

The subject's minute ventilation during the measurement time period is based on the following calculation.

$$\dot{V}_E \text{ (BTPS)} = \frac{\text{Measured Exhaled Volume} \times 60}{\text{Seconds of Collection Time}} \times \text{BTPS Factor}$$

The value 60 is used to convert the measurement from seconds to minutes.

Different options are possible in relation to the complexity of how gas collection devices are used during the test. One gas collection bag can be used to collect a gas sample. It will then have its gas content analyzed and emptied prior to the next sampling time period. Another possibility is for several collection devices to be used with a valve system controlling the flow of expired gas to each device. With this method, while one bag is filling, the other two can either be having their contents analyzed or be in the process of being emptied.

As indicated earlier, once analysis of the collection device's contents is performed, it is important for the gas within the device to be emptied into the system's spirometer. This is done to make sure that the device's gas volume is included in the total minute volume exhaled by the subject during the test.

The data generated from this system permits evaluation of $\dot{V}O_2$ and $\dot{V}CO_2$ (from the $FEO_2$ and $FECO_2$ values), $\dot{V}_E$, and respiratory rate at various levels of exercise. Unfortunately, because of its simple configuration, the data management required while using the system is cumbersome.

## Systems Making Use of a Mixing Chamber

Figure 13–8 provides an example of an exercise testing system that includes a mixing chamber for expired gas analysis. Additionally, a pneumotachometer is used for measuring exhaled volumes in this example system. As in the previous system, the gas sampling port at the subject's breathing valve permits analysis of $FetO_2$ and $FetCO_2$ values.

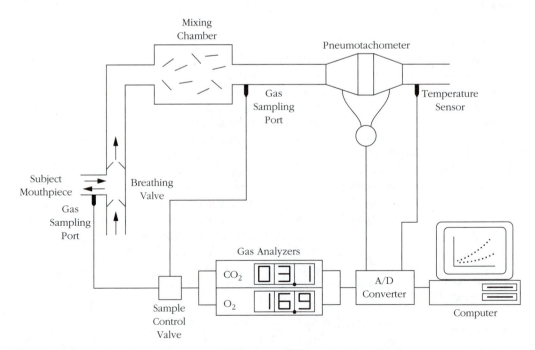

**Figure 13–8** *Cardiopulmonary stress testing system using a gas mixing chamber.*

The gas sampling port at the outflow connection of the mixing chamber is used for analysis of mixed expired gases.

An analog-to-digital signal converter and computer are also included in the sample diagram of Figure 13–8. This is to demonstrate that it is possible to include a computer to simplify the management of test data with these systems.

As with a gas collection system, this type of system also allows for periodic, noncontinuous sampling of expired gases. As before, at a series of planned exercise workload levels, two sets of measurements are taken at each level. The gas exiting from the mixing chamber is analyzed for determination of mixed expiratory $FEO_2$ and $FECO_2$ values. The subject's exhaled volume is measured over the period of time during which gas analysis is being done. The calculation of a value for $\dot{V}_E$ is performed in the manner described previously. The subject's $PetO_2$ and $PetCO_2$ values can be determined from the $FetO_2$ and $FetCO_2$ values. As described earlier, respiratory rate can be measured by use of a sensor at the subject's breathing valve.

As with the gas collection system, the data generated from this system permits evaluation of $\dot{V}O_2$ and $\dot{V}CO_2$ (from the $FEO_2$ and $FECO_2$ values), $\dot{V}_E$, and respiratory rate at different levels of exercise workload. The key difference between the two systems is the ease of operation. Use of the mixing chamber minimizes the amount of system manipulation that must be done by the operator during the test.

## Systems Making Use of Breath-by-Breath Analysis

Figure 13–9 provides an example of a stress testing system that makes use of breath-by-breath analysis for expired gas concentrations. A pneumotachometer is again used in this example system for measuring exhaled volumes.

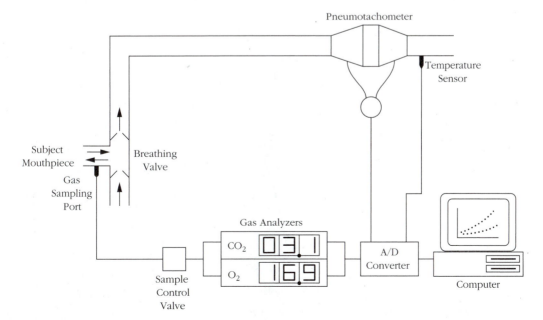

**Figure 13–9**  *Cardiopulmonary stress testing system using breath-by-breath analysis.*

*With this system, there is only a single port for sampling expired gas for analysis.* All gas analysis is performed at this one point in the breathing circuit. Values for $FO_2$ and $FCO_2$ are monitored continuously throughout the breathing cycle. This type of testing system is made possible because of the availability of modern, high-efficiency, rapid-response gas analyzers.

Values for $FetO_2$ and $FetCO_2$ and mixed expired $FEO_2$ and $FECO_2$ are based on the computer integrating the input from the gas analyzer and spirometer measurement systems. Integration of the gas analysis data by the computer allows values to be determined for $PetO_2$ and $PetCO_2$. Values for mixed expiratory $FEO_2$ and $FECO_2$ can also be determined by the computer. Using values for exhaled volume ($FEO_2$ and $FECO_2$), values for $\dot{V}O_2$ and $\dot{V}CO_2$ are determined for each breath. Mean values for $\dot{V}O_2$ and $\dot{V}CO_2$ are determined by averaging the breath-by-breath values during a specific time period.

The measurement data from the pneumotachometer and the gas analyzers can be displayed simultaneously by computer (Figure 13–10). As can be seen, there is a time lag between the changes in the subject's breathing volumes and changes in gas concentrations. This

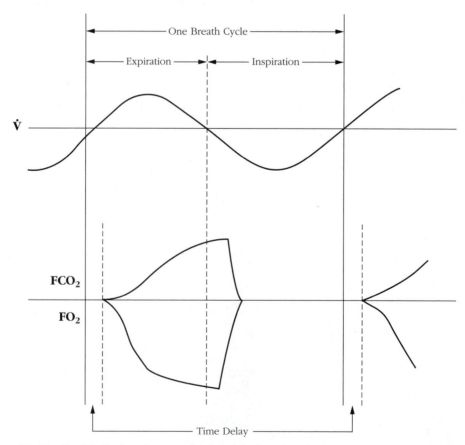

**Figure 13–10** *Graphic display of a test using breath-by-breath analysis.*

time lag is due to both the time needed to transport the sample gas from the breathing valve to the gas analyzers and the short additional time needed for analysis to be performed.

Calibration of the system and programming of a delay correction factor into the computer can compensate for the time lag. The result is correct simultaneous display of the changes in both the breathing volumes and the expired gas concentrations. Many computer systems will also allow display of an averaging of volume and gas analysis values over a short period of time (i.e., intervals of 10–60 seconds).

If a system such as this is functioning accurately, it provides the greatest capabilities for testing. Considerable data are made available, and operation, for the most part, is automated. The primary drawback of such a system is its complexity and expense.

## Review Questions

Please use the following review questions to evaluate your learning of information from this chapter. It might be helpful to write out your answers on a sheet of paper. If you are unsure of the answers to these questions, review the chapter to reinforce your learning.

1. Relating to treadmills:
   a. What is a treadmill, and how does it operate?
   b. What are benefits and drawbacks of treadmill use?
   c. How should a treadmill be used during exercise testing?
2. Relating to cycle ergometers:
   a. What is a cycle ergometer, and how does is operate?
   b. How do mechanical cycle ergometers and electromechanical cycle ergometers differ?
   c. What are benefits and drawbacks of cycle ergometer use?
   d. How are cycle ergometers used during exercise testing?
3. Relating to other types of exercise that can be used for exercise testing:
   a. What is an arm ergometer, and how can it be used for exercise testing?
   b. What are rowing/paddling exercises used for exercise testing?
   c. What is swimming ergometry?
4. Relating to spirometers that can be used for exercise testing:
   a. What a dry gas meter, and how can it be used during exercise testing?
   b. What is a Tissot spirometer, and how can it be used during exercise testing?
   c. How can a pneumotachometer be used during exercise testing?
5. What is a directional breathing valve, and how is it used during exercise testing?
6. Relating to gas collection and mixing systems:
   a. What gas collection systems are used during exercise testing?
   b. What are gas mixing chambers, and how are they used during exercise testing?
7. Relating to gas and blood gas analysis systems that can be used with exercise testing:
   a. What gas analysis systems are used during exercise testing?
   b. What invasive blood gas evaluation methods are used during exercise testing?
   c. What noninvasive blood gas monitoring systems are used?

8. Relating to cardiovascular monitoring performed during exercise testing:
    a. What types of electrocardiogram monitoring systems are used during exercise testing?
    b. How are electrocardiograms used during exercise testing?
    c. What types of noninvasive blood pressure monitoring systems are used during exercise testing?
    d. What types of invasive blood pressure monitoring systems are used during exercise testing?
    e. How can pulmonary artery catheterization be used during exercise testing?
9. Relating to the use of oxygen therapy equipment during exercise testing:
    a. What oxygen therapy equipment is used during exercise testing?
    b. How is oxygen therapy equipment used during exercise testing?
10. Relating to the systems used for exercise testing:
    a. What constitutes a "minimal" system for exercise testing?
    b. What constitutes a basic system (without expired gas analysis) for exercise testing?
    c. What are the basic operating characteristics of exercise testing systems with expired gas analysis and exhaled volume measurement?
    d. How do the basic systems and the systems using expired gas analysis and exhaled volume measurement differ from each other?
    e. What is the basic design of a system that makes use of gas collection devices?
    f. How are systems that make use of gas collection devises used?
    g. What is the basic design of a system that makes use of a mixing chamber?
    h. How are systems that make use of a mixing chamber used?
    i. What is the basic design of a system that makes use of breath-by-breath analysis?
    j. How are systems that make use of breath-by-breath analysis used?

# CHAPTER FOURTEEN

# ADMINISTRATION OF CARDIOVASCULAR STRESS TESTING

## RELATED LEARNING

Prior knowledge of the following related information will facilitate understanding and learning of the material in this chapter. The learner will be aided by being able to

1. Recall exercise physiology concepts from Chapter 12.
2. Recall equipment concepts from Chapter 13.

## LEARNING OBJECTIVES

Upon successful completion of this chapter, the learner should be able to

1. State indications and contraindications for cardiopulmonary stress testing.
2. Describe the different types of testing methods used for cardiopulmonary stress testing.
3. Describe the preliminary evaluation that must be performed on a subject before cardiopulmonary stress testing.
4. Describe the preparation that must be performed prior to cardiopulmonary stress testing in regard to
   a. laboratory
   b. subject
5. Describe the administration of cardiopulmonary stress testing, including
   a. preparation
   b. measurement of resting values
   c. test administration
   d. data reporting
6. Explain the calculation of physiologic test data related to cardiopulmonary stress testing, including
   a. exhaled minute ventilation
   b. exhaled tidal volumes

    c. oxygen consumption
    d. calculation of METS
    e. carbon dioxide production
    f. ventilatory equivalents for oxygen and carbon dioxide
    g. oxygen pulse
    h. physiologic deadspace and deadspace to tidal volume ratio
7. Explain the interpretation of cardiopulmonary stress tests in relation to
    a. poor conditioning
    b. pulmonary disorders
    c. cardiovascular disorders

## ———— KEY TERMS ————

lactate                                       neurocirculatory asthenia

Cardiopulmonary stress testing has, in one form or another, become a part of most clinical laboratories. There are many variations of exercise testing. Some of these variations will be discussed in this chapter. Regardless of the particular test procedure, certain facets of stress testing are the same.

## INDICATIONS AND CONTRAINDICATIONS FOR CARDIOPULMONARY STRESS TESTING

In general, cardiopulmonary stress testing serves three basic roles:

- Diagnosis of physical disorders.
- Quantification of impairment.
- Evaluation of therapy.

There are a number of more specific, clinical indications for stress testing, however, as shown in Table 14–1. In subjects who have multiple health disorders, the dominant disorder can be identified through stress testing.

    Serial stress testing over a period of time can be helpful in evaluating the response of COPD patients to reconditioning programs and/or the use of oxygen therapy. Evaluation of the response of an interstitial lung disorder to the use of anti-inflammatory medications can also be aided by serial stress tests.

    Cardiopulmonary stress testing, as its name implies, is stressful for the subject to undergo. For this reason, contraindications to the testing can be clearly identified. Table 14–2 provides a list of contraindications to stress testing.

**TABLE 14–1  Indications for Cardiopulmonary Stress Testing**

### General Indications for Stress Testing

- Assessment of general physical fitness.
- Evaluation of dyspnea (both with and without related chest pain and fatigue).

### Evaluation of Certain Pulmonary Disorders

- Chronic obstructive pulmonary disorders, including exercise-induced asthma.
- Interstitial lung disease.

### Evaluation of Certain Cardiovascular Disorders

- Pulmonary vascular disorders.
- Coronary artery disease.
- Other vascular disorders.

### Other General Disorders

- Neuromuscular disorders.
- Obesity.
- Anxiety-induced hyperventilation.

# TYPES OF TESTING METHODS

Procedures for cardiopulmonary stress testing can vary considerably. They differ not only in their purposes but also in their complexity and implementation. Cardiopulmonary stress test procedures can be broken down into three basic categories:

- Tests for evaluating the general fitness of a subject.
- Testing for evaluating the effects of exercise on oxyhemoglobin desaturation.
- Tests for evaluating a subject's exercise tolerance.

## TESTS FOR EVALUATING GENERAL FITNESS

A variety of simple tests can be administered to evaluate the general fitness of a subject. Two basic methods are the 12-minute walking distance test and the Harvard step test.

The *12-minute walking distance* test offers a simple screening method for fitness that requires little in the way of equipment or physiologic monitoring. It involves having the subject walk a circuit that has a known distance for a period of 12 minutes. For example, the subject might walk around a gymnasium or up and down a long hallway.

## TABLE 14–2 Contraindications for Cardiopulmonary Stress Testing

### General Contraindications

- Limiting neurologic disorders.
- Limiting neuromuscular disorders.
- Limiting orthopedic disorders.

### Pulmonary Contraindications

- $FEV_1$ of less than 30% of predicted value.
- $PaO_2$ of less than 40 mm Hg with subject breathing room air.
- $PaCO_2$ of greater than 70 mm Hg.
- Severe pulmonary hypertension.

### Cardiovascular Contraindications

- Acute pericarditis.
- Congestive heart failure.
- Recent myocardial infarction (within the last four weeks).
- Second- or third-degree heart blocks.
- Significant atrial or ventricular tachyarrhythmias.
- Uncontrolled hypertension.
- Unstable angina.
- Recent systemic or pulmonary embolism.
- Severe aortic stenosis.
- Thrombophlebitis or intracardiac thrombi.

The subject is encouraged to walk as fast and as far as possible during the 12-minute time period. Slowing down the pace of walking as fatigue develops during the test is acceptable. It is important, though, that the subject is left feeling she or he has walked as great a distance as was possible. The degree of a subject's fitness or exercise tolerance is based on how great a distance was covered. Greater distances walked within the available time indicate a greater tolerance to physical activity.

The *Harvard step test* is a long-used test that has undergone many modifications over the years. In the original test, the subject steps up onto and back down from a 20-inch high platform at a rate of 30 stepups per minute. This is done for five minutes. The subject is then allowed to rest for one minute, after which the pulse is taken for a 30-second time period. This pulse value is referred to as the *recovery heart rate*. The level of the recovery heart rate can be used to indicate the subject's level of fitness. Lower recovery heart rate values indicate a greater degree of fitness.

Modifications that can be made in performing this test include

- The wearing of a weighted backpack during the test. The pack weight should be approximately one third of the subject's body weight.
- Differences in step height from the original 20 inches or changes made in step height during the test.
- Changes in the duration of the exercise.
- Measurement of heart rate during the exercise.

Both the 12-minute walking distance test and the Harvard step test offer at least a limited ability to assess the amount of work that a subject is capable of performing. They offer a simple screening method for fitness evaluation that requires little in the way of equipment or physiologic monitoring. These tests are also useful for follow-up testing for subjects who are active participants in pulmonary or cardiac rehabilitation programs.

It is impossible with either test method to actually control and/or quantify the subject's muscle workload level during the exercise. With the walking distance test, such factors as walking speed and stride length can affect the actual quantity of muscle power being used by the subject. For the step test, both the height of the step and the step rate can be established in an attempt to regulate the workload performed by the subject. However, it is difficult to quantify accurately the amount of power used by the subject in stepping down off the platform.

An additional problem with both test methods is that it is difficult to have the subject perform a maximum power output level of exercise during the test. Without this performance, it is impossible to determine certain key physiologic parameters that are related to exercise tolerance.

## TESTING TO EVALUATE THE EFFECTS OF EXERCISE ON OXYHEMOGLOBIN DESATURATION

Testing can be done to evaluate the effects of exercise on arterial blood oxygen levels. Such testing is particularly helpful in the management of subjects who have pulmonary disorders. The goal for the test is to exercise the subject at a level of exertion that is performed by the subject during daily activities. During the exercise, measurements are made to evaluate effects on arterial blood oxygenation levels. The results of this testing can be used to evaluate the severity or progress of any pulmonary dysfunction and to evaluate the benefits of oxygen therapy during exertion.

The most direct method of evaluation is to sample arterial blood during exercise and to measure $PaO_2$ values directly. However, direct sampling and analysis of arterial blood is an invasive procedure that is not always easily performed. Fortunately, it is possible to use pulse oximetry during exercise as a substitute for direct analysis of arterial blood. Changes in $SpO_2$ values can indicate relative changes in arterial blood oxygenation.

At the time of testing, the subject should continue to take all prescribed medications. Either a treadmill or cycle ergometer can be used as a source of exercise. The treadmill may be a better choice only because it more appropriately simulates the type of exertion that is normal for the subject. During the test, three physiologic parameters are monitored: $SpO_2$ and blood pressure are measured, and an electrocardiogram (ECG) is performed. Measurement of $SpO_2$ during exercise is the point of the test. The ECG and blood pressure measurements are for monitoring the subject for potential adverse reactions to the exercise workload.

Before the test is performed, with the subject sitting at rest and wearing the pulse oximeter sensor, an arterial blood sample should be drawn for measurement of the $SaO_2$ value. There are two reasons for doing this:

- To note and record the amount of variation between the subject's $SpO_2$ and $SaO_2$ values.
- To ensure that the subject begins the test with an arterial $SaO_2$ that is $\geq 90\%$.

If the subject's room air $SaO_2$ is less than 90%, then before the test is performed, the subject must be placed on a liter flow of oxygen by nasal cannula that will raise the $SaO_2$ to a level that is $\geq 90\%$. This can be done without having to draw any additional arterial blood.

The $SaO_2$ value is obtained before the test so that the subject's $SpO_2$ value changes can be monitored during the test as an indication of the subject's $SaO_2$ values. This is based on the previously determined difference between the subject's $SpO_2$ and $SaO_2$.

Once these measurements are made, the subject should be asked to stand up. After one to two minutes of standing by the subject, the $SpO_2$ should be checked again. This must be done because in some instances the change in body position can cause a change in oxyhemoglobin saturation values. If the $SpO_2$ values indicate that the subject's $SaO_2$ has fallen below 90%, then adjustments should again be made in the amount of supplemental oxygen the subject is receiving.

With these preparations made, the test can be performed. The subject should be started on the treadmill or cycle ergometer at a minimal level of exertion. Slowly, the workload should be increased to a level judged to be equal to that experienced during daily activities. Once this level of exertion is reached, it should be continued for approximately six minutes. One of two possible things will occur during the test time period:

- The subject's $SaO_2$ values (based on $SpO_2$ measurement) will remain $\geq 90\%$ for the entire six minutes. In this case, the test can be terminated at the end of this time.
- The subject will experience an $SpO_2$ decrease of more than 5%, or the $SaO_2$ (based on $SpO_2$ measurement) will drop below 85%. In either case, regardless of how little time the test has progressed, the test should be terminated immediately.

The first outcome indicates that there is no significant desaturation of arterial oxyhemoglobin when the subject makes a change from rest to exertion. The second outcome indicates that significant desaturation does occur for the subject under conditions of normal exertion.

As an addition to the test, it is possible to determine a level of supplemental oxygen administration that will benefit the subject during exertion. There are two ways this can be done: One is to add (or increase the level of) supplemental oxygen at the first sign of significant desaturation (a drop of greater than 5% or a decrease to less than 85%) while the test is being performed. The oxygen delivery can be adjusted upward in increments of 1–2 l/min. One to three minutes of stabilization and assessment of $SaO_2$ ($SpO_2$) value changes must be permitted before the next increase in oxygen flow rate is made. Although seemingly convenient, this procedure can present problems:

- It is sometimes difficult to make up for the $SaO_2$ deficit and to determine a beneficial level of oxygen administration once the subject reaches a significant level of oxyhemoglobin desaturation.
- The procedure places the subject at some risk. This is due to the significant decrease in $SaO_2$ that can occur and the fact that it is not known how quickly or well the changes in supplemental oxygen levels will benefit the subject.

The alternative method for determining a beneficial level of supplemental oxygen is to first, as described previously, terminate the test at the first sign of significant desaturation. Then, with the subject at rest, add or increase the level of supplemental oxygen in an increment of 1–2 l/min. After one to three minutes of time for stabilization, the exercise test can be repeated to evaluate the effectiveness of that level of oxygen administration. This process can be repeated several times in an effort to find a beneficial level of oxygen administration. The testing should probably be limited to no more than three trials without the approval of the subject's physician, however. This procedure places the subject at less risk but is a more time-consuming method for establishing a therapeutic oxygen level.

## TESTS FOR EVALUATING EXERCISE TOLERANCE

Testing for the evaluation of exercise tolerance requires a greater control over the subject's exercise workload and a much greater degree of physiologic monitoring. Either a treadmill or a cycle ergometer can be used as a source of exercise for these tests. The types of monitoring and measurements made in conjunction with the testing include

- Physiologic monitoring. This can include heart and respiratory rate, blood pressure, ECG, oximetry, possibly arterial blood sampling and analysis, and pulmonary artery blood pressures.
- Measurement of breathing volumes and exhaled gas analysis. This is performed in order to make $\dot{V}O_2$ and $\dot{V}CO_2$ determinations.

Two tests for evaluating exercise tolerance are *constant work rate tests* and *incremental work rate tests*. Although these tests can be performed using the same equipment and monitoring measurements, they do differ in two significant ways:

- How the exercise workload is managed during the test.
- How the test end-point is determined.

## Constant Work Rate Tests

In the constant work rate test, the subject performs an exercise at a constant workload for a prolonged period of time (five to eight minutes). Physiologic monitoring is performed and measurements are made during the exercise time period.

The exercise is continued by the subject until a physiologic steady-state is achieved. This steady-state is generally based on the subject maintaining a constant elevated pulse level. If computerized instrumentation is used during the test, then constant elevated levels of $\dot{V}O_2$ and $\dot{V}CO_2$ can also be used to identify that a steady-state has been achieved. Once a steady-state is identified as being achieved, breathing volumes are measured and exhaled gas analysis is performed to make a final determination of $\dot{V}O_2$ and $\dot{V}CO_2$.

There are two ways in which a constant work rate test can be used:

- Determination of a subject's $\dot{V}O_2$max value.
- Follow-up studies to evaluate either the benefits of a form of therapy or a subject's progress in improving exercise tolerance.

For $\dot{V}O_2$*max determination*, a series of separate constant work rate tests, each at a progressively higher workload level, are performed. The $\dot{V}O_2$max determination is based on the $\dot{V}O_2$ value measured during the steady-state test at a workload level that produces either exhaustion for the subject or symptoms of physiologic distress.

Because a steady-state is achieved with this type of test before the final measurements are taken, the value for $\dot{V}O_2$ that is measured is most likely to be a correct assessment of the subject's maximum attainable exercise capacity ($\dot{V}O_2$max). An additional benefit is that the longer duration of exercise allows for less sophisticated, slower operating measuring systems to be used in collecting the test data. Unfortunately, this method of determining a value for $\dot{V}O_2$max is very time-consuming and can be very exhausting for the subject. A long recovery time is required before retesting can be performed.

Besides being used to determine a value for $\dot{V}O_2$max, constant work rate testing can be used in making *follow-up studies*. These follow-up studies are generally performed to monitor either:

- The benefits of a form of therapy.
- Progress in improving exercise tolerance.

Both of these uses are based on having an initial constant work rate test performed at a submaximal level of exercise. This test will serve as a basis for comparison with later tests. Values for $\dot{V}O_2$ and other parameters are measured. Follow-up tests are performed at the same submaximal level that was used during the initial test. When tests are performed to evaluate therapeutic benefit improvements should be seen in the measured parameters of follow-up tests if the therapy the patient is receiving is beneficial.

For subjects in a program to improve exercise tolerance, lower $\dot{V}O_2$ values on follow-up measurement indicate an improvement in the subject's conditioning and exercise tolerance. Use of constant work rate testing for this purpose allows monitoring of the subject's progress in improving exercise tolerance while not requiring the subject to perform exercise to a point of exhaustion or physiologic distress.

## Incremental Work Rate Tests

Incremental work rate tests differ significantly from constant work rate tests and are more commonly performed. They involve having the subject start exercise at a low workload level. Workload levels are then increased in brief, plateau-like increments throughout the test.

Reasonably fit individuals can begin at a workload level of 15 watts. Subjects with pulmonary or cardiovascular disorders will have to start at a lower workload level, possibly as low as 5 watts. Each workload level is maintained for a time interval of one to three minutes before the workload is increased to the next level. The workload level increases can be made in increments of 5, 10, 15, 20, 25, or 30 watts. The size of the increment chosen depends on the general fitness of the subject. Smaller incremental increases should be used for subjects in poor physical condition.

Physiologic measurements, breathing volume measurement, and exhaled gas analysis are all performed at the end of the time period for each workload level. This procedure is continued until a workload level is reached where one of the two following events occurs:

- The subject becomes exhausted (because of muscle fatigue and possibly breathing fatigue) and is unable to continue the exercise.
- The subject demonstrates some adverse reaction to the exercise. The nature of these adverse reactions will be described later.

With the occurrence of either of these events, final test measurements should be made and the stressful exercise portion of the test should be terminated.

Ideally, based on the size of the incremental workload increases, *the test should reach an end-point within approximately eight to ten minutes of when it was started.* With this type of test, a true steady-state may not be achieved at any of the workload levels used during the test. This is especially true for high workload levels. Fortunately, achieving a true steady-state is not necessary for being able to measure useful values for the highest $\dot{V}O_2$, heart rate, and ventilation levels the subject will attain with exercise.

When longer incremental workload time periods (four to six minutes) are used, it is more likely that a steady-state will be achieved. This is especially true for low or moderate workload levels. These longer incremental time periods may, however, result in premature muscle fatigue that can artificially shorten the test and limit the usefulness of the data.

When the stressful portion of the test is terminated, it is important that the subject not be permitted to become motionless in either the standing or sitting position for more than 10 seconds. This is necessary in order to avoid the significant postexercise drop in blood pressure that can occur with the sudden cessation of a high workload level of exercise. After the stressful exercise is over, the subject should either

- Stop exercising entirely and rest in a supine position, or
- Perform a continuation of the exercise at a minimal workload (zero workload at 50–60 pedal cycles/minute on the cycle ergometer or 0% grade at 2 mph on the treadmill) for at least two minutes. This serves as an exercise cool-down period.

The subject's ECG and blood pressure should be monitored during the cool-down period. After the cool-down period is completed, the subject should be permitted to stop exercising.

This type of test is designed primarily to test the exercise limits of the subject efficiently and to determine a measured value for the subject's $\dot{V}O_2$max. But this test method requires that the subject must perform exercise either to a point of exhaustion or to demonstrating physiologic distress each time the test is administered. This can be an intimidating prospect to a subject who already has a history of exercise limitations.

A variation of the incremental work rate test is the *ramp-type test*. With a ramp test, the increase in workload during the test is smooth and continuous instead of being incremental and in a series of plateaus. Other than the difference in how the workload is increased, the ramp test is the same as the incremental work rate test in all other aspects.

# PRELIMINARY EVALUATION OF THE SUBJECT

A certain amount of preliminary evaluation of the subject must be performed before cardiopulmonary stress testing can be administered. This evaluation serves two purposes:

1. To identify any potential contraindications to administration of the stress test.
2. To add to the body of knowledge that will be available on the subject for use in evaluating the subject's response to exercise.

The preliminary evaluation should, minimally, include the following components:

- *History taking.* This should relate particularly to tobacco use, medications taken, tolerance of normal physical activity, and correlation of activity with angina pectoris, dyspnea, and/or other symptoms of distress.
- *Physical examination.* Measurement should be made of the subject's shoeless height and weight. The examination should particularly include assessment of the subject's heart, lungs, peripheral pulses, and blood pressure measured from each arm.
- *Resting 12-lead ECG.*

Usually, routine pulmonary function studies are also performed on the subject. These tests generally include

- Lung volumes.
- Forced expiratory flow rates (before and after bronchodilator).
- Maximum voluntary ventilation.
- Carbon monoxide diffusing capacity.
- Resting room air or normal oxygen administration arterial blood gases.

These tests do not necessarily have to be done on the same day as the stress test but should be done recently enough to still be clinically significant.

# PREPARATION FOR THE TEST PROCEDURE

## PREPARATION OF THE LABORATORY

Certain preliminary concerns should be addressed on the day that stress testing is to be performed. The laboratory should be air-conditioned and temperature regulated to be comfortable for an exercising subject. The view that the subject has during the test should be relatively uncluttered with technical medical equipment, especially if it appears invasive or threatening. All necessary equipment should be organized and laid out in preparation. This is especially true for any blood sampling equipment. Operational checks of the equipment should have already been performed.

A "crash cart" with resuscitation equipment should be available in or near the laboratory facility. The technologists responsible for administering cardiopulmonary stress testing should be tested and certified for performing CPR.

## PREPARATION OF THE SUBJECT

### Prior to the Day of the Test

The subject should be given the following instructions before the day of the test:

- The subject should wear loose-fitting clothing to the laboratory on the day of the test. Low-heeled or athletic-style shoes are best suited for use during the test.
- The subject should be instructed that it is acceptable to eat a light meal prior to the test. However, the meal should be eaten at least two hours before the test.
- The subject should abstain from coffee and cigarettes for at least two hours before the test.
- Generally, the subject should continue on any medications that have been prescribed for routine use.

### On the Day of the Test

Once at the laboratory on the day of the test, the subject should have all of the test equipment explained and demonstrated. If a cycle ergometer is to be used, it should be adjusted to fit the subject properly. The subject should practice riding the cycle. During the practice, the cycle ergometer should be set at a low workload level and the subject should pedal within the required pedaling frequency range.

If a treadmill is to be used for testing, the subject should practice getting on the moving belt and walking without use of the handrails. Several trial practices at this may be needed to make the subject comfortable with use of the device. It is a good idea, with both devices, for the subject to practice while breathing on the breathing-valve and circuit assembly.

## ADMINISTRATION OF TESTING

The specific test procedure chosen for use will depend on

- The equipment that is available for use in testing.
- The need for diagnosis of a particular disorder.
- The need for quantification of a particular illness or infirmity.
- The need to evaluate the subject's response to a particular form of treatment.

The following discussion assumes that the test procedure is an incremental work rate study using a cycle ergometer and breath-by-breath analysis of the subject's breathing.

## PREPARATION

A final review of instructions relating to the test should be given to the subject. *It should be emphasized that a maximum work effort by the subject will be necessary for the test to be successful.* A system of hand signals should be agreed on with the subject.

If a resting arterial blood gas sample is to be taken as part of the test, it should be drawn at this time. Later, even at rest, being attached to the monitoring systems and/or the breathing circuit may cause the subject to change his or her breathing pattern. A resting value for **lactate** can also be determined from this blood sample.

The monitoring systems that are to be used during the test must be connected to the subject. Generally, the monitoring equipment will minimally include the mouthpiece for the breathing valve/circuit (nose clips must also be worn), blood pressure cuff, and ECG leads. A pulse oximeter may also be connected to the subject. If an arterial line is to be inserted, it must be done at this time.

The subject's comfort with the equipment is important. She or he should be questioned as to any problems or discomfort. The subject's seal around the mouthpiece and nose clips should also be checked.

An estimated value for the subject's HRmax should be calculated if it has not already been done.

## MEASUREMENT OF RESTING VALUES

With the preliminary preparation completed, actual measurement of test data should begin. The first measurements to be made are of the subject's resting values. These measurements should be made with the subject in a resting steady-state. This is best done if the subject is sitting quietly in a chair and breathing on the mouthpiece assembly. Generally, resting steady-state measurements can be made after the subject has been sitting quietly for approximately five minutes.

The parameters measured at rest should be the same ones that will be measured during exercise, that is,

- *Pulmonary parameters*—respiratory rate (f), minute ventilation ($\dot{V}_E$), end-tidal oxygen and carbon dioxide ($PetO_2$ and $PetCO_2$), and data to establish mixed expired gas values for oxygen and carbon dioxide.
- *Cardiovascular parameters*—heart rate (HR), blood pressure (BP), ECG.

From these measurements, determinations can be made for resting values for oxygen consumption ($\dot{V}O_2$) and carbon dioxide production ($\dot{V}CO_2$).

## TEST ADMINISTRATION

With all of the monitoring equipment connected to the subject, a practice run should be made with the subject operating the cycle ergometer at a *minimal* workload. This is to make sure that all of the monitoring equipment is going to function effectively while the subject is exercising.

Once all of the test systems check out, the stressful exercise portion of the test can be started. The subject should begin to exercise at the initial low workload. Increases in workload should occur at the preplanned time intervals. Monitoring data for expired gases, breathing volumes, heart and respiratory rates, blood pressure, and possibly blood gases (and lactate) should be collected at the end of the time period (last 30 seconds) for each workload level. Most modern computerized test systems permit a continuous graphic display of the test results as they are measured during the test.

A useful graphic to follow during the test is a display of the ventilatory equivalents for $\dot{V}O_2$ and $\dot{V}CO_2$ ($\dot{V}_E/\dot{V}O_2$ and $\dot{V}_E/\dot{V}CO_2$) as plotted against either workload levels or $\dot{V}O_2$. Figure 14–1 provides an example of this type of display. The appearance of the plotted figures would be the same regardless of whether workload or $\dot{V}O_2$ is used for the X axis of the graph.

As can be seen in Figure 14–1, once exercise has begun, the values for $\dot{V}_E/\dot{V}O_2$ and $\dot{V}_E/\dot{V}CO_2$ remain relatively stable until the anaerobic threshold is achieved. Until the

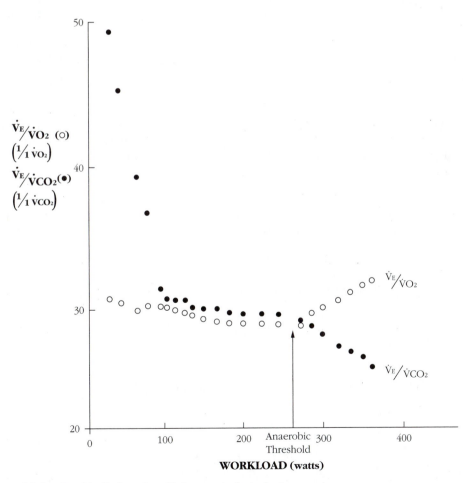

**Figure 14–1** *Graphic display of ventilatory equivalents during exercise.*

anaerobic threshold is reached, values for $\dot{V}_E/\dot{V}O_2$ normally remain in the range of 20–30 liters/liter $\dot{V}O_2$. $\dot{V}_E/\dot{V}CO_2$ values are generally in the range of 25–35 liters/liter $\dot{V}CO_2$.

After the anaerobic threshold is achieved, the buffering of the lactic acid from anaerobic metabolism causes a significant increase in $CO_2$ production. The result is a compensatory increase in ventilation needed to eliminate the increases in blood $CO_2$. These increases in $\dot{V}CO_2$ and $\dot{V}_E$ have an effect on the values for $\dot{V}_E/\dot{V}O_2$ and $\dot{V}_E/\dot{V}CO_2$.

Figure 14–1 demonstrates that, *after the anaerobic threshold has been reached, there is*

- *An increase in $\dot{V}_E/\dot{V}O_2$ values. This is because the rate of increase in $\dot{V}_E$ values is greater than the increases in $\dot{V}O_2$ values.*
- *Either a continuation of $\dot{V}_E/\dot{V}CO_2$ values being relatively stable and unchanged or, as shown on the example display, a decrease in $\dot{V}_E/\dot{V}CO_2$ values. This is because, normally, either the subject's ventilation increases keep pace with the increases in $\dot{V}CO_2$, or $\dot{V}CO_2$ levels increase at a rate faster than the subject's $\dot{V}_E$ increases can compensate.*

Based on these relationships, use of a display such as the one shown in Figure 14–1 provides a convenient tool for identifying the point at which the subject reaches the anaerobic threshold during exercise.

During the test, proper use of the exercise equipment may need to be reinforced with the subject. For the cycle ergometer, this means that the subject should pedal within the required frequency range for that device. The subject should receive encouragement to continue exercising until a maximal effort is achieved.

Monitoring of the subject during the test is extremely important. The subject should be observed closely and questioned regarding any adverse reactions to the exercise. The ECG tracing should be observed for the development of arrhythmias. Blood pressure measurement results should also be evaluated as an indicator of how well the subject is tolerating the test.

As described earlier, the test should be terminated when the subject either

- Achieves physical exhaustion due to a maximum work effort, or
- Demonstrates adverse reactions to the exercise.

The subject normally experiences exhaustion soon after having passed the anaerobic threshold (AT). The sense of exhaustion felt by the subject is a combination of two factors that are related to anaerobic metabolism:

1. The rapid consumption and depletion of glucose needed for muscle-cell metabolism.
2. An extremely elevated need for ventilation necessary for eliminating the excessive $CO_2$ produced by lactic acid buffering.

It is likely that the subject did in fact exercise to her or his maximum level if one or more of the following was demonstrated by the test measurement at the end of the test:

- $\dot{V}O_2max \geq 85\%$ of predicted.
- $\dot{V}_Emax \geq 70\%$ of MVV.
- HRmax $>90\%$ of predicted.
- Blood lactate $>8$ mM.

Adverse reactions displayed by the subject are generally due to pulmonary or cardiovascular disorders that are present. Table 14–3 lists the indications for stopping an incremental work rate test. The signs of distress listed in this table are also appropriate for indicating the need to terminate a constant work rate test.

---

**TABLE 14–3  Indications for Stopping a Cardiopulmonary Stress Test**

---

**General Indications**

---

• Testing or monitoring system failure

---

**Based on Normal Reaction to an Incremental Stress Test**

---

• Exhaustion or fatigue

---

**Based on Clinical Signs and Symptoms of Physiologic Distress**

---

• Dizziness or faintness
• Marked apprehension, mental confusion, loss of coordination, or headache
• Muscle cramping
• Nausea and/or vomiting
• Onset of sweating and pallor
• Severe claudication or other pain
• Unusual or severe fatigue
• Severe claudication or other pain
• Unusual or severe fatigue
• Onset or increase in cyanosis*
• Progressive chest pain that is suspected of being angina*
• Severe dyspnea*

---

**Based on Signs of Significant Hypoxemia**

---

• A decrease in $SaO_2$ of greater than 5%*
• A decrease in $SaO_2$ to less than 85%*
• A decrease in $PaO_2$ to less than 55 mm Hg*

---

**Based on Electrocardiogram Signs of Physiologic Distress**

---

• Atrial arrhythmias—paroxysmal atrial tachycardia, atrial fibrillation when it was absent at rest.
• Ventricular arrhythmias—frequent premature ventricular contractions (especially where they are occurring in a T-wave), paroxysmal ventricular tachycardia.
• Second- or third-degree heart block.
• Left or right bundle branch block when it was absent at rest.

---

**TABLE 14–3  (Continued)**

---

- ST segment changes—2 mm or more horizontal depression or down-sloping of the ST segment, 2 mm or more horizontal elevation of the ST segment.
- T-wave changes—symmetrical inversion of the T-wave when it was absent at rest.

---

### Based on Blood Pressure Signs of Physiologic Distress

---

- Systolic blood pressure changes—increases to greater than 250 mm Hg or failure of systolic pressure to increase with exercise or a decrease by more than 10 mm Hg.*
- Diastolic blood pressure changes—increases to greater than 120 mm Hg.*

---

*Indicates a particularly significant indication.*

If the test end-point is reached as a result of normal exhaustion, the subject should go through a cool-down period, have final measurements made, and then the exercise should be fully terminated. Subjects who demonstrate physiologic distress during the test should immediately terminate exercise and be monitored carefully (primarily for vital signs and ECG). The monitoring should continue until the subject returns to a normal resting state.

If, after a review of the test results, it is evident that the subject terminated the test prematurely without achieving a maximal effort, the test should be repeated. The repeat test can generally be performed after 30–45 minutes of having the subject rest. The goals and needs for the subject's exercise effort during the test should be reinforced before the retest.

## DATA REPORTING

After the test is completed, results should be reported and interpreted. The final report for the test should include the following key elements:

- A short clinical history of the subject. This should include the factors that indicated the need for testing.
- A description of how the test procedure was administered.
- A description of the subjective and objective clinical observations that were made of the subject during the test.
- Both tabular and graphic presentations of the data accumulated during the test. This generally includes results for f, HR, blood pressure, $\dot{V}_E$, $\dot{V}O_2$, $\dot{V}CO_2$. Other values, such as for blood gases or oximetry, $V_D/V_T$, etc., can also be presented.
- A summary presentation of the data measurements from the resting and maximal exercise time periods.
- Copies of the ECG and/or blood pressure tracings, especially if some abnormality is demonstrated by them.
- An interpretation of the test results.

# CALCULATION OF PHYSIOLOGIC TEST DATA

A number of parameters must be calculated in order to generate the data needed to evaluate a subject's exercise tolerance. The values that must be calculated include exhaled minute ventilation, exhaled tidal volume, oxygen consumption, carbon dioxide production, ventilatory equivalents for oxygen and carbon dioxide, respiratory quotient, oxygen pulse, and physiologic deadspace to tidal volume ratio. The calculations for each of these parameters will be presented here. The study section of this textbook provides examples of the calculation of these values.

## EXHALED MINUTE VENTILATION

Exhaled minute ventilation ($\dot{V}_E$) (l/min) at BTPS is calculated as follows:

$$\dot{V}_E = \frac{\dot{V}_{Meas} \times 60}{T_{Meas}} \times \text{BTPS Conversion Factor}$$

where $\dot{V}_{Meas}$ (l/sec at ATPS) is the measured volume displayed by the spirometer, $T_{Meas}$ (sec) is the amount of time that volume measurement was performed, 60 is used to convert the final value from l/sec to l/min, and the BTPS conversion factor is an approximate method for converting the ATPS $\dot{V}_{Meas}$ value to BTPS conditions.

A more accurate method would be to convert the $\dot{V}_{Meas}$ value to BTPS before $\dot{V}_E$ is calculated. Appendix B provides a table of ATPS-to-BTPS conversion factors based on gas temperature. Appendix B also provides an equation for converting a volume value directly from conditions of ATPS to conditions of BTPS.

## EXHALED TIDAL VOLUME

Exhaled tidal volume ($V_T$) (liters at BTPS) is calculated as follows:

$$V_T = \frac{\dot{V}_E}{f}$$

where $\dot{V}_E$ is the previously calculated exhaled minute ventilation (l/min at BTPS) and f is the respiratory rate (breaths/minute) during the time that the $\dot{V}_E$ was being measured.

## OXYGEN CONSUMPTION

Oxygen consumption ($\dot{V}O_2$) must be calculated. It should be noted that the units used for $\dot{V}O_2$ during exercise testing are l/min STPD. This differs from the units of ml/min that were used as an example in Chapter 12 (e.g., the 250 ml/min value for $\dot{V}O_2$ stated in Chapter 12 would now be expressed as 0.250 l/min). There are two possible methods for calculating $\dot{V}O_2$. The methods differ in whether values for both the subject's inspired and exhaled minute ventilation are measured during the test.

## Oxygen Consumption Calculation When Both Inspired and Exhaled Minute Ventilation Are Measured

If both inspired and exhaled minute volumes are measured, then the following equation can be used to calculate oxygen consumption:

$$\dot{V}O_2 = (FIO_2 \times \dot{V}_I) - (FEO_2 \times \dot{V}_E)$$

where the value used for $FIO_2$ is 0.2093, $FEO_2$ is measured from the mixed expired gas sample, and $\dot{V}_I$ and $\dot{V}_E$ (both l/min) are the inspired and exhaled minute ventilations at STPD. These minute ventilation values at STPD can be converted either from their directly measured ATPS values or from the previously calculated BTPS values. Appendix B provides equations that can be used for ATPS to STPD and BTPS to STPD conversions.

## Oxygen Consumption Calculation When Only Exhaled Minute Ventilation Is Measured

If only the exhaled minute volume is measured, then the following equation can be used for calculating oxygen consumption:

$$\dot{V}O_2 = \left\{ \left[ \left( \frac{1 - FEO_2 - FECO_2}{1 - FIO_2} \right) \times FIO_2 \right] - FEO_2 \right\} \times \dot{V}_E$$

where $FEO_2$ and $FECO_2$ are measured mixed expired gas values from the test, the value used for $FIO_2$ is 0.2093, and $\dot{V}_E$ (l/min) is the value measured during the test but converted to STPD. This value can be derived from either an ATPS or a BTPS value for $\dot{V}_E$ by use of one of the two methods described previously.

The following portion of the equation just stated,

$$\frac{1 - FEO_2 - FECO_2}{1 - FIO_2}$$

which is multiplied by the $FIO_2$ value, is included in the equation in order to correct for the difference between the subject's inspiratory and expiratory volumes. This difference in volumes is due to the effects of the respiratory exchange ratio (R).

## Calculation of METS

A value for METS can be calculated as follows:

$$METS = \frac{\dot{V}O_2 max}{0.0035 \text{ l/min/kg} \times Wt_{sub}}$$

where 0.0035 l/min/kg is the normal resting value of $\dot{V}O_2$, and $Wt_{sub}$ is the subject's actual body weight in kilograms.

## CARBON DIOXIDE PRODUCTION

A value for carbon dioxide production ($\dot{V}CO_2$) (l/min at STPD) can be calculated as follows:

$$\dot{V}CO_2 = (FECO_2 - FICO_2) \times \dot{V}_E$$

where $FECO_2$ is measured from the subject's mixed expired gas, a value of .0003 can be used for $FICO_2$ or an accurate measurement of $FICO_2$ can be made, and $\dot{V}_E$ (l/min) is the value measured during the test but converted to STPD. This value can be derived from either an ATPS or a BTPS value for $\dot{V}_E$ by use of one of the two methods described previously.

## VENTILATORY EQUIVALENTS FOR OXYGEN AND CARBON DIOXIDE

The ventilatory equivalents for oxygen ($\dot{V}_E/\dot{V}O_2$) and carbon dioxide ($\dot{V}_E/\dot{V}CO_2$) can be calculated by the following equations:

$$\dot{V}_{E\dot{V}O}2 = \frac{\dot{V}_E - (f \times V_D valve)}{\dot{V}O_2}$$

$$\dot{V}_E/\dot{V}CO_2 = \frac{\dot{V}_E - (f \times V_D valve)}{\dot{V}CO_2}$$

where $\dot{V}_E$ (l/min at BTPS) is the value calculated previously, f (breaths/min) is the respiratory rate during the measurement time period, $V_D valve$ (liters) is the amount of deadspace per breath that existed in the breathing valve, and $\dot{V}O_2$ and $\dot{V}CO_2$ (l/min at STPD) are the previously calculated values.

## RESPIRATORY EXCHANGE RATIO

A value for respiratory exchange ratio (R) can be calculated as follows:

$$R = \frac{\dot{V}CO_2}{\dot{V}O_2}$$

where $\dot{V}O_2$ and $\dot{V}CO_2$ (l/min at STPD) are the previously calculated values. The value calculated for R can generally be assumed to represent a value for the respiratory quotient (RQ).

## OXYGEN PULSE

A value for oxygen pulse ($O_2pulse$) (ml $O_2$/beat at STPD) can be calculated as follows:

$$O_2pulse = \frac{\dot{V}O_2 \times 1000}{HR}$$

where $\dot{V}O_2$ (l/min at STPD) is the value that was previously calculated, HR (beats/min) is the heart rate measured during the same time period, and 1000 is needed to convert the final value from liters $O_2$ to millileters $O_2$.

## PHYSIOLOGIC DEADSPACE AND DEADSPACE TO TIDAL VOLUME RATIO

Values for physiologic deadspace and the ratio of deadspace to tidal volume can be calculated if values for either $PaCO_2$ or $PetCO_2$ are available for the time period for which the deadspace values are being determined.

## Physiologic Deadspace Volume

A value for physiologic deadspace volume ($V_D$) (liters at BTPS) can be determined if a value for either $PaCO_2$ or $PetCO_2$ is available for substitution as a value for $PACO_2$. It can be calculated as follows:

$$V_D = \left( V_T \times \frac{PACO_2 - PECO_2}{PACO_2} \right) V_D value$$

where $V_T$ (liters at BTPS) is the previously calculated value, and $PACO_2$ (mm Hg) is the alveolar partial pressure of carbon dioxide. As described in Chapter 5, this can be substituted for by using values for either $PaCO_2$ or $PetCO_2$. $PECO_2$ (mm Hg) is the value for the subject's partial pressure of carbon dioxide in the mixed expired gas.

## Physiologic Deadspace to Tidal Volume Ratio

A value for physiologic deadspace to tidal volume ratio ($V_D/V_T$) can be calculated as follows:

$$V_D/V_T = \frac{V_D}{V_T}$$

where both the $V_D$ and the $V_T$ values (both at liters at BTPS) are taken from previous calculations.

# INTERPRETATION OF CARDIOPULMONARY STRESS TESTING RESULTS

In normal subjects, exercise performance is limited primarily by the function of the cardiovascular system. At the point where a normal subject becomes exhausted and achieves a normal $\dot{V}O_2max$, it is because the cardiovascular system has reached its limit of being able to supply enough oxygenated blood to the muscles to maintain their level of metabolism.

## NORMAL RESPONSE TO CARDIOPULMONARY STRESS TESTING

Generally, *the results of a cardiopulmonary stress test can be considered normal if the subject achieves a $\dot{V}O_2max$ that is within the 95% confidence limit for the subject's predicted normal.* Equations for predicting a normal value for $\dot{V}O_2max$ and the 95% confidence limits are presented in Table 14–4.

For the normal subject, the following will be true regarding his or her key monitored parameters at the end of an incremental work rate test. With the maximum exercise workload at the end of the test, the subject's

- $\dot{V}O_2max$ will be within the predicted normal range.
- $\dot{V}_Emax$ will be approximately 70% of the previously measured MVV (or, if not measured, approximated by $FEV_1 \times 35$). This represents a $\dot{V}_Emax/MVV$ of 0.70.

**TABLE 14–4  Predictive Equations for Normal $\dot{V}O_2$ Values (ml/min at STPD)**

### Cycle Ergometer Studies: Lower 95% Confidence Limit = 85% of Predicted $\dot{V}O_2$max

#### Male Subjects

| | |
|---|---|
| Normal or Underweight | $\dot{V}O_2max = Wt \times [50.72 - (0.372 \times A)]$ |
| Overweight[1] | $\dot{V}O_2max = [(0.79 \times Ht) - 60.7) \times (50.72 - (0.372 \times A))]$ |

#### Female Subjects

| | |
|---|---|
| Normal or Underweight | $\dot{V}O_2max = [(42.8 + Wt) \times (22.78 - (0.17 \times A))]$ |
| Overweight[2] | $\dot{V}O_2max = Ht \times [14.81 \times (0.11 \times A)]$ |

### Treadmill Studies: Lower 95% Confidence Limit = Predicted $\dot{V}O_2$max − (8.2 × Wt)

#### Male Subjects

| | |
|---|---|
| Normal or Underweight | $\dot{V}O_2max = Wt \times [56.36 - (0.413 \times A)]$ |
| Overweight[1] | $\dot{V}O_2max = [0.79 \times (Ht - 60.7)) \times (56.36 - (0.413 \times A))]$ |

#### Female Subjects

| | |
|---|---|
| Normal or Underweight | $\dot{V}O_2max = Wt \times [44.37 - (0.413 \times A)]$ |
| Overweight[3] | $\dot{V}O_2max = [0.79 \times (Ht - 68.2)] \times [44.37 - (0.413 \times A))]$ |

As referenced above for the predictive equations, a subject is considered to be overweight if

1. $Wt > [(0.79 \times Ht) - 60.7]$ for all male subjects.
2. $Wt > [(0.65 \times Ht) - 42.8]$ for female subjects undergoing cycle ergometer studies.
3. $Wt > [(0.79 \times Ht) - 68.2]$ for female subjects undergoing treadmill subjects.

*Wt = body weight in kilograms.*
*Ht = height in centimeters.*
*A = age in years.*
*Source: Modified from K. Wasserman, J.E. Hansen, D.Y. Sue, and B.J. Whipp, Principles of Exercise Testing and Interpretation (Philadelphia: Lea & Febiger, 1987).*

- $O_2$ saturation (and $PaO_2$) values will remain within the normal range.
- $V_D/V_T$ values will be normal in that they will have decreased in the manner that normally occurs with exercise.
- HRmax will closely approach the predicted HRmax ($\geq$ 90% of predicted).

- $O_2$ pulse values will be normal in that they will have increased in the manner that normally occurs with exercise.

A measured $\dot{V}O_2max$ value that is less than predicted can be due to the subject not performing a maximum work effort during the test. If this problem is identified, the test should be repeated.

## ABNORMAL RESPONSE TO CARDIOPULMONARY STRESS TESTING

Excluding a submaximal effort by the subject, *a measured $\dot{V}O_2max$ value that is below the 95% confidence limit for the subject's predicted normal value indicates that some factor is responsible for limiting the subject's ability to perform exercise.* There are three basic factors that can produce a limitation to exercise:

- Poor conditioning.
- Pulmonary disorders.
- Cardiovascular disorders.

Table 14–5 provides a comparison of the effects that these abnormalities have on key parameters measured during exercise testing.

The severity of a subject's exercise limitations can to some degree be quantified based on the $\dot{V}O_2max$ value that was achieved. The subject can be identified as having a mild to moderate impairment if the measured $\dot{V}O_2max$ is 60%–80% of the predicted normal

**TABLE 14–5  General Patterns for the Effects of Abnormalities on Key Stress Testing Parameters**

| Parameters at Maximal Exercise | Poor Conditioning | Pulmonary Disorders | Cardiovascular Disorders |
|---|---|---|---|
| $\dot{V}O_2max$ | Low | Low | Low |
| METS | Low | Low | Low |
| $\dot{V}_Emax/MVV$ | Low | **HIGH** | Low |
| $O_2Sat$ | N | **LOW** | N |
| $V_D/V_T$ | N | N or High | N |
| HRmax/Workload | High | N | High* |
| $O_2$pulse | **N** | N | **LOW** |

Low = *measured value is less than normal.*
High = *measured value is greater than normal.*
  N = *measured value is within the normal range.*
*In addition to the HR/Workload values being elevated, there are corresponding ECG arrhythmias.*
Note: *Physiologic responses in* **BOLD** *type are key parameters for interpretation.*

value. A severe impairment can be interpreted from a $\dot{V}O_2$max value that is less than 60% of the predicted normal.

## Poor Conditioning

Poor conditioning is often a contributor to limited exercise performance. This is true even if pulmonary or cardiovascular disorders are present. With poor conditioning, *the key factor limiting exercise is that the cardiovascular system is less capable than normal of being able to supply oxygenated blood to the working muscles.* This is evidenced by the following:

• HRmax is achieved at a lower than normal workload level (i.e., a high HRmax/workload value).

• $\dot{V}O_2$ is low as a result of the subject's cardiovascular system reaching its maximum level of performance (HRmax) earlier than normal during the test and at a lower workload.

• $\dot{V}_E$max/MVV is low as a result of the subject becoming fatigued before reaching an exercise level that challenges the need for ventilation.

As can be seen in Table 14–5, the pattern of test results for a subject with poor conditioning is similar to that of a subject with a cardiovascular disorder. This is because, as stated previously, the primary factor limiting exercise with poor conditioning is a less than normal performance by the cardiovascular system.

## Pulmonary Disorders

Obstructive and restrictive pulmonary disorders can both limit a subject's ability to perform and maintain increased levels of muscular work. As can be seen in Table 14–5, in addition to the reduced $\dot{V}O_2$ value, the abnormal test results all relate to pulmonary parameters measured during the test.

*An elevated value for $\dot{V}_E$max/MVV indicates that a ventilatory limitation to exercise performance is very likely to be present in the subject.* Increased values for $\dot{V}_E$max/MVV occurs primarily in subjects with obstructive disorders. The increase is due largely to the pre-exercise reduction in MVV that these subjects often have. Because of their reduced overall ability to generate a high level of ventilation, the ventilation that takes place during exercise requires use of a greater portion of the subject's ventilatory reserve.

A normal subject's $\dot{V}_E$max value during maximum exercise will be approximately 70% of her or his measured or predicted MVV. This means that even during a maximum exercise performance, the subject does not have to perform a maximum level of ventilatory work. There still exists approximately a 30% reserve in ventilatory potential.

Conversely, an obstructed subject's $\dot{V}_E$max during maximum exercise may approach or be equal to his or her measured or predicted MVV value. The subject is performing a nearly maximal level of ventilatory work, leaving little or no ventilatory reserve. Because of this limit in ventilation, some of these subjects may experience a maximum level of exercise tolerance before the anaerobic threshold is reached.

The reduction in $SaO_2$ ($SpO_2$) and $PaO_2$ values and the increase in $P(A-a)O_2$ values in these subjects occur because exercise generally worsens any pulmonary disorder that is capable of producing hypoxemia. Disorders such as ventilation/perfusion abnormalities, diffusion defects, and right-to-left shunting can all contribute to a worsening of hypoxemia during exercise. In some subjects who are hypoxemic and have elevated $P(A-a)O_2$ values at rest, these values improve with exercise. These improvements can be due to one or both of the following mechanisms:

- Reduction in $PACO_2$ values. These reduced $PACO_2$ values can result from the increases in ventilation that occur during moderate or high levels of exercise. The reduced values in turn increase $PAO_2$ values and therefore blood oxygenation.
- Increases in cardiac output and/or redistribution of ventilation. These changes can improve ventilation/perfusion relationships within the lung.

Pulmonary vascular disorders such as pulmonary hypertension can cause significant abnormalities in test results. Subjects with these disorders often have elevated $V_D/V_T$ values at rest. Because of this elevation, when these subjects perform exercise, the normal pattern of $V_D/V_T$ decreases with exercise does not occur. Instead there is an abnormally elevated $V_D/V_T$ value during exercise.

Because of the high levels of deadspace ventilation in these subjects, $\dot{V}_E/\dot{V}CO_2$ values can also be elevated (greater than 50 liter/liter $\dot{V}CO_2$). Significant $HbO_2$ desaturation and hypoxemia during exercise are also demonstrated in subjects with pulmonary vascular disorders.

## Cardiovascular Disorders

Many cardiovascular disorders can limit a subject's ability to perform and maintain increased levels of muscular work. These disorders include cardiomyopathy, coronary artery disease, peripheral vascular disorders, increased systemic vascular resistance, cardiac valvular disorders, and **neurocirculatory asthenia**.

Table 14–5 shows how cardiovascular disorders can affect the results of exercise testing. A key point is that *many subjects who have cardiovascular disorders will reach their maximum tolerated exercise level before the anaerobic threshold is reached.* This can be a diagnostic sign for exercise limitations that are due to cardiovascular disorders.

The reduced value for $\dot{V}_E max/MVV$ is not the result of a pulmonary dysfunction caused by the cardiovascular disorder. The subject's ability to perform an MVV maneuver and ventilation during exercise may well be normal. Instead, the reduced $\dot{V}_E max/MVV$ value is due to the level of the subject's exercise performance being prematurely limited by cardiovascular factors. The exercise was limited before there was a physiologic need to increase the level of ventilation significantly. This physiologic need results in a measured $\dot{V}_E max$ value that is less than the subject's actual capability and an artificially reduced value for $\dot{V}_E max/MVV$.

The cardiovascular disorders listed previously all can have the effect of reducing the stroke volume of the heart. For this reason, the increased cardiac output needs of exercise must be met, even more so than normally, by increases in heart rate. The heart rate increases and reaches a maximum level more quickly and at lower workloads than normal.

This same set of factors also results in the value for $O_2$pulse being reduced in these subjects. Stroke volume is reduced, and higher heart rates are needed to respond to a given $\dot{V}O_2$ level. The result is a reduction in $O_2$pulse. *The low $O_2$ pulse value may be interpreted directly as an indication that the subject's stroke volume is limited during exercise.*

A key factor in identifying cardiovascular limitations to exercise is the fact that the elevated $HR_{max}$/workload relationship also corresponds to arrhythmias and/or ST segment changes being demonstrated on ECG as the heart rate increases. Premature ventricular contractions (PVCs) are often demonstrated during exercise by subjects with cardiovascular disorders. They are often induced by myocardial ischemia and can appear with a frequency of 10 or more per minute. PVCs are significant because their presence can be a precursor to more serious, life-threatening arrhythmias such as ventricular tachycardia and ventricular fibrillation. Coupled PVCs or strings of PVCs often precede the start of more serious arrhythmias.

ST segment depression indicates that myocardial ischemia is likely to be present. ST segment depression by more than 1 mm for a time duration of 0.08 second is a significant sign for myocardial ischemia. When the ST segment reduction occurs at low workloads and continues after exercise has been stopped, it is very likely that a multiple-vessel coronary artery disorder is responsible for the ischemia.

The presence of exertional hypotension or a marked increase in diastolic blood pressure during exercise can also indicate the presence of a severe coronary artery disorder. The subject's clinical history and correlation with coronary artery disease risk factors must be taken into consideration before a final judgment is made.

In the case of some cardiovascular disorders, it is possible for reduced HRmax values to be demonstrated during exercise. Subjects with complete heart block and subjects receiving medications that inhibit stimulation from the sympathetic branch of the autonomic nervous system (beta-blocking agents) are in this category. Pathophysiologic impairment of the autonomic nervous system or denervation of the heart (as associated with heart transplantation) can also result in reduced HRmax values. At times, ischemic myocardial disorders can cause reduced HRmax values. This occurs when the test is terminated early because of the presence of significant arrhythmias.

When reduced HRmax values occur during an exercise test, it is possible to quantify the degree of impairment. HRmax values of 90%–94% of predicted indicate a borderline disorder, 85%–89% a mild disorder, 75%–84% a moderate disorder, and values 74% or less a severe disorder. It should be noted that these are arbitrarily chosen values. They can be used as guidelines for interpretation but do not provide a definitive identification of impairment.

## Review Questions

Please use the following review questions to evaluate your learning of information from this chapter. It might be helpful to write out your answers on a sheet of paper. If you are unsure of the answers to these questions, review the chapter to reinforce your learning.

1. What are indications and contraindications for cardiopulmonary stress testing?
2. Relating to different types of exercise tests:
   a. What is the 12-minute walking distance test?
   b. What is the Harvard step test?
   c. How is testing to evaluate the effects of exercise on oxygemoglobin desaturation performed?

    d. How can testing to evaluate the effects of exercise on oxyhemoglobin desaturation be used to evaluate the need for supplemental oxygen during exercise?

    e. What are constant work rate tests?

    f. What are incremental work rate tests?

3. Relating to preparation for exercise testing:

    a. What preliminary evaluation should be performed before cardiopulmonary stress testing is performed on a subject?

    b. How should the laboratory be prepared for the test?

    c. How should the subject be prepared for the test?

4. Relating to the time that cardiopulmonary stress testing is performed:

    a. What preparation is required?

    b. What resting measurements should be made?

    c. What monitoring should be performed during the test?

    d. At what point is the test terminated?

    e. What are adverse reactions that a subject may demonstrate during cardiopulmonary stress testing?

    f. What data should be reported?

5. Relating to what is done after cardiopulmonary stress testing is completed:

    a. How is a value for exhaled minute ventilation determined?

    b. How is a value for exhaled minute volume determined?

    c. How is a value for oxygen consumption determined?

    d. How is a value for carbon dioxide production determined?

    e. How are values for ventilatory equivalents for oxygen and carbon dioxide determined?

    f. How is a value for respiratory exchange ratio determined?

    g. How is a value for oxygen pulse determined?

    h. How are values for physiologic deadspace and deadspace to tidal volume ratio determined?

6. Relating to the interpretation of cardiopulmonary stress testing results:

    a. Under what conditions are the results of cardiopulmonary stress testing considered normal?

    b. What effect does poor conditioning have on the results of cardiopulmonary stress testing?

    c. What effects do pulmonary disorders have on the results of cardiopulmonary stress testing?

    d. What effects do cardiovascular disorders have on the results of cardiopulmonary stress testing?

# CHAPTER FIFTEEN

# ADMINISTRATION OF TESTS FOR METABOLIC AND NUTRITIONAL ASSESSMENT

## RELATED LEARNING

Prior knowledge of the following related information will facilitate understanding and learning of the material in this chapter. The learner will be aided by being able to

1. Recall cardiopulmonary stress testing concepts from Chapter 14.
2. Describe the basic operation and use of positive-pressure, volume-controlled mechanical ventilators.

## LEARNING OBJECTIVES

Upon successful completion of this chapter, the learner should be able to

1. State the need for bedside metabolic and nutritional assessment in the clinical setting.
2. Describe the test procedures used for metabolic and nutritional assessment.
3. Describe the methods for performing indirect calorimetry, including
   a. closed-circuit calorimetry
   b. open-circuit calorimetry
   c. special considerations for performing indirect calorimetry
4. Describe the administration of metabolic/nutritional assessment tests.
5. Describe the calculations required for metabolic/nutritional assessment.
6. Explain the significance of metabolic/nutritional data.

## KEY TERMS

enteral
kilocalorie

neutral thermal environment
parenteral

Metabolic and nutritional assessment at the bedside has become an important part of providing care for critically ill or injured patients. Many of the measurement techniques and determinations made during cardiopulmonary stress testing can be modified for use in metabolic and nutritional assessment. Much of the difference is in how the techniques are applied and in additional calculations that are performed.

# THE NEED FOR BEDSIDE METABOLIC AND NUTRITIONAL ASSESSMENT

Critically ill and injured patients can experience significant changes in their metabolic processes. These metabolic changes can have a direct impact on nutritional needs. Despite the fact that critically ill or injured patients are confined to a bed, their levels of metabolic activity are usually significantly greater than those of a normal individual who is resting in bed.

Ensuring that these patients' nutritional intake is adequate to meet their metabolic needs is an important part of care. A complication to this situation is that these patients are generally not able to take solid food by mouth. They often must have their nutritional needs met by use of **parenteral** nutritional procedures. The combination of the changes in metabolic activity levels and special nutritional requirements greatly complicates the management of critically ill and traumatized patients.

Both undernourishment and overnourishment are problems for critical care patients. If a patient's caloric expenditure, based on metabolic activity levels, exceeds the available caloric intake of nutrients, *undernourishment* or starvation can occur. Fat stores in the patient may be used to compensate for the undernourishment. More importantly, the protein in muscle tissue may also be consumed as a source of "nutrition." The breakdown of the body in this way, at a time when it is trying to fight infection and/or repair itself, is counterproductive to the patient's recovery.

*Overnourishment* is also a problem. Caloric intake in excess of metabolic needs and caloric expenditure will result in storage of the excess calories in the form of body fat. Accumulation of fat stores can be a source of physiologic stress to the organ systems and can hinder the patient's recovery.

# TEST PROCEDURES FOR METABOLIC AND NUTRITIONAL ASSESSMENT

Measurement of a patient's body weight changes and evaluation of body fat levels through upper arm skinfold measurements can be used to assess the effects of a patient's nutrition. *Calorimetry* provides another method of assessing a patient's metabolic and nutritional status. This is the measurement of the amount of body heat in units of *calories* that is generated by the body during metabolism. A greater number of calories measured by calorimetry directly indicates that there is a greater rate of metabolism and consumption of nutrients occurring within the body.

## TYPES OF CALORIMETRY PROCEDURES

There are two basic types of calorimetry procedures: direct calorimetry and indirect calorimetry.

### Direct Calorimetry

*Direct calorimetry* makes use of a chamber that completely encloses the test subject and directly measures the quantity (calories) of heat released by the body. Unfortunately, such a device is not practical for use at the bedside.

### Indirect Calorimetry

*Indirect calorimetry* provides a more practical approach to bedside metabolic and nutritional testing. The exhaled volume measurement and expired gas analysis principles used in exercise testing are applied with indirect calorimetry procedures. Measurement of values for $\dot{V}O_2$, $\dot{V}_E$, and, in many cases, $\dot{V}CO_2$ is performed. Use of these values in a series of calculations makes it possible to use indirect calorimetry to derive some clinically significant metabolic and nutritional data on a patient. These data include determination of values for

- The patient's estimated *resting energy expenditure* (REE) level. This is the amount of body heat generated by the patient's metabolic processes within a 24-hour period with the body in a stable, quiet resting state. The unit of measure for REE is the **kilocalorie** (kcal). The REE for a normal individual represents approximately two thirds of his or her daily caloric energy requirements.
- The number of kilocalories generated by the patient through metabolism of each of the three main nutritional substrates: carbohydrates, lipids, and protein.
- The patient's *respiratory exchange ratio* (R), which can be used as an indicator of the patient's *respiratory quotient* (RQ).

Availability of these data can greatly improve the nutritional management of critically ill and injured patients.

# METHODS FOR PERFORMING INDIRECT CALORIMETRY

There are two methods that can be used for performing indirect calorimetry: closed-circuit calorimetry and open-circuit calorimetry.

## CLOSED-CIRCUIT CALORIMETRY

*Closed-circuit calorimetry* is a method of directly measuring the rate of a subject's oxygen consumption from within a closed breathing system. It permits determination of a value for $\dot{V}O_2$ without obtaining values for a subject's $FIO_2$ and $FEO_2$. Two techniques can be used for closed-circuit calorimetry. One involves measurement of $\dot{V}O_2$ by oxygen depletion and the other by oxygen replacement.

Both techniques involve having the subject rebreathe for a period of time on a closed breathing system. The closed breathing system consists of a mouthpiece and tubing that connect directly to a volume-displacement spirometer. Values for $\dot{V}_E$, $V_T$, and f can be determined from spirometer measurements made during the test. A canister containing a carbon dioxide-removing compound, such as soda lime, must be included in the breathing circuit to permit rebreathing without the risk of hypercapnia. Nose clips must be worn by the subject.

## The Oxygen-Depletion Technique for Closed-Circuit Calorimetry

The *oxygen-depletion technique* involves having the subject rebreathe for a period of time on the closed breathing system. Because of the subject's metabolism, oxygen will be consumed from the system during the time of rebreathing. The carbon dioxide produced by metabolism and exhaled by the subject is absorbed from the rebreathing system by the soda lime. Thus, as the subject consumes oxygen from within the spirometer during rebreathing, a decreasing volume will be registered on the spirometer tracing. A value for $\dot{V}O_2$ can be determined by dividing the amount of the spirometer volume decrease (in milliliters) by the time period (in minutes) that rebreathing was performed.

## The Oxygen-Replacement Technique for Closed-Circuit Calorimetry

The *oxygen-replacement technique* involves having a connection added to the closed breathing system that permits the addition of oxygen as the subject rebreathes. The goal is to establish a rate of oxygen addition to the breathing circuit that matches the rate of the subject's oxygen consumption. This is done by adjusting the rate of oxygen flow into the system in order to maintain the spirometer at a constant volume level. The oxygen flow rate (in ml/min) that is required for volume maintenance can then be considered to be equal to the subject's rate of oxygen consumption.

The system as presented does not permit a method for measuring the subject's $\dot{V}CO_2$. If desired, the $\dot{V}CO_2$ can be measured by adding a $CO_2$ analyzer to the system and making measurements of expired $CO_2$ values. A value for $\dot{V}CO_2$ can also be estimated. For example, if the subject's value for respiratory quotient is 0.85, the value for the subject's $\dot{V}CO_2$ would be approximately equal to 0.85 times the measured $\dot{V}O_2$ value.

## Closed-Circuit Calorimetry for Mechanically Ventilated Patients

The description so far has referred only to making measurements on spontaneously breathing subjects. This same method can be used for making measurements on patients receiving mechanical ventilatory support. However, it involves making significant changes in the rebreathing circuit system and in how the patient is supported by the ventilator.

- The spirometer of the rebreathing system (it must be a bellows-type spirometer) is enclosed within a chamber that has a fixed, constant volume.

- The ventilator is connected to the chamber that contains the spirometer of the rebreathing system.
- The patient's artificial airway is connected to the subject connection of the rebreathing system.
- The patient is ventilated by having the positive pressure volume that is delivered by the ventilator compress the bellows of the spirometer. This in turn forces air from the spirometer into the subject.

This method can be used with either the oxygen-depletion technique or the oxygen-replacement technique. There are two points to be considered, however:

1. Care must be taken in establishing the $FIO_2$ of the gas contained within the rebreathing system before the patient is connected. It should reasonably match the $FIO_2$ that was being delivered by the patient's ventilator.
2. An increase will have to be made in the volume delivered by the ventilator. This increase compensates for the volume of gas compressed within the spirometer chamber as pressure builds up there to force gas from within the spirometer into the patient.

The amount of ventilator volume increase that is needed can be judged by monitoring the $V_T$ excursions of the spirometer. If the spirometer volume excursions are less than the pre-set ventilator volume, the ventilator volume control setting will have to be increased. The compensatory increase often results in being approximately 1 ml of volume increase for each cm $H_2O$ generated by the ventilator during inspiration. Once adequate ventilation has been established, the patient's $\dot{V}O_2$ can be measured.

## OPEN-CIRCUIT CALORIMETRY

*Open-circuit calorimetry* involves measuring $\dot{V}O_2$, $\dot{V}CO_2$, and $\dot{V}_E$ in a manner similar to that used during exercise testing. Systems with either a mixing chamber or breath-by-breath analysis can be used. Spontaneously breathing subjects can use a mouthpiece, nose clips, and breathing valve as described previously for exercise testing.

A subject who is ill and lying in bed may not be comfortable breathing on such an apparatus. For this reason, *head enclosure systems* have been developed to make measurements more comfortable for reclining subjects.

These systems operate as follows: A hood or canopy encloses the subject's head. A constant flow of air is maintained through the hood. This is done by having the system draw a flow of air into the hood that exceeds the subject's inspiratory flow rate. Generally, air flow rates through the hood of approximately 40 l/min are adequate. The subject's ventilatory parameters ($\dot{V}_E$, $V_T$, and f) are determined by having the system measure the cyclic changes in the total gas flow into and out of the hood during breathing. This can be referred to as using "bias" flow measurement to determine ventilation volumes. Expired gas analysis is performed on the gas exiting the hood.

Open-circuit calorimetry can be performed with patients receiving mechanical ventilatory support. The requirements for doing this are the ability to determine values for the patient's $FIO_2$ and $FEO_2$, $FICO_2$ and $FECO_2$, and exhaled volumes. Generally, the gas analysis is performed through breath-by-breath analysis at the patient's artificial airway/ventilatory circuit connection.

## SPECIAL CONSIDERATIONS FOR PERFORMING INDIRECT CALORIMETRY

Patients who are receiving supplemental oxygen or are receiving mechanical ventilatory support (probably with supplemental oxygen) present special problems for performing indirect calorimetry.

### Considerations for Subjects Receiving Supplemental Oxygen

Systems have been previously described for use in exercise or metabolic/nutritional testing. With these systems, while a measured value for $FEO_2$ is needed for determining a value for $\dot{V}O_2$, it is assumed that the value for $FIO_2$ is 0.21. This is because the subject is described as inspiring room air while breathing on the test system.

Subjects who are receiving supplemental oxygen create a change in this situation. The $FIO_2$ is going to have a value that is something greater than 0.21. Additionally, the oxygen/air gas mixing systems used to establish an $FIO_2$ often do not maintain an absolutely constant $FIO_2$ level. At least minor fluctuations in $FIO_2$ can occur. For this reason, the subject's $FIO_2$ cannot be assumed to be what is set on the mixing system.

*As a result of these considerations, for subjects who are receiving supplemental oxygen, measurements must be made of $FIO_2$ values during the test in addition to the $FEO_2$ measurements that are typically made.* The only exception to this is when closed-circuit calorimetry is used. With closed-circuit calorimetry, determination of a value for $\dot{V}O_2$ is not based on a calculation using values for $FIO_2$ and $FEO_2$.

### Considerations for Subjects Receiving Mechanical Ventilatory Support

Patients who are on mechanical ventilatory support by positive pressure ventilation also present a special problem for testing. The problem relates to gas analysis. It is based on the fact that the operation of many gas analyzers is affected by changes in total gas pressure and/or the partial pressure of gases. The cyclic pressure increases during inspiration and decreases during expiration within the breathing circuit of a positive pressure ventilator are the source of this problem. These increases and decreases affect the total pressure of the gases within the breathing circuit and therefore the partial pressures of the gases. The result is that, depending on the gas analysis sampling techniques used, the pressure increases during inspiration will produce falsely elevated gas analysis readings. *It is important that the lower gas analysis value, taken when positive pressure is not exerted within the circuit, be recorded.*

## ADMINISTRATION OF METABOLIC/NUTRITIONAL ASSESSMENT TESTS

The indirect calorimetry test performed for metabolic/nutritional assessment generally involves a measurement time period of no more than a half hour. However, the primary purpose for performing the test is to establish an estimation of what the subject's *resting energy expenditure* (REE) will be over an extended period of time—usually a 24-hour period. The manner in which the subject is prepared and how the test is administered both have a significant impact on how accurate this estimation will be.

## PREPARATION FOR TESTS

In preparation for a test, there are certain key points that should be considered:

- Drugs or other substances that affect metabolism should be avoided prior to the test. Caffeine, methylxanthine-type medications, and nicotine all can have a stimulating effect on metabolism.
- The subject should fast for two to four hours prior to the time the test is scheduled to start. If the subject is receiving either **enteral** or parenteral feedings, the feedings should be administered by a continuous method instead of being given by bolus.
- Patients receiving mechanical ventilatory support should be in a reasonably stable medical condition. If possible, no ventilator control adjustments should be made within one to two hours before the start of the test. This is because control changes that affect $FIO_2$ or $\dot{V}_E$, especially in subjects who have pulmonary disorders, can significantly affect the patterns of gas exchange within the lung.

## TEST ADMINISTRATION

There are also two points of concern that should be addressed during administration of a test:

- A **neutral thermal environment** should be maintained for the subject during the test. This may mean that special arrangements will have to be made for subjects who are febrile or hypothermic.
- Once test measurements are begun, they should continue to be made until it can be confirmed that they represent a steady-state level for metabolism. This is demonstrated if the subject's measured values for $\dot{V}O_2$, $\dot{V}CO_2$, $\dot{V}_E$, and heart rate remain reasonably stable and do not vary more than $\pm 5\%$ over a reasonable period of time.

    In some cases, the subject may not demonstrate steady-state conditions within the usual time interval for the test. If this problem occurs, the test interval can be extended to allow for sampling over a longer period of metabolic activity. The longer period may allow an accumulation of data that are more representative of what the subject's average metabolic state will be over a 24-hour period.

# CALCULATIONS REQUIRED FOR METABOLIC/ NUTRITIONAL ASSESSMENT

The first thing that must be done with the test data is to calculate values for the subject's $\dot{V}O_2$ and $\dot{V}CO_2$ during the test time period. This is done by use of the equations described previously for exercise testing in Chapter 14. It should be noted that only a value for exhaled minute ventilation is measured during this test. As a result, the equation used for calculating $\dot{V}O_2$ should be the one presented earlier that makes use of only a $\dot{V}_E$ value and not the one previous to that which makes use of both $\dot{V}_E$ and $\dot{V}_I$ values.

In addition to the values for $\dot{V}O_2$ and $\dot{V}CO_2$, a value for the subject's *urinary nitrogen* (UN) must be established. A UN value is determined through measurements on a 24-hour collection of urine and has a unit of gm/24 hours. With all of this data available, it is possible to calculate the subject's metabolic and nutritional status.

## CALCULATION OF RESTING ENERGY EXPENDITURE

The subject's REE (kcal/24 hours) can be calculated by use of the following equation:

$$REE = \{1.44 \times [(3.941 \times \dot{V}O_2) + (1.106 \times \dot{V}CO_2)]\} - (2.17 \times UN)$$

The number 1.44 is needed to change the $\dot{V}O_2$ and $\dot{V}CO_2$ contributions to the calculation from ml/min to l/24 hours. Note that if the UN portion of the equation were excluded, the calculation of REE from the $\dot{V}O_2$ and $\dot{V}CO_2$ values alone would result in an error of only 2% at most.

If a value for $\dot{V}CO_2$ is not available, as might be the case when closed-circuit indirect calorimetry is performed, it is possible to use the preceding equation to calculate REE using only the values for $\dot{V}O_2$ and UN. This is demonstrated in the following modified equation:

$$REE = \{1.44 \times [(3.941 \times \dot{V}O_2) + (1.106 \times (\dot{V}O_2 \times 0.85))]\} - (2.17 \times UN)$$

The modification assumes that with a normal respiratory quotient of 0.85, the subject's $\dot{V}CO_2$ value is equal to the $\dot{V}O_2$ times 0.85. If the subject's actual respiratory quotient varies from the normal value of 0.85, the REE calculation will be in error by no more than 5% at most.

As a source of comparison, it is possible to calculate predictive values for REE for normal subjects who are at complete rest. For male subjects, the equation is

$$REE = 66.47 + (13.75 \times Wt) + (5.00 \times Ht) - (6.76 \times A)$$

For female subjects, the equation is

$$REE = 655.10 + (9.56 \times Wt) + (1.85 \times Ht) - (4.68 \times A)$$

where Wt is the subject's weight in kilograms, Ht is height in centimeters, and A is the subject's age in years. Under the conditions of this calculation, the REE of the subject is based on the metabolism of the subject's lean body mass. In the past, the parameter predicted by these equations was referred to as the subject's *basal metabolic rate* (BMR).

## CALCULATION OF THE NUMBER OF KILOCALORIES PRODUCED BY METABOLIC SUBSTRATES

It is possible to calculate the number of kilocalories of body heat generated by the metabolism of carbohydrates, lipids, and proteins. First the caloric equivalent (in grams) of each substrate is calculated as it contributes to metabolism. For carbohydrates, the equation is

$$\text{Carbohydrate Caloric Equivalent} = (4.12 \times \dot{V}O_2) - (2.91 \times \dot{V}CO_2) - (1.94 \times UN)$$

For lipids, the equation is

$$\text{Lipid Caloric Equivalent} = (1.69 \times \dot{V}O_2) - (1.69 \times \dot{V}CO_2) - (2.54 \times UN)$$

For proteins, the equation is

$$\text{Protein Caloric Equivalent} = (6.25 \times UN)$$

It should be noted that these equations were originally intended for applications where the subject presented reasonably normal respiratory quotient values. Subjects who have respiratory quotient values less than 0.71 or greater than 1.0 will produce negative values for either the carbohydrate or lipid caloric equivalent.

Once a value for the caloric equivalent has been calculated for each substrate, it is possible to calculate the contribution of each to body heat production in kilocalories:

$$\text{Carbohydrate Caloric Contribution} = 4.18 \times \text{Carbohydrate Caloric Equivalent}$$

$$\text{Lipid Caloric Contribution} = 9.46 \times \text{Lipid Caloric Equivalent}$$

$$\text{Protein Caloric Contribution} = 4.32 \times \text{Protein Caloric Equivalent}$$

A value for the total number of kilocalories of body heat produced by the subject in a 24-period can be calculated by adding up the caloric contributions of carbohydrate, lipid, and protein substrates.

The percentage that each substrate contributes to metabolism can be calculated as in the following example for carbohydrates:

$$\% \text{ Carbohydrate Contribution} = \frac{\text{Carbohydrate Caloric Contribution}}{\text{Total Calories in 24 Hours}}$$

## ESTIMATION OF RESPIRATORY QUOTIENT

The subject's respiratory quotient can be estimated based on calculation of the respiratory exchange ratio. The respiratory exchange ratio can be calculated in the same manner as described in Chapter 14 for exercise testing. The value for the respiratory quotient can generally be accepted as being equal to the value for the respiratory exchange ratio.

It is possible to calculate the amount of the respiratory quotient that was produced by the metabolism of carbohydrates and lipids. This is based on the fact that the value for urinary nitrogen reflects the quantity of proteins that have undergone metabolism. The following equation can be used to calculate the metabolic contribution of carbohydrate and lipid metabolism to the respiratory quotient [RQ(Car-Lip)]:

$$RQ(\text{Car-Lip}) = \frac{(1.44 \times \dot{V}CO_2) - (4.8 \times UN)}{(1.44 \times \dot{V}O_2) - (5.9 \times UN)}$$

As before, the value 1.44 is used to convert the $\dot{V}O_2$ and $\dot{V}CO_2$ values from units of ml/min to units of l/24 hours.

# SIGNIFICANCE OF METABOLIC/NUTRITIONAL DATA

The test results produced by indirect calorimetry can be very useful in the clinical setting. The data are often used either for the general nutritional management of critically ill patients or to manage the nutrition of patients who have or are at risk for experiencing ventilatory failure.

## GENERAL NUTRITIONAL MANAGEMENT FOR CRITICALLY ILL PATIENTS

A primary application of the measurement data from indirect calorimetry is in the nutritional management of critically ill patients. Although they are "resting" in bed, their rate of metabolism is far greater than that of a normal resting individual. The amount of this metabolic rate increase can vary considerably, depending on the nature of the patient's illness or injury.

Higher levels of metabolism result in more kilocalories of body heat being produced. The caloric heat energy released by the body is directly linked to the amount of energy that is consumed by metabolism. This is significant because a primary purpose of feeding is to provide nutrients that will satisfy the caloric needs of the body. The caloric input value of the feedings must match the caloric heat energy produced by the body, that is, the amount of energy input needed to support the body's metabolism.

In the past, an equation such as the one described previously was used to estimate a value for REE for the patient as if he or she were normal. This normal value was then adjusted by use for certain "factors" that were based on the nature of the patient's illness or injury. The outcome of these calculations was an estimate of the subject's caloric requirements that needed to be met through feeding.

*Indirect calorimetry eliminates the need for estimation of a subject's caloric needs.* It allows for actual measurements of what caloric needs a particular patient has at that point in her or his illness. Given this knowledge, a more specific dietary plan can be made for the patient.

## NUTRITIONAL MANAGEMENT FOR PATIENTS WHO HAVE OR ARE AT RISK FOR VENTILATORY FAILURE

Another benefit of indirect calorimetry is the management of patients with pulmonary disorders that can or have produced ventilatory failure. The reason for this is that different nutritional substrates result in different values for a subject's respiratory quotient. This is based on the following relationships between nutritional substrates and the corresponding respiratory quotient values they produce.

- Carbohydrate metabolism results in an RQ of 1.0.
- Lipid metabolism results in an RQ of 0.71.
- Protein metabolism results in an RQ of 0.82.

A patient receiving nutrition from a diet consisting primarily of carbohydrate compounds will have an RQ closer to 1.0. This will result in a greater level of $CO_2$ production for a given level of $O_2$ consumption. The outcome is that the subject will have to work harder at ventilation in order to respond to the greater quantity of $CO_2$ being produced. Conversely, a subject having a diet consisting largely of lipid compounds will have an RQ closer to 0.71. This will result in less $CO_2$ production from metabolism and a lesser burden for ventilation.

These relationships are especially important in patients who have difficulty maintaining an adequate level of ventilation. A diet consisting primarily of carbohydrate compounds may increase the patient's $CO_2$ production to a point where ventilatory failure may occur. Also, under the same conditions, weaning a patient from mechanical ventilatory support can also be made more difficult.

One approach to managing this type of patient is to perform indirect calorimetry and to make calculations of RQ(Car-Lip) values. Adjustments in the patient's diet can then be made. With these changes, the relative quantities of lipids are increased while carbohydrates are decreased. These changes should be balanced in an attempt to maintain the correct amount of total feeding calories being provided the subject. The idea is to lessen the subject's work of ventilation.

Once the dietary changes have been made, indirect calorimetry can be repeated and RQ(Car-Lip) recalculated. This is done to evaluate the effectiveness of the feeding adjustments in terms of a more beneficial RQ being produced and total caloric input being maintained.

## Review Questions

Please use the following review questions to evaluate your learning of information from this chapter. It might be helpful to write out your answers on a sheet of paper. If you are unsure of the answers to these questions, review the chapter to reinforce your learning.

1. Relating to the used of bedside metabolic and nutritional assessment:
   a. What purpose is served by the clinical use of bedside metabolic and nutritional assessment?
   b. What are methods that can be used for bedside evaluation of a subject's metabolic and nutritional condition?
2. Relating to calorimetry:
   a. What is closed-circuit calorimetry?
   b. How does the oxygen-depletion technique differ from the oxygen-replacement technique?
   c. What is open-circuit calorimetry?
   d. What are special considerations for performing indirect calorimetry?

3. Relating to the administration of metabolic/nutritional assessment tests:
   a. What preparation is needed before metabolic/nutritional assessment tests are performed?
   b. What are concerns that must be addressed during metabolic/nutritional assessment tests?
4. Relating to the determination of results for metabolic/nutritional assessment tests:
   a. How is resting energy expenditure (REE) determined?
   b. How are the number of kilocalories produced by metabolic substrates determined?
   c. How is respiratory quotient (RQ) estimated?
5. Relating to the use of metabolic/nutritional assessment measurements:
   a. How is metabolic/nutritional assessment applied to the nutritional management of critically ill patients?
   b. How is metabolic/nutritional assessment applied to the nutritional management of patients who have or are at risk for ventilatory failure?

# CHAPTER SIXTEEN

# QUALITY ASSURANCE FOR PULMONARY FUNCTION TESTING

## ———— RELATED LEARNING ————

Prior knowledge of the following related information will facilitate understanding and learning of the material in this chapter. The learner will be aided by being able to

1. Recall equipment concepts covered in Chapters 1, 3, and 10.
2. Recall the concepts of pulmonary function testing covered in Chapters 2, 4, 5, 6, and 11.
3. Recall the statistical "Key Terms" in Chapter 7.

## ———— LEARNING OBJECTIVES ————

Upon successful completion of this chapter, the learner should be able to

1. State the components of a quality assurance process for pulmonary function testing.
2. Describe the calibration and quality control for spirometers and plethysmographs, including
   a. general principles for calibration and quality control of volume, flow, and pressure measuring equipment
   b. calibration and quality control for spirometers
   c. calibration and quality control for body plethysmographs
3. Describe the calibration and quality control for gas and blood gas analysis instruments, including
   a. general principles for calibration and quality control for gas and blood gas analysis instruments
   b. the intended range for measurement and performance challenges
   c. calibration and quality control for gas analyzers
   d. calibration and quality control for blood gas analyzers

--------- **KEY TERMS** ---------

gain                              isothermal                         sensitivity

The whole purpose for pulmonary function testing is to generate physiologic measurement data that correctly reflect the current state of a subject's pulmonary system. Once available, the data are often used to make important evaluations and decisions regarding a subject's health. *Unless a great effort is made in maintaining quality in all factors that affect the measuring process, the measurement data that is generated is worthless.*

# COMPONENTS OF A QUALITY ASSURANCE PROCESS

Quality assurance practices serve two needs relating to the quality of measurement for physiologic data. These needs relate to the quality of:

- the procedures used during pulmonary function testing.
- the equipment used during pulmonary function testing.

Both must work effectively together in the process of supplying correct physiologic measurement data on a subject.

## TEST QUALITY ASSURANCE

Test quality assurance is something that is performed with each test administration. In order to assure quality, there are three things that must be evaluated with each test:

- Technologist performance.
- Equipment performance.
- Subject performance.

*Technologist performance* relates to how correctly the technologist followed the approved laboratory procedure for administering the test. *Equipment performance* relates to whether the equipment functioned as intended during the administration of a test. *Subject performance* relates to how effectively the subject understood, cooperated, and performed during the test procedure.

*The technologist is the key to test quality assurance.* Honest, critical self-evaluation should accompany the technologist's performance of each test. It is also the responsibility of the technologist to evaluate the performance of the equipment and the subject during each test. This requires critical observation and evaluation of the equipment, subject, and data produced during a test. Also, as part of the overall quality assurance for the laboratory, a technologist's performance should be evaluated routinely by an objective observer.

*The basis for performing test quality assurance has been provided in the previous chapters where the various test procedures were described.* Before the results for any test are finalized for reporting, there are three concerns that must be evaluated by the technologist:

- Did the equipment perform optimally?
- Did the subject perform optimally?
- Do the test results satisfy the criteria for acceptability for the particular test(s) performed?

If the responses to all three of these questions are *yes*, then the test results should be reported. If the response to even one of the questions is *no*, then, depending on the extent and specific nature of the situation, the technologist should do one or more of the following:

1. Attempt to correct the equipment and/or subject difficulty and repeat the affected test(s).
2. Decide that the measurements at least acceptably reflect the subject's capabilities and report the data. However, the report should specify the concerns the technologist has regarding the test procedure and/or the test results.
3. Report that testing was attempted but acceptable results could not be generated.

Especially in the case of the second choice, it is extremely important for the technologist to use good judgment in making the decision. A safe maxim in pulmonary function testing is that *it is better to report no results than to report incorrect results.*

## EQUIPMENT QUALITY ASSURANCE

The quality of any effort to make measurements can be only as good as the measuring tools that are used. This is especially true in pulmonary function testing, where so many complex measurements are made. *Equipment quality assurance is a process to ensure that the measuring tools used in pulmonary function testing are functioning at minimally acceptable levels of performance or better.* The American Thoracic Society has established standards for pulmonary function testing equipment performance. These are presented in Appendix C.

Equipment quality assurance is based on certain key factors: good maintenance of the equipment and routine performance of calibration and quality control procedures.

### Maintenance

Two types of maintenance procedures must be performed on pulmonary function testing equipment: preventative maintenance and corrective maintenance. *Preventative maintenance* consists of procedures performed on a scheduled basis in order to *avoid* breakdowns or problems with the equipment. An example is the regular checking of the water level in a water-sealed spirometer. Doing this at appropriately regular intervals ensures that the water level will not drop below a point that could possibly allow the bottom of the bell to lose contact with the water. The policy and procedure manual for a laboratory must include schedules and requirements for preventative maintenance. The manufacturer(s) of a laboratory's equipment can generally be used as a resource for developing these guidelines.

*Corrective maintenance* is performed whenever there is a breakdown in a piece of equipment. Again, the equipment's manufacturer(s) generally provide(s) guidelines for servicing the equipment. These guidelines can include adjustments and/or repairs that may be made by the laboratory personnel. Some servicing, however, may have to be performed by biomedical technologists from within the institution or by service staff from the manufacturer.

With any equipment maintenance that is performed, it is important that adequate records be kept. These records should contain the dates and types of preventative maintenance procedures that are performed. The dates and nature of corrective maintenance procedures should also be recorded. *Following any maintenance, a calibration and/or quality assurance check of the equipment should be made.* This will ensure that the equipment is operating within specifications after maintenance.

## Calibration and Quality Control

Having well-maintained equipment does not guarantee that a laboratory's measurements will correctly reflect the actual condition of the subject's lungs. In order to be effective, the measuring systems must be both precise and accurate in relation to how they are to be used.

*Precision* refers to how reproducible measurements are when testing is repeated. In other words, a precise instrument will, with each attempt at measurement, consistently provide the same result, even if it is the wrong value. At first, this seems to be an odd quality for an instrument to have. What good is an instrument that consistently provides a result that is wrong? However, if a precise instrument can be adjusted to provide a correct result, the outcome will be an instrument that consistently provides the correct result.

*Accuracy* refers to how close the results of measurement are to the correct *actual* value of what is being measured. For example, you have an object with a known actual weight of 6 grams. When the object is weighed with a scale, the scale is accurate if it correctly displays the object's weight as being 6 grams.

Accuracy is judged in a slightly different way for pulmonary function measuring systems. This is because of the complexity of the measurements being made. Such factors as a slight variation in the subject's effort, change in body position, or fatigue can cause measurement results to vary slightly, even if the condition of the subject's lungs has not changed. For this reason, *accuracy is based on how closely the mean of a series of measurements approximates the actual value of what is being measured.*

There is one other important aspect of accuracy. In order to be most useful, *a measuring system must continue to be accurate over a range of values.* When a wider value range is measured by a system, it is more difficult to maintain the same level of accuracy over the entire range.

The goal of any measurement system manufacturer is to produce instruments that are precise in making measurements. *Given a precise instrument, calibration performed prior to the instrument's use will make the instrument accurate. Once the instrument is calibrated, quality control is periodically done to test the instrument to evaluate how well it is functioning.*

*Calibration.* Calibration is a process that makes a precise measuring instrument function so that the results correctly reflect the actual value of what is measured. Calibration of a measuring instrument consists of two steps:

1. Using the instrument to make a measurement of a sample that has a known, fixed value. This sample can be referred to as a *test signal*.
2. If necessary, making a calibration adjustment on the instrument so that the measurement results are equal to the fixed, known test signal value that is being measured.

An example can be provided with a nonspecific description of calibration of a spirometer (a more complete explanation of spirometer calibration will be provided later). Using a large, syringelike device, a *known* volume of air is moved into and out of the spirometer in order to provide a test signal. During this volume challenge, the readout of measured volume is observed. If a discrepancy exists between the known test signal volume and the displayed measurement, the spirometer must be adjusted to display the correct measured volume. Once the instrument is calibrated in this way, later measurement of a subject's volumes with the spirometer should produce results that are correct for the subject.

*Quality Control.* The periodic challenging of a calibrated instrument to confirm the accuracy of the measurements that are being made is called *quality control*. Once an instrument is calibrated, it can be assumed that the instrument is making correct measurements. But there is no room for assumption when measuring physiologic parameters. Quality control procedures serve as a double check of instrument performance and eliminate any assumptions. As with calibration, having an appropriate test signal is important to the success of a quality control procedure.

A simple example of quality control for a spirometer is to have a healthy subject with known, stable lung volumes periodically tested on the instrument. The subject serves as the "test signal" for the quality control procedure. The results of the quality control testing of the subject should remain consistent with the results of previous testing for that subject.

The remainder of this chapter will be a presentation of the calibration and quality control requirements for the equipment used in a pulmonary function laboratory. The equipment will be divided into two categories. One category consists of instruments used for making measurements of volume, flow, and pressure. The second category consists of instruments used for gas and blood gas analysis.

It should be noted that the manufacturer of the equipment used in a laboratory will have specific recommendations for calibration and quality control procedures. The purpose for the remaining material is to provide a general basis for understanding the procedures that are recommended.

# CALIBRATION AND QUALITY CONTROL FOR SPIROMETERS AND PLETHYSMOGRAPHS

Spirometers and plethysmographs have some similarities in the instrumentation they employ. Spirometers can make use of either primary volume measuring (PVM) or primary flow measuring (PFM) instrumentation. Plethysmographs (variable-pressure, constant-volume type) include use of PFM and pressure measuring instrumentation. Because of the similarity of the instrumentation used, spirometers and plethysmographs will be discussed together.

## GENERAL PRINCIPLES FOR CALIBRATION AND QUALITY CONTROL OF VOLUME, FLOW, AND PRESSURE MEASURING INSTRUMENTS

Taken as a category, spirometers and plethysmographs together include three basic types of instrumentation:

- Volume measuring instrumentation.
- Flow measuring instrumentation.
- Pressure measuring instrumentation.

There are some general principles that can be applied to the calibration and quality control of these instruments.

### Equipment for Generating an Appropriate Calibration or Quality Control Test Signal

Described here are sources of test signals for volume, flow, and pressure measuring instruments. As will be seen, some test signal sources may be useful in more than one application.

*Calibrated Syringe.* A calibrated syringe is a precise, manually operated large-volume syringe that has a known volume. For calibration and quality control purposes, the volume of the syringe must be 3.0 liters or greater. The syringe must have an accuracy of at least 15 ml or at least 0.5% of full scale (which is 15 ml for a 3.0 liter syringe). For some calibrated syringes, the volume output can be changed.

Calibrated syringes can provide test signals for both PFM and PVM spirometer systems. A variation of the calibrated syringe is the "computerized" syringe. This is a calibrated syringe that includes a microprocessor and a timing mechanism. The microprocessor integrates the volume output of the syringe with the time taken during the output. A display on the syringe then reveals the flow rate of the gas that exited the syringe during the maneuver. The flow rate displayed by the syringe can be compared against the flow rate measured and displayed by the spirometer.

*Automated Syringe.* Automated syringes are calibrated syringes that are motor-driven to provide automated control of both the volume output and flow rate. They are generally computerized and display the output flow rate. Automated syringes can be used in the same calibration and quality control situations as other calibrated syringes.

*Explosive Decompression Devices.* Explosive decompression devices contain a known quantity of gas ($CO_2$ or air) that is held at a fixed pressure. The gas is released through a fixed orifice. The benefit to this type of device is that it generates both reproducible volumes and flow rates.

Explosive decompression devices can be used to provide precise volume and flow test signals. They are useful for evaluating volume and flow rate measurements made by both PVM and PFM spirometer systems. One drawback is that this type of device offers only an "expiratory maneuver." Some spirometer systems require both "inspiratory" and "expiratory" signals for calibration and quality control.

When $CO_2$ is used as the gas in this type of device, there can be limitations to its use. $CO_2$ has different physical characteristics than the air normally measured by a spirometer. For some types of PFM spirometers (e.g., thermal anemometer), this difference in gas composition can affect the accuracy of the volume readings.

*Weighted Volume-Displacement Spirometer.* A precise, accurate volume-displacement spirometer can be used to evaluate flow measurements made by PFM and by other PVM spirometers. A simple water-sealed spirometer is excellent for this purpose.

The flow signal is generated by adding a weight to the bell of the water-sealed spirometer. The weighted spirometer bell starts in the elevated position. When the bell is released, it will fall at a constant rate. This in turn produces a constant flow rate of air out of the spirometer. Given a constant, fixed weight, a very reproducible "expiratory" flow rate test signal will be generated by this method.

*Rotameter.* A rotameter is a gas flow metering device that consists of a spherical float in a tapered tube. The tapered tube is marked with flow-rate graduations. It is essentially similar to the Thorpe-type flowmeters used in medical gas therapy. Rotameters may or may not be designed to provide the capability of adjusting the output flow rate. The precise gas flow rates made available by an accurate rotameter can be used to evaluate the flow measuring capability of a spirometer.

*Rotary Sinusoidal Pump.* A sinusoidal pump consists of an electrical motor-driven wheel that is connected, by a rod, to the plunger of a calibrated syringe. As the motor turns the wheel, the plunger is pulled back and forth within the calibrated syringe. The movement of the wheel and plunger produces rapidly repeating "inspiratory" and "expiratory" volume and flow signals. Adjustments of the motor's speed can increase or decrease the frequency of syringe plunger movement. The syringe volume may also be adjustable. Use of this type of device can provide three types of test signals:

- Fixed, reproducible "inspiratory" and "expiratory" volumes.
- Fixed, reproducible "inspiratory" and "expiratory" flow rates.
- High and low frequencies of alternating "inspiratory" and "expiratory" volumes and flows.

A rotary sinusoidal pump can be used to test the frequency response of a measuring device and its ability to remain accurate.

*Water or Mercury Manometer.* A precise, accurate water or mercury manometer can be used to evaluate the function of a pressure transducer in a pulmonary function testing system. The manometer is used by injecting air into a port on the manometer. The same air pressure is also transmitted to the instrument being evaluated. This pressurizes both the manometer and pressure transducer to the same level. The pressure reading of the measuring instrument should be equal to the pressure displayed on the manometer.

## Basic Procedures for Instrument Evaluation

For the most part, the devices described here are used primarily for instrument calibration procedures. However, they can also be used for quality control procedures.

With calibration, the test signal from the device serves as a basis for making an adjustment of the measuring instrument that will make it more accurate. Quality control procedures involve using a device's test signal as a "test" to determine whether a calibrated instrument is still accurate at some point in time after calibration.

## CALIBRATION AND QUALITY CONTROL OF SPIROMETERS

Many problems can occur with spirometers that can affect their operation and accuracy. Table 16–1 provides a list of these problems. Routine maintenance, calibration, and quality control procedures can either prevent these problems from occurring or can identify their presence.

---

**TABLE 16–1  Problems Affecting Spirometer Operation**

### Problems Affecting the Operation of Any Spirometer

- Leaks in the spirometer's tubing or tubing connections.
- Incorrect timing calibration of the spirometer's recording mechanism.
- Defective analog-to-digital interfacing between the spirometer and the computer or its software.
- Incorrect calibration of the spirometer. This could relate to incorrect establishment of the spirometer's analog signal gain adjustment, ATPS/BTPS correction, or software correction factor.

### Problems Relating Specifically to Primary Volume Measuring Spirometers

- Cracks or leaks in the structure of a volume-displacement spirometer.
- Mechanical resistance to the movement of a spirometer's components.
- A low water level in water-sealed spirometers.
- Incorrect translation by the system's potentiometer of the spirometer's movement into an analog signal.

### Problems Relating Specifically to Primary Flow Measuring Spirometers

- Obstruction of the spirometer's flow sensor by dirt or other material.

With spirometers, there is a blurred distinction between calibration and quality control. Spirometer volume accuracy should be checked daily for systems that remain stationary in a laboratory setting. In essence, this volume accuracy check is a form of quality control assessment. However, at the time of the volume accuracy check, if the spirometer's volume accuracy is not acceptable, then a calibration adjustment must be made.

Some systems are used for performing industrial screenings or other larger epidemiologic studies. In this case, the system is moved to a different location, and large numbers of tests are performed. For these systems, volume accuracy checks and, if needed, calibration adjustments should be performed daily before testing and each time the system is moved to a new site. If large numbers of tests are being performed, the volume checks and calibration should be performed at least every four hours during the course of testing.

The quality control/calibration adjustment procedure will be described under the "Calibration of Spirometers" heading. Other types of quality control procedures for spirometers will be presented later.

## Calibration of Spirometers

Regardless of whether a spirometer is a PFM or a PVM system, the equipment and procedures used in calibration are the same. The only exception is that volume-displacement spirometers must have a volume leak test performed each day prior to any volume accuracy check or calibration adjustment. This is done by placing a weight or applying a constant force against the spirometer when it is filled to one half its volume. The volume level of the spirometer should remain constant during the time that the weight or force is applied. Once the weight or force is removed, the spirometer should return to its original resting volume position.

A spirometer must be accurate to within ±3% or 50 ml of the actual volume that is being measured, whichever is greater. An appropriate test signal is required in order to perform spirometer calibration procedures. Generally, a large-volume (3.0 liters or greater) calibrating syringe is used. If a 3.0 liter syringe is used, the maximum permitted spirometer error during calibration is ±90 ml. Either a manually operated or automated-type syringe can be used.

In calibrating a spirometer, a predetermined volume of air (3.0 liters, in this example) is injected into (or through) the spirometer. With water-sealed spirometers, it is a good idea to inject and withdraw air to and from the spirometer several times before the actual volume challenge is performed. This will permit equilibration between the syringe air and the moist air within the spirometer.

PFM spirometers may require the use of a length of tubing between the syringe and the flow sensor. This is to minimize flow artifact that can be produced by the syringe. PFM spirometers should also have the calibrating volumes from the syringe introduced into the spirometer at different flow rates. Flow rates should be varied between 2 l/sec and 12 l/sec. This can be done with a 3.0 liter calibrating syringe by using the following injection times over a series of three volume injections:

- One volume injection with a duration time of 1 second (flow rate = 3.0 l/sec).

- One volume injection with a duration time of 6 seconds (flow rate = 0.5 l/sec).
- One volume injection with a duration time between 2 and 6 seconds (flow rate between 1.5 l/sec and 0.5 l/sec).

It is important to note that the syringe volume used for calibration is at ATPS. This differs from the BTPS volume that is normally measured and is compensated for by the spirometer. Therefore, any BTPS-to-ATPS compensation must be eliminated prior to comparison of the syringe volume with the spirometer's measured volume.

If, using a 3.0 liter syringe, a measured volume displayed by the system is within ±90 ml of the test signal volume, then no calibration adjustment is necessary. If the displayed volume is outside this range, then there are three possible sources of the error:

- If the calibrated syringe is an adjustable type, it is set at the wrong volume.
- There was a leak at the connection between the calibrated spirometer and the spirometer.
- A calibration adjustment needs to be made on the spirometer.

The first two possibilities should be investigated before calibration adjustments are made on the spirometer.

If a spirometer calibration adjustment is required, the nature of the adjustment depends on how volumes are measured and displayed/recorded by the spirometer. A spirometer may require one of the three following possible adjustments:

1. Adjustment of the **gain** of the analog output signal from the measurement system (e.g., potentiometer on a primary volume measuring spirometer or flow sensor from a primary flow measuring spirometer). This is done as a simple electrical control adjustment so that the displayed spirometer volume is changed to reflect the test signal volume.
2. Establishment of a computer software correction factor. Once established, this factor will then be used by the software when making future analysis of the analog signal from the spirometer. Table 16–2 demonstrates the method the computer uses in determining a software correction factor.
3. Adjustment of the **sensitivity** of the recording system response to the analog signal from the measuring system. As with the analog output gain adjustment, this is a simple electrical control adjustment that will make the recorded volume equal to the test signal volume.

Note that the calibration procedure just described involves a test signal that has a single volume (3.0 liters). With calibration at one volume, it is *assumed* that the spirometer will be accurate over its entire range of measurement. This may or may not be true. A spirometer that has a very linear performance over its range of operation will be reasonably accurate at all volumes. But if the spirometer has poor linearity, the greatest accuracy will be at volumes nearest to the calibration volume. The spirometer will be less accurate at volume ranges that are above and below the calibration volume.

---

**TABLE 16–2  Calculation of a Software Correction Factor**

---

A software correction factor is calculated by use of the following equation:

$$\text{Software Correction Factor} = \frac{\text{Test Signal Volume}}{\text{Measured Volume}}$$

As an example of how this equation is used, given a test signal volume of 3.0 liters, the spirometer being challenged measures and displays the test signal volume as being 3.04 liters. As a result, the spirometer's computer establishes a software correction factor as

$$\text{Software Correction Factor} = \frac{3.00 \text{ liters}}{3.04 \text{ liters}} = .987$$

This means that future volume determinations by this spirometer will be "corrected" by being multiplied by .987 before they are displayed as a final value.

---

## Quality Control for Spirometers

Various aspects of spirometer performance should be checked as a part of quality assurance. The daily volume accuracy challenge just described is a cornerstone to spirometer quality control. Flow accuracy and frequency response can also be checked to assess the quality of spirometer performance.

*Assessment of Volume Accuracy.*   There are certain things that can be done to make volume accuracy quality control procedures more challenging for the spirometer. For example, as stated earlier, challenging the spirometer at different flow rates is helpful. Also, the use of different volume levels (e.g., 1.0 liter, 3.0 liters, or 5.0 liters) provides even greater challenges to spirometer measurement quality.

The linearity of PVM spirometers should be checked at least quarterly. This is done by checking the calibration of the spirometer over the entire range of its measuring capability. The calibration check can be performed in 1.0 liter increments using a 1.0 liter calibrating syringe. PFM spirometers should have linearity checks performed at least weekly. This is done using a series of several different flow rates as described previously. If the spirometer meets volume accuracy requirements for all of the flows and/or volumes tested, then it satisfies the requirement for linearity.

*Assessment of Flow Accuracy.*   Flow accuracy checks are actually more useful for PVM spirometers than for PFM spirometers. A PFM spirometer that is accurately measuring volumes is doing so because it is accurately measuring air flow rates. If the flow-rate measurements were inaccurate, then the volumes displayed by the spirometer would also be inaccurate. In contrast, a calibrated PVM spirometer that is accurately measuring volumes is not necessarily accurately measuring flow rates.

A variety of methods can be used to evaluate spirometer flow accuracy. Computerized syringes and explosive decompression devices can be used. The flow rates generated by these devices can be compared against the flow rates measured by the spirometer.

Spirometer flow accuracy can be assessed by other methods as well. One is use of a rotameter to establish a fixed flow rate of gas. The gas flow output from the rotameter is then passed into the spirometer for measurement and comparison. As described earlier, an accurate, weighted water-sealed spirometer can also be used to generate a flow for assessing the accuracy of other spirometers.

*Assessment of Flow Resistance.* A spirometer should create a minimum of resistance to the subject's effort to move air into or through it. The flow resistance created by a spirometer is felt by the subject as the amount of work (pressure) required to produce a certain rate of gas flow (i.e., cm $H_2O$/l/sec). The standard for spirometers is that a pressure of no more than 1.5 cm $H_2O$ should be required to produce a flow of 0 to 14 l/sec into or through the spirometer.

Normally spirometer flow resistance is not checked unless there is reason to question the spirometer's performance. It can be evaluated, however. First, some method must be used to establish a constant flow of 14 l/sec into or through the spirometer. This may be done by one of the methods described previously. By connecting a manometer between the flow source and the spirometer, the amount of pressure needed to produce the flow can be measured.

*Assessment of Frequency Response.* During measurement of a maneuver such as the MVV, the rapid changes in flow direction and rate of flow presents a special challenge for a spirometer. Assessment of a spirometer's frequency response can be used to evaluate this ability.

A rotary sinusoidal pump can be used to assess a spirometer's accuracy under these conditions. The goal for spirometer frequency response is to measure a 2.0 liter sine wave volume exchange (with a volume exchange rate of 250 l/min) with an accuracy of ±10% or 15 l/min, whichever is greater.

This quality control measure is not routinely applied to spirometers. Generally, a spirometer's frequency response is evaluated only if there is reason to suspect that an inaccuracy exists.

*Assessment of Recorder Function.* The accuracy of a spirometer system's recorder timing speed should be checked at least quarterly. This can be done by running the recorder and, at regular fixed time intervals, applying a volume signal to the spirometer for recording. The interval timing between volume signals (two seconds, for example) can be measured by use of a stop watch. Once the tracing is made, the intervals as recorded by the recorder can be measured. The recorder is accurate if the recorded time intervals are equal to the intervals established by the stop watch.

# CALIBRATION AND QUALITY CONTROL OF BODY PLETHYSMOGRAPHS

Many problems can affect the operation and accuracy of body plethysmographs. Table 16–3 provides a list of these problems. As with spirometers, routine maintenance, calibration, and quality control procedures can either prevent these problems from occurring or can identify their presence.

With body plethysmographs, there is a clear distinction between calibration and quality control procedures. Body plethysmograph function is based on data input from more than one measuring instrument. Flow transducers, pressure transducers, and other instruments may be included, depending on the plethysmograph's design. Calibration procedures must be performed separately for each of the measurement instruments in the plethysmograph. However, quality control procedures are based on the overall performance of the plethysmograph for determining values for lung volumes and airway resistance.

Calibration procedures for the plethysmograph measuring instruments should be performed at least once a day. Quality control procedures may be done less often but should still be performed with frequent regularity.

## Calibration of Body Plethysmographs

The calibration procedures described here are primarily for use with a constant-volume, variable-pressure body plethysmograph. These procedures include calibration of the mouth pressure transducer, flow transducer, and the cabinet pressure transducer. A non-constant-volume plethysmograph requires the same type of calibration procedures for the mouth pressure and flow transducers. The manufacturer's recommendations must be followed for calibration of this type of plethysmograph's cabinet volume measurement system.

Specific calibration procedures follow. Two things should be noted, however:

- The manufacturer of a plethysmograph system will have specific recommendations for its calibration.
- Computer-based plethysmograph systems will generally perform automatic calibration adjustments once an appropriate test signal is applied.

---

### TABLE 16–3  Problems Affecting Body Plethysmograph Operation

- Leaks in the plethysmograph's door seals or tubing connections.
- Incorrect calibration of the plethysmograph's pressure or flow transducers.
- Obstruction or damage to the plethysmograph's pressure or flow tranducers.
- Poor flow or pressure transducer performance as a result of vibration from being loosely mounted.
- Poor frequency response of the plethysmograph's measurement systems.
- Excessive thermal drift within the plethysmograph's cabinet.

*Calibration of the Mouth Pressure Transducer.* The mouth pressure transducer can be calibrated by use of a mercury or water pressure manometer. The pressure range of the manometer should be approximately that of the pressures normally measured by the transducer ($\pm 25$ cm $H_2O$).

The manometer is attached to the pressure transducer, and air is injected into the manometer to apply a constant pressure (e.g., 10 cm $H_2O$) to the transducer. With this known, constant pressure applied against the transducer, calibration adjustments should be made as required. The adjustments are to the displayed pressure deflection reading on the graphic display of the plethysmograph. In the example used, this would mean adjustment so that the displayed pressure deflection is to a pressure calibration factor ($P_{Mo}$ Cal) of 10 cm $H_2O$/cm on the graphic display. With computer-based systems, a software correction factor, as described earlier, will be established.

*Calibration of the Flow Transducer.* The goal for flow transducer calibration is the same as for pressure transducer calibration. The graphic display should be calibrated so that the deflection of the flow reading is to a known, fixed value. Some systems require that a known constant flow be applied through the transducer. This can be done using a rotameter or a weighted water-sealed spirometer. Given a flow of 2 l/sec, for example, the deflection will be adjusted to 2 cm at this flow level. This will result in a flow calibration factor ($\dot{V}$Cal) of 1 l/sec/cm of deflection.

Computer-based systems can permit flow transducer calibration by use of a 3.0 liter calibrated syringe. This is similar to the calibration described for PFM spirometers. Based on the introduction of the syringe's test signal, the computer will establish a correction factor.

*Calibration of the Cabinet Pressure Transducer.* Calibration of the cabinet pressure transducer is based on the goal of having the pressure measured by the transducer represent a certain specific change in cabinet volume. This calibration is done with the cabinet empty.

A rotary sinusoidal pump device is used with a calibrated syringe that has a smaller volume, generally 25–50 ml. With the pump/syringe device attached to a port on the empty cabinet, a panting-like volume change test signal, 30 ml for example, is generated. Using this signal, a calibration adjustment should be made to the graphic display of the cabinet pressure reading. In the example provided, if a 2-cm deflection is adjusted for a 30 ml signal, then the result would be a volume calibration factor (V Cal) of 15 ml per centimeter of deflection. It is useful to recheck this calibration by using different frequencies of volume change by the sinusoidal pump. Calibration checks can be made at volume change frequencies from 0.5–5.0 cycles/sec (Hertz).

Nonconstant-volume plethysmographs can make use of a similar arrangement for calibration. The difference is that the calibration is of a cabinet flow or volume transducer rather than a pressure transducer.

Because the box is empty at the time of calibration, a subject volume correction factor ($F_{Sub}$) is applied to the final calculations made during use of the plethysmograph. This factor was described in Chapter 4.

*Determination of a Value for $F_{Cal}$.* Also mentioned in Chapter 4 was a $\Delta P/\Delta V$ calibration factor ($F_{Cal}$) for the plethysmograph cabinet. This factor is required for the calculation of $V_{TG}$. A value for $F_{Cal}$ is calculated based on the values for $P_{Mo}$ Cal and V Cal that were described earlier. The following equation demonstrates the calculation of a value for $F_{Cal}$.

$$F_{Cal} = \frac{V\,Cal}{P_{Mo}\,Cal}$$

## Quality Control for Body Plethysmographs

Quality control for body plethysmographs is based on use of a device called an **isothermal** lung analog (Figure 16–1). A glass flask with a volume between 3.0 and 5.0 liters is used. The flask must have a stopper in the top that will permit two connections to the flask. One connection is for a rubber squeeze bulb. Generally squeeze bulbs with a volume between 60 and 100 ml are used. The other connection is for an adapter that will per-

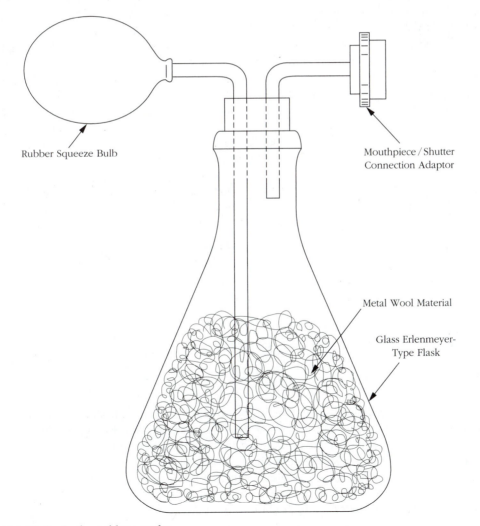

Rubber Squeeze Bulb

Mouthpiece / Shutter
Connection Adaptor

Metal Wool Material

Glass Erlenmeyer-
Type Flask

**Figure 16–1** *Isothermal lung analog.*

mit attachment of the flask to the mouthpiece shutter/transducer assembly of the plethysmograph.

There are two important characteristics of the isothermal lung analog. First, the device is intended to have isothermal properties. As will be described, the lung analog is used by having the technologist create pressure changes within the flask by squeezing the squeeze bulb. Unfortunately, these pressure changes can inadvertently result in changes in gas temperature and therefore in the relative gas volume within the flask. The physical properties of the metal wool material allow it to serve as a heat sink that will, it is hoped, eliminate variations in flask gas temperature.

The second characteristic of the lung analog is that it has a fixed, known volume. The volume of the flask, squeeze bulb, the connector to the mouthpiece shutter/transducer, and related tubing must be measured in advance of use. Filling these parts with water and measuring the volume of the water is a method of doing this. The accuracy of the measurement of the lung analog's volume must be within ±2%.

Once the volume of the lung analog is known, the volume of the metal wool material that is placed in the lung analog must be subtracted from the volume of the lung analog. The volume of the metal wool is determined by first weighing the quantity of material used. Then, the weight (gm) of the metal wool material is divided by the value for its density (gm/ml). The resulting value is the volume of the metal wool material.

The lung analog is used by an individual who sits within the closed plethysmograph cabinet with the analog attached to the mouthpiece pressure/shutter assembly (shutter closed). While holding her or his breath, the user squeezes and releases the lung analog bulb in the simulation of a panting maneuver. This is meant to produce a test signal that will result in a $\Delta P_A / \Delta V_A$ tangent value.

Given a tangent value for this simulated panting maneuver, the normal method for determining $V_{TG}$ can be used to arrive at a measured value for the lung analog's volume. Two modifications to normal calculations must be made:

- The value for BTPS water vapor pressure (47 mm Hg) should not be subtracted from the value for $P_{atm}$.
- The value for $F_{Sub}$ used in the calculation must include both the actual volume of the lung analog ($V_{LA}$) and the volume of the technologist who is operating the analog.

The following equation demonstrates how this is done:

$$F_{Sub} = \frac{[V_{Cab} - (W_{Sub}/1.07) - V_{LA}]}{V_{Cab}}$$

Once a value for the lung analog's $V_{TG}$ has been determined, it should be compared with the actual predetermined volume of the lung analog. Accuracy of the plethysmograph's operation is demonstrated when the two volumes are within ±5% of matching. This procedure for quality assessment should be performed at different frequencies of simulated panting with the lung analog squeeze bulb. Frequencies used should range from 0.5 to 5.0 cycles/sec (Hertz). The accuracy of lung analog volume determination should not change with changes in "panting" frequency.

## Assessment of Spirometer and Plethysmograph Function Using Known Subjects

The American Thoracic Society recommends the use of known subjects as "test signals" for quality control. This can be done for both spirometers and plethysmographs. The first step is the selection of at least three healthy subjects who are representative of the population normally tested by the laboratory. Laboratory and other institutional personnel can be used for this purpose. Once the subjects are selected, baseline tests should be performed on them using the equipment that will later undergo quality assurance testing. The results of these tests should be logged. Before the tests are performed, the equipment should first be correctly calibrated and other measures of quality assurance should also be performed.

A program for quality assurance is based on having these same healthy subjects retested on the equipment on a quarterly basis or at any time that the equipment's performance is questioned. Satisfactory equipment quality is demonstrated if the results of repeat testing of the subjects is within two standard deviations of the mean value for the subjects. A problem is identified when the results for any one of the subjects are more than two standard deviations from the mean value for that subject. If this occurs, a complete check of the instrument's operation should be made. The testing should be repeated after any repairs are made.

As an additional check for quality assurance, these same subjects should be tested in other laboratories at least annually. Significant deviations between the values measured in the original laboratory and measurements from other laboratories should prompt an investigation of the equipment's performance.

# CALIBRATION AND QUALITY CONTROL FOR GAS AND BLOOD GAS ANALYSIS INSTRUMENTS

Gas analyzers are designed to analyze gases in the gaseous state. They are generally used as components of a larger measuring system. As described earlier in the book, they are often included in spirometer systems for measurement of such parameters as FRC and $D_LCO$. Different types of gas analyzers may be included in a measurement system. The ones used depend on the specific types of tests being performed.

Blood gas analyzers are stand-alone systems that contain a $PO_2$ electrode, pH electrode, and $PCO_2$ electrode. They are capable of measuring the partial pressure of $O_2$ and $CO_2$ in either a liquid or a gaseous sample. The value for pH can be measured only for a liquid sample.

## GENERAL PRINCIPLES FOR CALIBRATION AND QUALITY CONTROL OF GAS AND BLOOD GAS ANALYSIS INSTRUMENTS

Gas and blood gas analyzers share similarities in respect to calibration and quality control procedures that are performed. Information on these similarities will be presented before the specifics of gas and blood gas analyzer calibration and quality control are described.

## Intended Range for Measurement and Performance Challenges

The measurement systems used for gas and blood gas analysis present a challenge to making accurate physiologic measurements. By their nature, it is unlikely that these systems will be accurate in making measurements over a wide range of values. This is especially true with the electrochemical electrodes used in blood gas analyzers.

One response to this problem, as will be described, is the use of two points of calibration—a low and a high value. The assumption is that this improves the quality of measurement of values in the range between these two points of calibration. This is not a safe assumption, however. The high point value and low point value may be accurate, *but if the measurement system is not linear, measurements made between these two points can be incorrect.* Unfortunately, many gas and blood gas analysis sensors have poor linearity over a wide range of values.

The best way to deal with this problem is to use the narrowest two-point calibration range possible for the type of measurement being made. This requires two actions:

- The range of values most likely to be encountered during use of the instrument or the range where there is the greatest concern for accuracy must be identified.
- The high and low test signals chosen for calibration and quality control must represent the high and low extremes of the range that has been identified.

For example, the $PO_2$ electrode of a blood gas analyzer can be calibrated using a range of 0% (0 mm Hg) to 20% (approximately 140 mm Hg) oxygen. This represents a reasonable range for the $PO_2$ values that are most likely to be encountered. However, if there is a greater concern for accuracy in measurement within the pathologic range of $PO_2$ values, a calibration range of 0% (0 mm Hg) to 12% (approximately 85 mm Hg) oxygen can be used.

## Sampling Conditions

Another major concern for the calibration and quality control of gas and blood gas analysis instruments is the conditions present during the measurement of a typical sample. One type of analyzer may normally make measurements under conditions where the sample gas is flowing. Another analyzer may be designed to measure a gas sample that is static (not moving) within the sensor chamber. Analyzers designed to measure the partial pressure of a gas may be affected by a change in the flow rate of the gas sample.

At the time of calibration for these instruments, the conditions must match those present when the instrument is being used on a subject. For example:

- In an instrument where changes in the partial pressure of the sample can affect the analysis process, the sample flow rate of the instrument must be checked and set before the analyzer sensor is calibrated.
- The test signal that is used during calibration should reasonably match the conditions of routine sample analysis.

Some systems include adjuncts to their gas analyzer's sampling circuit (i.e., $H_2O$ absorbers, $CO_2$ absorbers, filters). If these are normally present during the instrument's use, they should also be in place during calibration and quality control procedures.

# Methods Used for Generating an Appropriate Calibration or Quality Control Test Signal

Certain types of test signals can be used to challenge gas and blood gas analyzing instruments. Some test signal sources can be useful in more than one application.

*Gaseous Samples.* Calibration and some quality control procedures can be performed using precise, calibration-grade gas mixtures as a test signal. As described earlier, the concentrations of the gases selected should be within a proper range for the typical application of the instrument.

These gas mixtures are supplied in pressurized cylinders. The fractional concentration of each gas in the mixture is listed on the cylinder's label. The gas concentrations should be certified by the manufacturer as being correct. Even with this certification, the concentrations of the contents of these cylinders should not be taken for granted. Either mass spectrometry or a method called the *Scholander technique* can be used to assay a cylinder's contents. If mass spectrometry is used, the mass spectrometer must be correctly calibrated before the gas concentrations are assayed.

The actual concentration of the gas must be ±0.03% of the concentration stated on the cylinder's label. Each laboratory should develop a policy and procedure for confirming the concentrations of test signal gas cylinder contents.

Some analyzers are designed only to measure gaseous samples. The CO and He analyzers used in a $D_LCO$-SB procedure, and the He and $N_2$ analyzers used in the two types of gas-dilution FRC determination methods are of this type. They are all challenged only with gaseous sample test signals. Analyzers of this type generally make their measurements as a percent value. Therefore, the gases selected as test signals will be supplied as also having a certain known percent value.

Gaseous samples can be used as calibration test signals for blood gas analyzers as well. They present a problem in this application, however. The measurements made by the $PO_2$ and $PCO_2$ electrodes are of the partial pressure of those gases. In both cases, the value for partial pressure is affected by both the percent concentration of the sample gas and the current barometric pressure. The gases used for blood gas analyzer calibration must be humidified prior to being sent to the measuring chamber. Table 16–4 demonstrates the method for determining the partial pressure of a test gas used for a blood gas analyzer.

As will be discussed, there are differences in how, especially, a $PO_2$ electrode will respond to a gaseous sample than it will to a blood sample. Given the same actual $PO_2$ value, a $PO_2$ electrode will measure the $PO_2$ of the blood sample as being less than the same $PO_2$ of the gaseous sample. This fact has some impact on how gaseous test signals can be used for blood gas analyzer calibration.

*Commercial Buffered-Solution Samples.* Commercial buffered-solution samples are used only with blood gas analyzers. These are buffered solutions, with a known pH value that can also be supplied with known $PO_2$ and $PCO_2$ values. Three different types of these solutions are available: aqueous buffer solutions, fluorocarbon emulsions, and blood-based solutions.

---

**TABLE 16–4  Calculation of the Partial Pressures in a Test Gas Sample**

---

The cylinder(s) of precision source gas being used will state the fractional concentration ($F_{SG}$) of each of the gases in the mixture.

The barometric pressure ($P_{Atm}$) must be determined at the time of calculation and 47 mm Hg is subtracted to account for the partial pressure of water vapor at body temperature.

The partial pressure of any particular gas contained within the mixture ($P_{Gas}$) is calculated in the following manner:

$$P_{Gas} = (P_{Atm} - 47 \text{ mm Hg}) \times F_{SG}$$

The calculation must be performed immediately before each time the gas sample is going to be used. This is to account for the effects of the current $P_{Atm}$.

---

*Aqueous buffer solutions* generally consist of a bicarbonate buffer solution. This type of solution, when prepared only with a known pH value, is the primary method for calibration of a blood gas analyzer's pH electrode. Similar solutions are also available with known $PO_2$ and $PCO_2$ values.

Unfortunately, as described for the gaseous test signals, the performance of the $PO_2$ electrode with aqueous solutions is not consistent. A wide variation in measured values can be demonstrated when test signal sample measurements are made and compared between two or more different analyzers (interinstrumental comparisons). This is true even when the same solution sample is tested and compared between instruments. The measurement inconsistency is far greater than would be demonstrated with a blood sample used for interinstrumental comparison of $PO_2$ values. Because of this inconsistency, the suppliers of the solutions are forced to state a wide range of expected $PO_2$ values for a given sample.

The pH and $PCO_2$ electrodes of a blood gas analyzer respond with a greater relative consistency to aqueous buffered solutions. This results in the suppliers of the solutions being able to state more narrow ranges for the expected measured pH and $PCO_2$ values.

*Fluorocarbon emulsions* are a type of perfluorinated compound. This gives them enhanced oxygen-dissolving characteristics when compared with buffered aqueous solutions. Fluorocarbon emulsions provide a closer range of interinstrumental comparison values for $PO_2$. The range is still more broad than would be demonstrated by interinstrumental comparison of blood $PO_2$ values.

Both the aqueous buffered solutions and the fluorocarbon emulsions are available commercially in 2–3 ml vials. They are intended for use as blood gas analyzer quality control samples for all three electrodes. Although expensive, they are relatively easy to use. Both types of preparations can be stored refrigerated for long periods of time. They can be left at room temperature for shorter periods of time to allow easy access and use.

Generally, all that is required before use of these solutions is that they be shaken for 10–15 seconds prior to analysis. The vial should be held at its ends by the thumb and first finger of the user when it is shaken. Holding the vial around its middle can increase the temperature of the solution and adversely change the partial pressures of the gases in solution.

*Blood-based solutions* are also available. They may be supplied as small vials of hemoglobin/buffer solutions or as denatured red cell/buffer solutions. Of the three types of commercial buffered-solution samples, the blood-based solutions provide the narrowest range of intended $PO_2$ values. The range is still not as narrow as that found with actual whole blood samples, however. These solutions are much more sensitive to changes in temperature than are the other commercial solutions. They require refrigeration for storage. Additionally, vials of blood-based solution must be agitated and warmed to 37°C in a water bath for several minutes prior to being opened and analyzed.

## Tonometered Blood Samples

A tonometer is a device that permits blood to come in contact and equilibrate with a gas that has known $PCO_2$ and/or $PO_2$ values. This results in the blood containing a known $PCO_2$ and $PO_2$. Unfortunately, when whole blood is used, tonometry cannot be employed to establish a known pH for the blood. As with commercial buffer solutions, tonometered blood samples are used only for evaluating the operation of blood gas analyzers.

Tonometered blood samples provide the best test signal for challenging the $PO_2$ electrode while still providing an acceptable test signal for use with the $PCO_2$ electrodes. This is due to the fact that real blood is used in making the test signal. Tonometered blood samples create the narrowest range of expected $PO_2$ values when interinstrumental comparisons are made. $PO_2$ values in the range of 20–150 mm Hg provide optimal test signal values. In this range, the $PO_2$ values measured by a calibrated, functional blood gas analyzer should be within ±5 mm Hg of the tonometered $PO_2$. $PO_2$ values greater than 150 mm Hg can begin to demonstrate a greater range of variation in expected measured values.

Generally, commercially prepared source gases are used for tonometry. The gases are supplied having precise, known fractional concentrations of $CO_2$ and $O_2$. With given fractional quantities of the gases, the corresponding $PCO_2$ and $PO_2$ values are calculated in the manner described in Table 16–4.

The key to tonometer operation is that a large contact area must be created between the blood sample and the source gas. This large area allows for more efficient partial pressure equilibration.

Two basic types of tonometers are available. One causes the blood to be spun in a chamber so that it is spread into a thin film. At the same time, the chamber is flooded with a precision gas that has known $CO_2$ and/or $O_2$ partial pressure values. This type of tonometer offers the advantages of using smaller quantities of precision gas and causing very little foaming of the blood sample.

Another type of tonometer operates by bubbling the source gas through the blood sample. Ideally, the bubbles should be 2–7 mm in size in order to create a large surface area for gas/blood equilibration. Larger quantities of precision gas are used by this process. Foaming of the blood can be a problem with some tonometers of this type.

The blood used for tonometry should be less than 24 hours old. The patients supplying the blood should be free of hepatitis and HIV infection. The blood should be checked by a laboratory and rejected if it demonstrates significant hemolysis, an elevated white count (greater than 20,000), or elevated lipid levels.

During its operation, the tonometer must be kept at 37°C. The source gas must be humidified in order to minimize dehydration of the blood. The amount of time needed for equilibration to take place depends on the gas flow rate and the quantity of the blood sample. The manufacturer of a tonometer will have guidelines for making this determination. If the flow rate of the source gas is too great, it can cause dehydration and cooling of the blood sample.

Once the blood has reached partial pressure equilibrium with the source gas, it is ready to be used as a test signal sample. Proper handling of the blood sample is crucial for it to work effectively as a test signal. The following steps should be taken in withdrawing the blood sample from the tonometer:

1. The sample syringe must be purged with the source gas three to five times before the blood sample is withdrawn from the tonometer.
2. A small quantity of blood should be drawn into the syringe and then expelled. This is to ensure that no gas bubbles will remain in the syringe when the actual sample is drawn.
3. The blood actually to be used as a test sample can then be withdrawn from the tonometer. Care should be taken when doing this. Too much force used in withdrawing the blood can result in bubbles forming in the syringe.

Variations in the technique of individual technologists can affect the quality of the sample as a test signal.

Tonometry is less costly than use of pre-tonometered commercial solutions. However, tonometry requires greater time and work on the part of the laboratory staff. Also, there are certain problems associated with the use of tonometers to prepare test samples. These are presented in Table 16–5.

---

**TABLE 16–5  Problems Associated with Preparing Tonometered Blood Test Samples**

---

- The laboratory staff can be exposed to the risk of infection with hepatitis and the HIV.
- Having tonometered blood samples prepared for $PO_2$ and $PCO_2$ challenges does not eliminate the need to purchase commercial buffered solutions needed to challenge the pH electrode.
- Errors in the partial pressure value of the blood sample can occur during preparation. These errors can be caused by
  Incorrect calculation of the expected $PO_2$ and $PCO_2$ values.
  Improper temperature control of the tonometer.
  Gas flow rates that are less than adequate for the time given for equilibrium.
  Poor technique when the blood sample is withdrawn from the tonometer.

---

A tonometer can be used to impart a specific gas partial pressure to fluids other than blood. Aqueous buffered solutions with known pH values can be tonometered to be given a specific $PO_2$ and/or $PCO_2$ value. As described earlier for aqueous buffered solutions, though, there will be a problem with having a wide range of expected $PO_2$ values with these tonometered samples.

## Basic Procedures for Instrument Evaluation

There are basic procedures for instrument evaluation that can be used on both gas and blood gas analyzers. These include two- and one-point calibration procedures and multiple-point linearity checks.

*Two-Point and One-Point Calibration.* In *two-point calibration*, two test signals are used, one with a low (possibly zero) value and the other with a higher value. As described earlier, these values should represent the high and low expected values for the analyzer's intended range of use.

Each test signal must have a known fractional concentration or partial pressure for which the analyzer will be challenged. For He or CO gas analyzers, a zero value can easily be achieved simply by drawing room air into the measuring chamber of the analyzer. This will work for any analyzer that is used to measure a gas that has a zero or near zero concentration in atmospheric air. The expression of "zeroing" an analyzer refers to calibrating the analyzer to the low value test signal. This is true regardless of whether the low value test signal is actually zero or is some low value.

When calibrating at two different levels, the goal is to both balance and slope the instrument's range of performance. The *balance* of the instrument is established when calibrating adjustments are made with the sensor exposed to the low-value test signal. Once the instrument is balanced, then the *slope* of the instrument can be established. This is done by making calibration adjustments while the instrument's sensor is exposed to the high-value test signal. Figure 16–2 provides a graphic demonstration of the effects of balancing and sloping calibration adjustments.

The degree of accuracy that is needed for calibration procedures differs with the intended range of measurement. In applications where the range is very broad, accuracy can be determined to a whole mm Hg or percent value. Conversely, analyzers used in metabolic studies or exercise testing require a finer degree of accuracy in calibration. For these instruments, calibration should be done to at least the hundredth of a percent.

The frequency with which two-point calibration must be performed is based on the stability of the instrument. Some instruments, such as gas chromatographs, are very stable and only require occasional two-point calibration. Others, such as the electrodes of a blood gas analyzer, are less stable and require much more frequent calibration.

*One-point calibration* is a simpler form of calibration than two-point calibration. The instrument is challenged with only one test signal. The value of the test signal selected for one-point calibration differs from instrument to instrument. One-point calibration is very useful for instruments such as blood gas analyzers that have a greater tendency for sensor drift. In order to keep an instrument fine-tuned, simpler one-point calibrations are performed more frequently than are two-point calibrations.

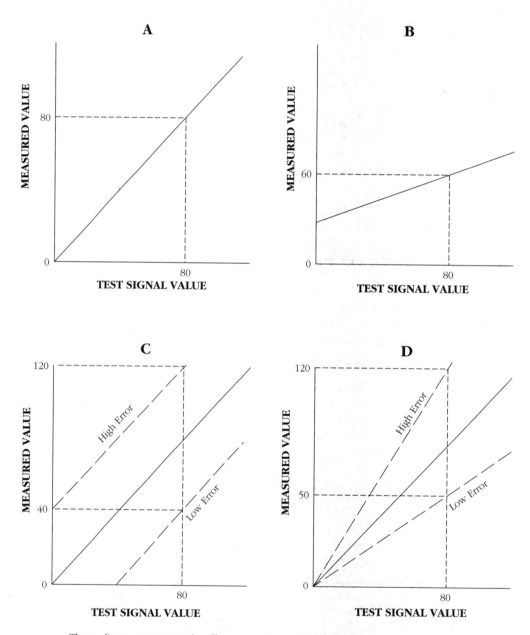

These diagrams represent the effects on analyzer measurement when:

**A** – Both the balance and the slope are calibrated correctly.
**B** – Neither the balance nor the slope are calibrated correctly.
**C** – The slope is correct but both a high balance error and a low balance error are demonstrated.
**D** – The balance is correct but both a high slope error and a low slope error are demonstrated.

**Figure 16–2**  *Examples of the effects of balancing and sloping a gas or blood gas sensor.*

*Multiple-Point Linearity Checks.* As stated earlier, having an instrument correctly calibrated at a high and a low value does not automatically ensure accuracy over the entire range of measurement. Even though a sensor is properly balanced and sloped, it may not be *linear* in its performance over the range. Figure 16–3 demonstrates the difference between an He analyzer, which tends to be linear in its operation, and a CO analyzer, which performs with less linearity.

In order to test an instrument for linearity, the instrument must be challenged at more than just two (the low and high) value points. Three or more different test signal values must be used to evaluate for linearity. This is done by analyzing a series of known test signals over the range of the instrument's operation. A statistical analysis can then be performed to develop a regression equation that relates the differences between the actual values and the pattern of measured values. Once available, the equation can serve to "correct" future measured values to a more linear level of performance. This correction equation can be used manually by the technologist, or it can be programmed into the software of a computer-based measuring system.

How often linearity should be checked depends on the instrument in question and how it is used. Analyzers used with gas dilution lung volume determinations (FRC), $D_LCO$ measurements, exercise studies, and metabolic studies should have linearity checks performed at least once every six months or when error in their measurements is suspected. CO analyzers may require even more frequent checks for linearity of measurements.

## CALIBRATION AND QUALITY CONTROL OF GAS ANALYZERS

Many problems can affect the operation and accuracy of gas analyzers. Table 16–6 provides a list of these problems. Routine maintenance, calibration, and quality control procedures can either prevent these problems from occurring or can identify their presence.

### Calibration of Gas Analyzers

Gas analyzers used for gas dilution lung volume (FRC) determinations, $D_LCO$ measurements, exercise testing, and metabolic studies should have a two-point calibration performed prior to each test administration. Calibration of continuous monitoring-type analyzers, such as capnographs, should be performed at least daily or as per the manufacturer's recommendations.

### Quality Control of Gas Analyzers

The frequency with which quality control procedures should be performed on gas analyzers depends on the type of instrument and how it is used. The manufacturer of a pulmonary function testing system will be able to provide guidelines for the frequency and procedures that should be used for quality control.

The methods that can be used for quality control of gas analyzers include:

- Challenges with known gas values.
- Use of a mechanical lung analog.
- Testing of known subjects.

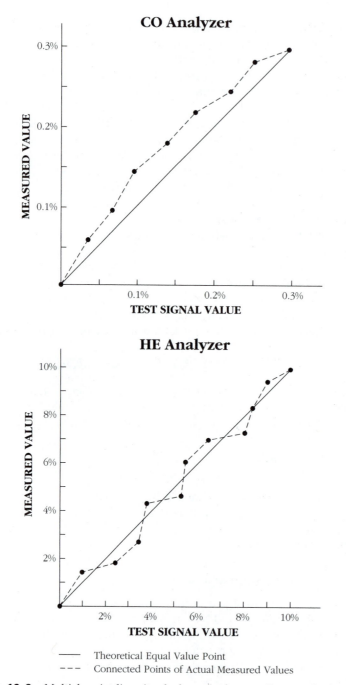

**Figure 16–3** *Multiple-point linearity check graphs for a nonlinear and a linear gas analyzer.*

---

**TABLE 16–6 Problems Affecting Gas Analyzer Operation**

---

The problems that can develop with an analyzer depend on the components the analyzer includes and how these are used to perform gas analysis. Depending on the analyzer, examples of problems that can occur include

- Inadequate warmup of the analyzer before use.
- Blockages in an analyzer's sampling port or tubing.
- Leaks in an analyzer's sample tubing or tubing connections.
- Exhausted carbon dioxide and/or water vapor absorbers.
- Contamination of the analyzer's electrode(s) or photocell(s).
- For gas chromatographs, deterioration and/or contamination of the column packing material.
- For mass spectrometers or nitrogen analyzers, poor vacuum pump performance.
- For infrared analyzers, malfunctions of the chopper motor, poor optical quality balance, and/or aging of the detector cells.
- For oxygen analyzers, electrolyte or fuel cell exhaustion.

---

*Challenges with Known Gas Values.* Challenging a gas analyzer with a gas sample having a known concentration is a simple and basic method for analyzer quality control. It is most helpful if an analyzer can be challenged with gas concentrations at different levels.

There are two ways in which a laboratory can challenge an analyzer at different gas levels. A collection of cylinders containing a series of different precise gas values can be purchased by the laboratory and kept on hand for quality control procedures. This may involve a significant expense in materials. It also presents the problem that these gases may still have to be assayed to confirm the precision of their contents.

Another, simpler method is to have just one precise gas cylinder that contains a high concentration (preferably 100%) of the desired gas. A gas sample is drawn from the high concentration source and is diluted with room air. A large-volume calibrated syringe can be used for measuring and holding the diluted gas sample. The syringe must have a valve at its inlet that can be connected to both the gas source cylinder and to the analyzer to be evaluated. The valve is necessary to limiting the gases that enter and exit the syringe. This is done to minimize the chances of contamination of the sample.

With a given, known quantity of a 100% concentration precision gas and a certain amount of air that is used to dilute the gas, a known percentage for the test sample can be calculated. Table 16–7 demonstrates how this is done. The volume of any valve mechanism connected to the syringe must be included in the syringe volume. The volume of the syringe's inlet connection should also be accounted for if it is not already considered by the manufacturer as part of the syringe's volume.

In challenging an analyzer, a series of diluted samples at different concentrations can be made. The analyzer should then be tested with a sample from each dilution and the

---

**TABLE 16-7  Calculation of the Concentration in a Diluted Test Sample**

---

The percentage of a gas that will be in a diluted test sample can be determined in the following way:

$$\text{Diluted Gas Sample \%} = \frac{\text{Volume of Precision Gas}}{\text{Volume of Precision Gas + Volume of Added Air}} \times 100$$

Using a 3.0 liter calibrated syringe, if 100 ml of the 100% precision gas is first aspirated into the syringe and then 1200 ml of room air is aspirated, the following final percent will result for the gas sample.

$$\text{Diluted Gas \%} = \frac{100 \text{ ml}}{100 \text{ ml} + 1200 \text{ ml}} \times 100$$

Diluted Gas % = 7.7%

Other combinations of 100% precision gas and room air volumes can be used (e.g., 100 ml gas + 900 ml air, 100 ml gas + 1100 ml air, etc.).

---

*Volume of the Precision Gas* = the volume of the 100% precision gas that is aspirated into the calibrated syringe.

*Volume of Added Air* = the volume of air that is aspirated into the syringe after aspiration of the 100% precision gas.

*Diluted Gas Sample %* = the final percent concentration of the gas that will be in the calibrated syringe after the dilution procedure is completed.

results plotted in the manner shown in Figure 16–3. Doing this permits two types of analyzer evaluations to be performed.

- The accuracy of the analyzer can be evaluated based on how close the analyzed values are to the actual values of the test signal mixtures.
- The linearity of the analyzer can be evaluated based on the pattern that the measured values follow in relation to the actual values of the test signal mixtures.

Together, these evaluations will strongly demonstrate the quality of the analyzer's performance.

*Mechanical Lung Analogs.*   Gas analyzers do not have to be evaluated individually as instruments in the manner just described. They can also be evaluated during their performance as part of a pulmonary function measuring system. For example, the gas analyzers used to perform either gas dilution lung volume determinations or $D_L CO$ studies can be challenged during the administration of a test. A mechanical lung analog can permit this because it will have

- A known volume that should be accurately measured by the system during an "FRC" determination.

- A $D_LCO$ value that should be accurately measured as zero because physiologic gas exchange (external respiration) cannot occur in the mechanical lung.

Errors in gas analyzer operation will be demonstrated when either the "FRC" volume is inaccurately measured or the $D_LCO$ is measured as having anything other than a value of zero.

A mechanical lung analog can be as simple as a calibrated syringe that is attached to the subject connection of the system. The plunger of the syringe will be manipulated during the test in a manner that simulates the way the subject should breathe.

When used for a gas dilution lung volume determination, the plunger of the syringe should initially be set at some volume in the middle of the syringe's range. This known volume setting is the volume that should be correctly determined by the system. Different initial spirometer settings can be used to test the system at different ranges of function.

When the syringe "lung" is used as part of a $D_LCO$-SB test, the procedure should begin with the syringe plunger pushed all the way in to the zero volume level. This empties the syringe and is the "RV" level for the lung analog. During the test, the syringe should be "ventilated" in the same manner as a real subject would breathe.

These types of evaluation procedures challenge more than just the system's gas analyzers. All measuring instruments involved in the test will have to function correctly in order for the expected results to be measured accurately. Problems with the spirometer, breathing circuit components, or a computer-based system's software can all result in inaccurate measurements.

During these evaluations, the system's automatic gas or temperature correction systems should be bypassed. This may be difficult with some computer-based systems. The software of the system may be set for testing human subjects without permitting an override of some correction functions.

As described earlier, a calibrated syringe can be used as a simple lung analog. Other more complex lung analogs can be made. Regardless of the configuration, though, the lung analog must have a known volume. The "lung" may be constructed with a fixed volume. However, variable lung analogs can also be made so that different known volumes can be pre-set by the operator.

*Testing of Known Subjects.*   As with spirometers and plethysmographs, data on known subjects can be used as part of the quality control of gas analyzers. Data on known subjects provide for the same overall system evaluation that occurs with the use of mechanical lung analogs.

The guidelines described earlier for using data on known subjects for spirometer and plethysmograph quality control can also be applied to gas analyzer quality control. In this application, known subjects are not as sensitive as a mechanical lung analog in identifying system errors. Human subjects present too much natural variability to be that precise. Despite this, gross abnormalities in system function can be identified. Human subjects are useful for evaluating the participation of gas analyzers in automated exercise testing and metabolic measurement systems. Systems of this sort do not lend themselves easily to the use of a mechanical analog.

## CALIBRATION AND QUALITY CONTROL OF BLOOD GAS ANALYZERS

Blood gas analyzers have a greater need for calibration and quality control than gas analyzers. Many problems can affect the operation and accuracy of blood gas analyzers. Table 16–8 provides a list of these problems.

Electrode malfunctions are the most frequent cause of analysis errors by blood gas analyzers. Regular maintenance to the electrodes is important for continued quality performance of the analyzer. Inadequate temperature control of the measuring system can also have a significant effect on blood gas analysis. With $PO_2$ levels in the range of 70–100 mm Hg, the measured $PO_2$ will increase by 7% for each 1°C increase in temperature. $PCO_2$ values will increase by 4% and pH values increase by 0.0146 for each 1°C temperature increase.

Another source of analysis errors can arise during manual calibration. Manual calibration problems are generally due to errors made by the operator in performing the calibration procedure.

Routine maintenance and properly performed calibration and quality control procedures can either prevent these problems from occurring or can identify their presence.

---

### TABLE 16–8  Problems Affecting Blood Gas Analyzer Operation

---

#### Problems Relating to Electrode Function

- Buildup of protein and other blood products on the electrode membrane surfaces.
- Leaks in the electrode membranes that can cause contamination or depletion of the electrolyte solution in the electrodes.

---

#### Problems Relating to Analyzer System Operation

- Inadequate temperature control of the sample/electrodes chamber.
- Incorrect calibration with automatic calibration procedures.
- Contamination or incomplete aspiration of calibrating solutions, gases, and blood samples into the measuring chamber because of system tubing leaks or pump malfunctions.

---

#### Problems Relating to Use of the Analyzer by the Operator

- Incorrect calibration with manual calibration procedures.
- Factors relating to preanalytic error, including
  air bubbles in the blood sample.
  delay in performing analysis.
  clotting of the sample because of inadequate addition of an anticoagulant.
  excessive quantities of liquid heparin that affect pH, $PCO_2$, and $PO_2$ values.

---

## Calibration of Blood Gas Analyzers

Of the electrodes in a blood gas analyzer, the pH electrode is the most stable in its operation. The electrode that is least stable and most sensitive to variations in operation is the $PO_2$ electrode. The stability of the $PCO_2$ electrode falls between that of the pH and $PO_2$ electrodes.

Table 16–9 provides the accuracy and common calibration test signal ranges that are used for the pH, $PCO_2$, and $PO_2$ electrodes. As described earlier in the chapter, the high/slope calibration point chosen for the $O_2$ electrode depends on the range of values where accuracy is most desired. If shunt studies are being performed, calibration at an even higher range of $PO_2$ may be advisable.

A regular schedule must be followed for performing one- and two-point calibration procedures. Minimally, two-point calibrations should be performed at least every eight hours. Two-point calibration should also be performed if one-point calibration demonstrates that excessive electrode drift has occurred. Many automated systems perform two-point calibrations at a greater frequency than the minimum guidelines.

One-point calibration should be performed just prior to the analysis of each sample if analysis is only occasionally performed. On instruments where samples are frequently analyzed, one-point calibration should be performed every 30 minutes.

Manual calibration procedures permit the operator to have full control of the calibration process. This includes permitting the operator to determine when the electrode has reached an end-point in measuring the sample value. With the operator being part of the process, it is more likely that contamination of the calibration gas or buffer samples will be detected. Calibration end-point values that are not acceptably close to the test signal values will alert the operator to an analysis problem.

Manual calibration also permits changes in the gases used in performing a calibration (e.g., a higher $O_2$ calibration level can be used prior to analysis of a shunt study sample).

**TABLE 16–9  Range of Accuracy and Common Ranges for Calibration of Blood Gas Analyzer Electrodes**

|  | Electrode Accuracy Range | Calibration Range |
|---|---|---|
| pH | ±0.01 | 6.840 (Low/Balance Value) 7.384 (High/Slope Value) |
| $PCO_2$ | ±2% (approx. ±1 mm Hg at 40 mm Hg) | 5% $CO_2$ (Low/Balance Value) 10% $CO_2$ (High/Slope Value) |
| $PO_2$ | ±3% (approx. ±2.5 mm Hg at 80 mm Hg) | 0% $O_2$ (Low/Balance Value) 12% or 20% $O_2$ (High/Slope Value) |

Unfortunately, manually calibrated analyzers are at risk of being less precise in making measurements. This is because variations, even minor, in how operators perform calibration procedures can affect the precision of the instrument.

Automatic calibrations permit an analyzer to attain a greater degree of precision. This is due to the fact that each calibration is performed in precisely the same manner. Sophisticated analyzer systems provide a series of displays that can indicate when a malfunction is discovered during calibration and what the nature of that malfunction is most likely to be. This information assists the operator in correcting a calibration problem.

There is a problem associated with automatic calibration procedures. The automation results in the operator being less aware of the calibration process. If contamination of the calibration gases or buffers occurs, it is less likely that the operator will detect the problem. This contamination can result in the analyzer being calibrated farther and farther from the value of the calibration test sample. Computer programming safeguards are generally built into an analyzer's software in order to minimize this problem.

An important calibration variable that must be discussed is the effect of the *gas/blood calibration factor* of $PO_2$ electrodes. As stated earlier, for a given actual $PO_2$ value, the measured $PO_2$ from a gaseous sample will be higher than the same $PO_2$ measured from a blood sample. This is due to the fact that reduction of the oxygen at the tip of a polarographic electrode occurs more rapidly within a gaseous medium than in a liquid. Blood especially, because of its physical properties, has an effect on the rate of reduction. The gas/blood calibration factor is more significant for $PO_2$ values that are greater than 100 mm Hg. It is especially significant with $PO_2$ values greater than 400 mm Hg.

It is possible to determine how significant the gas/blood calibration factor is for a given $PO_2$ electrode. A series of precise gases with different $PO_2$ values is used to tonometer a series of blood samples. For each $PO_2$ level, a sample of the precise gas and then a sample of the tonometered blood are analyzed. The gas and blood $PO_2$ values are plotted on a graph and used as a basis for determining a ratio to relate the two values in an equal way. With many automated systems, this factor has been determined by the manufacturer and is already compensated for in the system's software.

## Quality Control of Blood Gas Analyzers

Unlike with gas analyzers, quality control procedures for blood gas analyzers are a regular and frequent part of using the instrument. Minimally, quality control procedures should be performed at least every eight hours. Additionally, they should be performed immediately after any maintenance procedures have been performed on an electrode and whenever analyzer performance is in question.

A particular problem for blood gas analyzer quality control is the possibility of preanalytic error. (These problems were listed in Table 16–8.) It is important that every laboratory work to minimize the occurrence of these types of problems.

Three types of quality control procedures that can be used for blood gas analyzers are the:

- Analysis of test standard samples.
- Proficiency testing.
- Interinstrumental comparisons.

*Analysis of Test Standard Samples.*   Generally, as their primary blood gas analyzer quality control procedure, laboratories analyze test standard samples at least every eight hours. The samples used can be either blood/buffers tonometered on site or they can be commercially prepared samples.

Minimally, two different levels of pH, $PCO_2$, and $PO_2$ should be used to challenge the quality of analyzer performance. For example, one test standard sample can contain a pH value that is acidotic, a $PCO_2$ value that is hypercapnic, and a $PO_2$ value that is hypoxemic in comparison to normal physiologic values. The second sample can contain an alkalotic pH, a hypocapnic $PCO_2$, and a hyperoxemic $PO_2$. Many laboratories also use a third standard that contains values for pH, $PCO_2$, and $PO_2$ that are within the normal physiologic range.

When tonometered blood or buffered solutions are used to create quality control test standards, two to three different precise gas mixtures must be available for preparing the samples. These mixtures are needed to create samples for challenging the $PCO_2$ and $PO_2$ electrodes. Even with blood tonometered for use with $PCO_2$ and $PO_2$ electrodes, two to three different buffered solutions are still needed to challenge the pH electrode.

No single standard for blood gas analyzer performance can be equally applied to all analyzers in all laboratories. Even if the same test standard samples were used, over a series of measurements made and compared between two laboratories, there would be slight variations in the statistical records of the performance of the analyzers. This difference is the result of operator performance variations and the contribution of the factors that can create preanalytic error with regular blood samples.

Since a universal standard for analyzer performance is not possible, each laboratory must establish its own statistical history of analyzer performance. Once established, *the analyzer is then judged against its own quality control performance history.* Analyzer performance is judged to be poor when it is performing in error in relation to its history of good performance.

The statistical history is begun with a series of tests that are performed using quality control test standard samples. At the time of this test series, the analyzer must be at peak performance. This is based on its recent maintenance history and its having just had a two-point calibration performed.

Generally, 20 to 30 test standard samples are analyzed. A separate record of performance is maintained for the measurements from each electrode. Figure 16–4 provides an example of how the results of a 20-sample test series would be recorded for a $PO_2$ electrode. This type of graphic record is referred to as a *Levey-Jennings chart.* The actual $PO_2$ value for all of the test standard samples used in this example series was 100 mm Hg. Similar records would be made at the same time for the performance of the pH and $PCO_2$ electrodes during the test series.

Once the measurement series is completed, a statistical evaluation of the results is performed. The statistical analysis includes determining the mean value and standard deviation for the results of the test series.

Using the data in Figure 16–4, the *mean value* for an electrode's test series results is determined by the following equation:

$$\text{Mean Value} = \frac{(X_1 + X_2 + X_3 + \ldots + X_{20})}{20}$$

| Sample # | 1 | 2 | 3 | 4 | 5 | 6 | 7 | 8 | 9 | 10 | 11 | 12 | 13 | 14 | 15 | 16 | 17 | 18 | 19 | 20 |
|---|---|---|---|---|---|---|---|---|---|---|---|---|---|---|---|---|---|---|---|---|
| $PO_2$ | 98 | 103 | 99 | 101 | 98 | 102 | 100 | 97 | 101 | 100 | 98 | 97 | 102 | 98 | 102 | 103 | 99 | 102 | 98 | 102 |

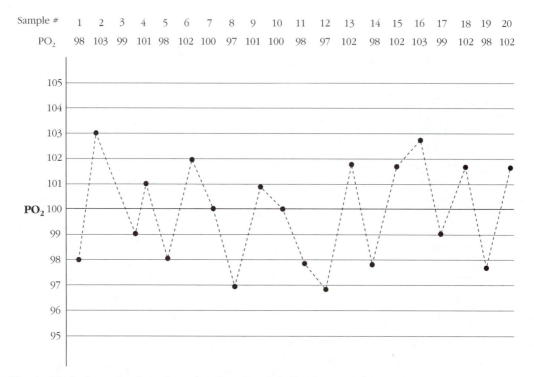

**Figure 16–4** *Levey-Jennings chart of quality control challenge test results.*

where X is the measured sample $PO_2$ value, and 1, 2, 3, . . . 20 relate to the number of each test sample in the series. For the data presented in Figure 16–4, the mean value for the test series was 100 mm Hg.

The *standard deviation* for the sample series is determined by use of the following equation.

$$\text{Standard Deviation} = \frac{[(X_1 - MV)^2 + (X_2 - MV)^2 + \ldots + (X_{20} - MV)^2]}{20}$$

where X is the measured sample $PO_2$ value; 1, 2, . . . 20 relate to the number of each test sample in the series; and MV is the mean value that was calculated previously. The final value from this calculation is expressed as a positive number. For the data presented in Figure 16–4, the standard deviation is 2 mm Hg.

The standard deviation (SD) value for a series of test values has a special statistical significance. For a "population" of properly measured samples that have a normal, bell-shaped distribution of values,

- 68.3% of the measured values will fall within 1 SD of the mean value (approximately 14 out of a population of 20 samples).
- 95.5% of the measured values will fall within 2 SD of the mean value (approximately 19 out of a population of 20 samples).

- 99.7% of the measured values will fall within 3 SD of the mean value (approximately 20 out of a population of 20 samples).

Once a statistical pattern, as just described, has been established for an analyzer, future analyzer performance can be evaluated against this standard. A standard for performance is useful for two reasons:

- It provides a statistical definition of what normal, *in-control* performance is for that particular blood gas analyzer.
- It provides a statistical framework that can be used to identify when analyzer performance is poor and an *out-of-control* situation exists.

Future quality control measurements of test standard samples are compared against the statistical history of analyzer performance. The relationship of the most recent test standard measurements compared to the past record provides the basis for determining whether an analyzer is in-control or out-of-control.

Each laboratory should have a specific written protocol for interpreting the results of quality control test standard measurements that occur during the routine quality control process. An example of a protocol system is presented in Table 16–10. Figure 16–5 demonstrates a hypothetical graphic representation of each of the possible error conditions described in Table 16–10.

The presence of these error patterns is confirmed if two or three test standard levels are measured for each electrode. If, for example, all of the two or three test standard levels run for an electrode during a quality control evaluation have values that are either 2 SD greater than or 2 SD less than the mean value, it is very likely that an *out-of-control* condition exists for that electrode.

A *warning* condition indicates that a statistically significant change in an electrode has occurred. No particular response on the part of the operator is required in this situation. It is a good idea, however, that subsequent quality control tests be performed with an awareness that a previous warning event had been recorded.

An out-of-control condition requires that the operator take certain actions. Table 16–11 describes the actions that should be taken when an out-of-control condition is demonstrated by an analyzer during a quality control evaluation. Table 16–12 provides a list of the types of problems that can cause an out-of-control condition to exist.

Putting the entire process into perspective, at least every eight hours a quality control evaluation should be performed on blood gas analyzers. At the time the evaluation is performed, each of the three electrodes in the analyzer should be challenged with two to three test samples, each with a different expected value. If commercially prepared samples are used, this means that two to three samples will need to be analyzed, each with its own pH, $PCO_2$, and $PO_2$ levels. If tonometered blood is used, then four to six samples will need to be analyzed: two to three tonometered blood samples for $PCO_2$ and $PO_2$ levels and two to three buffered solution samples for pH levels.

Assuming that three different levels are measured for each electrode, *each time that a quality control procedure is performed, nine different values will have to be recorded and made part of the statistical history of the analyzer.* This very quickly becomes a great deal of data

---

### TABLE 16–10 Protocol for Interpretation of Blood Gas Quality Control Data

---

This protocol is based on how a single current measurement result or series of recent measurement results relate to the mean value (MV) and standard deviation (SD) of past measurements.

---

#### Interpretations Based on Single Quality Control Test Standard Measurements

---

- When one measurement exceeds the range of ±2 SD from the MV, it indicates a *warning* condition for analyzer performance.
- When one measurement exceeds the range of ±3 SD from the MV, it indicates an *out-of-control* condition for the analyzer.
- When one measurement differs from the immediately previous test standard measurement by a value equal to 4 SD, it indicates an *out-of-control* condition for the analyzer.

---

#### Interpretations Based on a Pattern of Consecutive Quality Control Test Standard Measurements

---

- When two consecutive measurements both exceed the range of either +2 SD from the MV or −2 SD from the MV, it indicates an *out-of-control* condition for the analyzer.
- When four consecutive measurements all exceed the range of either +1 SD from the MV or −1 SD from the MV, it indicates an *out-of-control* condition for the analyzer.
- When ten consecutive measurements all have values that are either greater than the MV or are less than the MV, it indicates an *out-of-control* condition for the analyzer.

---

to manage. Fortunately there are a variety of computer-based quality control data management software programs available to assist in this process. This type of software program can simplify the process of maintaining and analyzing quality control data. The software can even assist in identifying analyzer/operator errors that are detected by the quality control process. Many accrediting agencies require that this type of record keeping system be used.

*Proficiency Testing.* The blood gas analyzer quality control procedures described so far have been largely *internal* mechanisms for quality assurance. The procedures and response mechanisms for the results of these quality control tests are determined within the institution.

*Proficiency testing* provides an *external* mechanism for blood gas quality control and is a significant requirement of the Clinical Laboratory Improvement Act (CLIA) of 1967, updated in 1988. Proficiency testing is a process whereby a laboratory enrolls with an agency

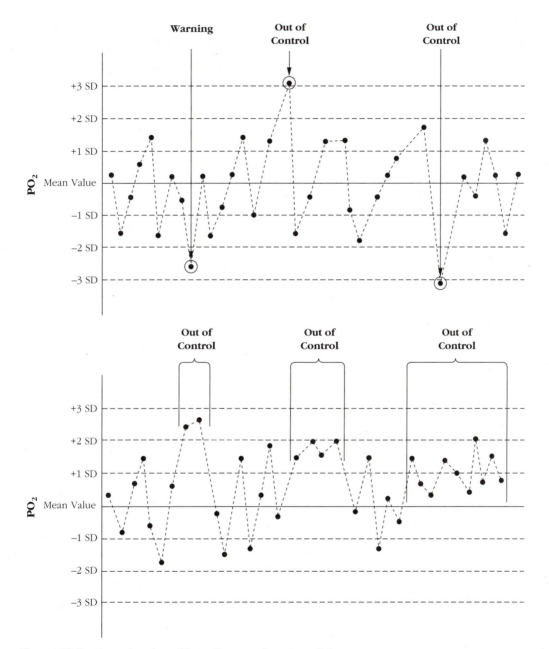

**Figure 16–5** *Examples of possible quality control error conditions.*

## TABLE 16–11 Response to an Out-of-Control Condition

### With an Out-of-Control Condition Based on a Random Error

- A two-point calibration should be performed, and then the quality control challenge should be repeated.
- If the follow-up quality control challenge is *in control*, no further action is needed.
- If the follow-up quality control challenge is *out of control*, then troubleshooting and corrective procedures should be performed as outlined by the instrument's manufacturer.

### With an Out-of-Control Condition Based on a Systematic Error

- Troubleshooting and corrective procedures should be performed as outlined by the instrument's manufacturer.

Troubleshooting and corrective procedures should be continued until, after two-point calibration, quality control test sample values are within ±2 SD of the mean value.

## TABLE 16–12 Problems That May Produce an Out-of-Control Condition

### Problems Associated With Operation or Use of Analyzer

- Contamination or misanalyzation of the calibration test signal buffer solutions or gas samples.
- Variations in analyzer electrode/measuring chamber temperature regulation.
- Electrode function problems (e.g., loss of membrane integrity, buildup of protein and blood products on the membrane, contaminated electrolyte, electrical circuit malfunction).
- Inconsistent calibration procedures.

### Problems Associated With Quality Control Process

- Changes in the storage and preparation of the quality control test standard samples.
- Inconsistent sampling of the quality control test standard samples.

that on a regular schedule supplies test samples with pH, $PCO_2$, and $PO_2$ values unknown to the laboratory. At the same time, identical samples are sent to all of the other laboratories enrolled with that agency. The samples must be analyzed by the participating laboratories and the results of testing sent back to the agency.

In order to satisfy CLIA requirements, the analysis of the proficiency testing samples must follow certain guidelines:

- The test samples must be analyzed as part of the routine of blood sample management.
- The test samples cannot be independently analyzed in another laboratory for comparison and confirmation of the test results.
- No interlaboratory communication regarding the sample or its analysis results is permitted.

Once the results of the proficiency testing sample analysis are returned to the agency, the data are compared and reported back to the participating institutions. The agency report for a laboratory compares that laboratory's results against its own past performance history and against laboratories with similar instrumentation. Comparisons are also made between all of the enrolled laboratories regardless of instrumentation. The comparative results include the mean and standard deviation values for each specific type of instrument used in the testing process.

The proficiency testing process provides an excellent means of challenging and evaluating the accuracy of blood gas analysis by a laboratory. Being an outside, objective process, it can detect systematic problems in the performance of the analyzer and its operator. Such problems as faulty calibration procedures and poor sample management by the operator can result in poor performance on proficiency testing.

The CLIA regulations for proficiency testing must be followed by all licensed laboratories. Otherwise the laboratory can lose its license. Most institutional accrediting agencies require that the laboratories within an institution be licensed under CLIA guidelines. The CLIA guidelines outline the circumstances under which poor performance can result in the loss of a laboratory's license. Guidelines are also provided for the process of license reinstatement.

*Interinstrumental Comparisons.*   Many laboratories operate more than one blood gas analyzer. Often, two analyzers are maintained, one for regular sample analysis and the other as a backup in case of failure of the primary analyzer. With two or more analyzers available, *interinstrumental comparisons* can be performed as a quality control procedure. Quality control is performed simply by analyzing the same subject blood sample or quality control test sample on both analyzers. As with any quality control process, the results of this joint analysis should be recorded.

Some difference in measured value is acceptable. However, based on the recorded history of the compared performance of the analyzers, significant variations may indicate an out-of-control condition in one or both of the analyzers. An evaluation of the instruments should be performed if an out-of-control condition is detected.

A variation of using interinstrumental comparisons for quality control is to have a particular value confirmed by use of different instrumentation. For example, the performance of a blood gas analyzer pH electrode can be compared to the pH determined on that sample by a standard pH-only measuring instrument.

## Review Questions

Please use the following review questions to evaluate your learning of information from this chapter. It might be helpful to write out your answers on a sheet of paper. If you are unsure of the answers to these questions, review the chapter to reinforce your learning.

1. Relating to the concept of test quality assurance:
   a. What is test quality assurance?
   b. How does test quality assurance relate to the technologist?
   c. How does test quality assurance relate to the equipment?
   d. How does test quality assurance relate to the subject?
   e. What should be done when test quality is questioned?
2. Relating to equipment quality assurance:
   a. What is equipment quality assurance?
   b. How does equipment quality assurance relate to equipment maintenance?
   c. How does preventative maintenance differ from corrective maintenance?
3. Relating to definitions for quality assurance:
   a. What is precision?
   b. What is accuracy?
   c. How do precision and accuracy differ?
   d. What is calibration?
   e. What is quality control?
   f. How do calibration and quality control differ?
4. Relating to equipment used for spirometer and body plethysmograph quality assurance:
   a. What is a calibrated syringe?
   b. What is an automated syringe?
   c. What is an explosive decompression device?
   d. What is a weighted volume-displacement spirometer?
   e. What is a rotameter?
   f. What is a rotary sinusoidal pump?
   g. What is a water or mercury manometer?
5. Relating to the quality assurance for spirometers:
   a. What are problems that can affect the function of spirometers?
   b. How can spirometers be calibrated?
   c. How accurate must a spirometer be?
   d. What must be done if a spirometer is found to be inaccurate?
   e. How can the volume accuracy of a spirometer be evaluated?
   f. How can the flow accuracy of a spirometer be assessed?
   g. How can the flow resistance of a spirometer be assessed?

h. How can the frequency response of a spirometer be assessed?

i. How can the recorder function of a spirometer be assessed?

6. Relating to quality assurance for body plethysmographs:

   a. What are problems that can affect the function of body plethysmograph?

   b. How can the mouth pressure transducer be calibrated?

   c. How can the flow transducer be calibrated?

   d. How can the cabinet pressure transducer be calibrated?

   e. How can $F_{Cal}$ be determined?

   f. How is quality control performed for body plethysmographs?

   g. What is a lung analog?

   h. How is a lung analog used with a body plethysmograph?

   i. How is body plethysmograph function assessed by the use of known subjects?

7. Relating to quality assurance for gas and blood gas analyzers:

   a. How does the intended range of measurement affect the calibration of electrodes?

   b. How can the nature of the test sample used affect the calibration of gas and blood gas analyzers?

   c. How can gaseous samples be used for calibrating test samples?

   d. What are different commercial buffered-solution samples available for use as calibrating test samples?

   e. How can commercial buffer-solution samples be used for calibration?

   f. What is tonometered blood?

   g. How can tonometered blood be used in calibration?

   h. What is a two-point calibration?

   i. What is a one-point calibration?

   j. What are multiple-point linearity checks?

8. Relating to quality assurance for gas analyzers:

   a. What are problems that can affect the function of a gas analyzer?

   b. How should gas analyzers be calibrated?

   c. How can challenges with known gas values be used for the quality control of gas analyzers?

   d. How can mechanical lung analogs be used for gas analyzer quality control?

   e. How can the testing of known subjects be used?

9. Relating to quality assurance for blood gas analyzers:

   a. What are problems that can affect the function of blood gas analyzers?

   b. How is blood gas calibration performed?

   c. When should two-point and one-point calibration be performed?

   d. How does the gas/blood calibration factor affect the calibration of $PO_2$ electrodes?

   e. How is quality control for blood gas analyzers performed?

   f. What is a Levey-Jennings chart?

   g. How is a mean value for blood gas analyzer electrode calibration results calculated?

   h. How is a value for standard deviation calculated?

   i. What is the special significance of standard deviation values in relation to a set of sample results?

   j. What is the significance of a warning condition for blood gas analyzer quality control?

   k. What is the significance of an out-of-control condition?

   l. What is proficiency testing of blood gas analyzers?

# EVALUATION OF THE GRAPHIC RESULTS OF A FORCED VITAL CAPACITY MANEUVER

## PURPOSE FOR THE DEMONSTRATION

This section provides a demonstration in making measurements on the graphic results of a forced vital capacity maneuver and performing calculations based on those measurements. From these calculations, values for such parameters as FVC, $FEV_{0.5}$, etc., will be determined. In the past, this was the method used for making determinations for a subject's test results. With today's testing system technology, however, the need for making these measurements and calculations has been all but eliminated as a regular routine.

Although it is no longer a skill used by a pulmonary function technologist, this demonstration is provided for several important reasons. They are to reinforce:

1. How the movement of a volume displacement spirometer relates to the dynamics of a forced expiratory maneuver.
2. How the structure of the volume/time graph provides a representation of the subject's performance of a forced expiratory maneuver.
3. How each of the determined parameters relates to a specific portion of the subject's expiratory maneuver.

New learning from this demonstration relates to the procedure for the measurements and calculations used in making parameter determinations from a graph.

## DESCRIPTION OF THE VOLUME/TIME FORCED EXPIRATORY MANEUVER TRACING

### HOW THE TRACING WAS CREATED

Figure 1 provides an example of a volume/time tracing from a forced expiratory vital capacity maneuver. It was created by using a 13.5 liter Collins water-sealed spirometer that has a bell factor (BF) of 41.27 ml/mm (0.04127 l/mm). The spirometer produced the tracing by use of pen attached to a chain-compensated type of system. The graph paper was attached to a drum that rotated the paper to the right at a constant speed during the time that the graph was recorded. The recording drum rotation speed was 1920 mm/min (32 mm/sec). As can be seen, the graph paper is laid out with horizontal lines that are marked in volume units and vertical lines that are unlabeled.

## SIGNIFICANCE OF THE TRACING

How is all of this information significant to the tracing and its use? It is significant in the following ways:

1. Because this is a volume-displacement spirometer, the distance of vertical movement by the spirometer bell is in direct proportión to the amount of volume exhaled by the subject. The speed of vertical bell movement is in direct proportion to the subject's expiratory flow rate.
2. The spirometer bell factor of 41.27 ml/mm (0.04127 l/mm) relates the amount the spirometer bell moves vertically to the air volume breathed by the subject. Given the volume of this particular spirometer bell, each millimeter of vertical bell movement results from 41.27 ml (0.04127 liter) of air entering or leaving the spirometer as the subject breathes. *This also means that each millimeter of vertical distance on the graph represents 41.27 ml (0.04127 liter) of volume.*

The horizontal lines on this particular graph paper happen to be calibrated to represent this ratio of vertical distance to volume. Although the lines of the graph paper are labeled with volume values, this information will not be used in performing either the measurements or calculations for this demonstration.

3. Because the spirometer used in creating the graph is a chain-compensated system, upward vertical movement of the spirometer bell resulted in downward movement of the tracing pen. As the subject exhaled air into the spirometer, it was represented by a downward tracing on the graph paper. A greater exhaled volume is shown by a greater downward movement. Inspiration is demonstrated by an upward tracing on the graph paper.
4. Rotation of the drum to which the graph paper was fastened produced a horizontal time component to the tracing. Because the paper was being rotated to the right, it means that the start of the maneuver is to the right of the paper and expiration progresses to the left. The rotation speed of 32 mm/sec is significant because it means that *each 32 mm of horizontal distance on the graph represents one second of time.* Because the vertical lines on the graph paper are 32 mm apart at this drum rotation speed, each vertical line represents one second of elapsed time.

## RELATING THE TRACING TO THE SUBJECT'S FORCED EXPIRATORY VITAL CAPACITY MANEUVER

How does all of this information relate to a tracing of a forced expiratory vital capacity maneuver? Looking again at Figure 1 we can see that

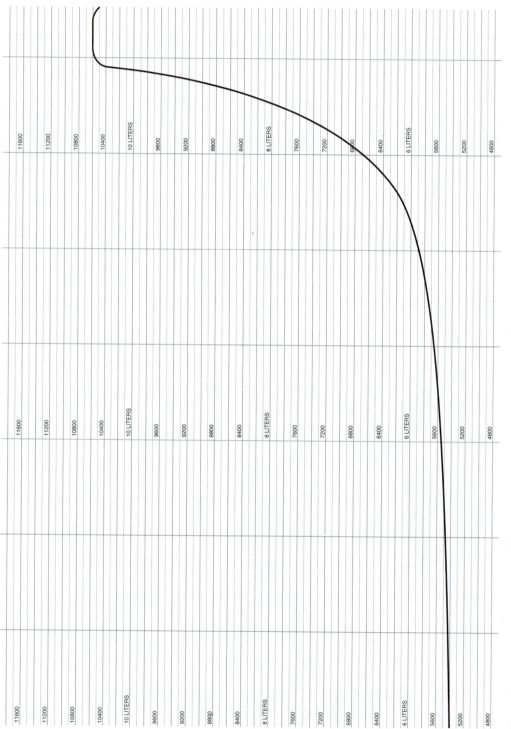

**Figure 1** *Example of a graphic tracing for a forced vital capacity maneuver.*

1. The end-inspiratory volume, just before the start of the forced expiratory maneuver, is represented by the highest vertical point the tracing line reaches at the upper right of the tracing.
2. The downward (to the left) line of the tracing demonstrates the exhaled volumes and flow rates of the subject. The early, fast expiratory flow rates of the expiration resulted in a sharp downward movement of the pen and tracing line. The later flattening of the curve represents the slowing of later flow rates during expiration.
3. The flat portion of the tracing line toward the lower left of the tracing represents the end of the last portion of the effort and the level of total volume exhaled by the subject during the maneuver.
4. The upward line at the far left of the tracing represents the subject's inspiration at the end of the maneuver.

# PROCEDURE FOR EVALUATION OF A VOLUME/TIME TRACING FOR DETERMINATION OF VOLUME AND FLOW RATE PARAMETER VALUES

## BASIC STEPS FOR TRACING EVALUATION

Tracing evaluation is performed in a series of three basic steps:

1. Identifying and marking certain key points on the tracing that are needed as a basis for making later measurements.
2. Making measurements on the tracing and performing the calculations that are needed for determination of *volume* parameters.
3. Making measurements on the tracing and performing the calculations that are needed for determination of *flow rate* parameters.

Each of these steps will be described and demonstrated in detail. Illustrations of the steps are provided.

## IDENTIFYING AND MARKING KEY POINTS ON THE TRACING

Before any meaningful measurements can be made on the tracing, certain key points must be identified and marked:

1. The volume level on the tracing that represents the maximal inspiratory volume performed by the subject just prior to the forced expiratory effort.
2. The time-zero point that represents where the subject first began the forced expiratory effort from the maximal inspiratory volume level.

### Identifying and Marking the Maximal Inspiratory Volume

A line that represents the maximal inspiratory volume achieved prior to the start of the expiratory maneuver is marked horizontally across the tracing. This volume level is indicated by the highest point reached by the tracing line at the upper right of the tracing.

In Figure 2 this level happens to correspond to the 10600 ml volume line on the graph paper. As a result of this coincidence, we can use the 10600 ml volume line to indicate the maximal inspiratory volume level.

## Identifying and Marking the Time-Zero Point

The exact time point at which the forced expiration was begun must be clearly identified and marked on the graph. If the expiration is begun sharply by the subject from the maximal inspiratory level, it is easy to identify this point. Unfortunately, with most subjects, there is usually at least a slight rounding of the curve at the point where expiration is begun. As a result, the *back-extrapolation method* must be used to identify the start of expiration.

The back-extrapolation method is demonstrated in Figure 2–4 (in Chapter 2), where the start of the forced expiration tracing is isolated and enlarged. It involves extending the forced expiratory line straight upward to intersect with the maximal inspiratory volume line. This is done by aligning with the first "straight" downward 5 mm of the forced expiration line. A line is then extended upward to intersect with the maximal inspiratory volume line. The intersection of these two lines is the time-zero point for the forced expiratory maneuver. This method should be used even when it appears that the start of expiration is relatively sharp. The time-zero point in Figure 2 has been marked.

## MAKING MEASUREMENTS ON THE TRACING AND PERFORMING CALCULATIONS FOR VOLUME PARAMETERS

The following volume parameters can be determined from a forced vital capacity volume/time curve: FVC, $FEV_{0.5}$, $FEV_1$, $FEV_2$, $FEV_3$. Determination of volume parameters is based on measurements of vertical distance (VD, in mm) at specific points on the tracing. All measurements are made to the nearest 0.5 mm. Figure 3 demonstrates the measurements needed for making volume determinations.

The value for the volume is calculated by the following equation:

**Volume = VD in mm × BF in l/mm × BTPS Conversion Factor**

The bell factor, as stated earlier, is 0.04127 l/mm of vertical distance on the graph. As described in the textbook, the volume measured by the spirometer is under conditions of ATPS. In order to report the volume exhaled by the subject accurately, the technologist must convert the volume measured from the tracing back to BTPS conditions. The tracing used for this example was measured with the spirometer having a temperature of 20°C. The BTPS conversion factor for this temperature is 1.102. Therefore, for the volume determinations for this tracing, the equation that will be used is

**Volume = VD in mm × 0.04127 l/mm × 1.102**

## Determination of FVC

Determination of FVC is based on the greatest downward vertical distance from the maximal inspiratory level demonstrated by the forced expiratory maneuver tracing. This occurs at the left end of the tracing where maximal expiration is demonstrated. Figure 3 demon-

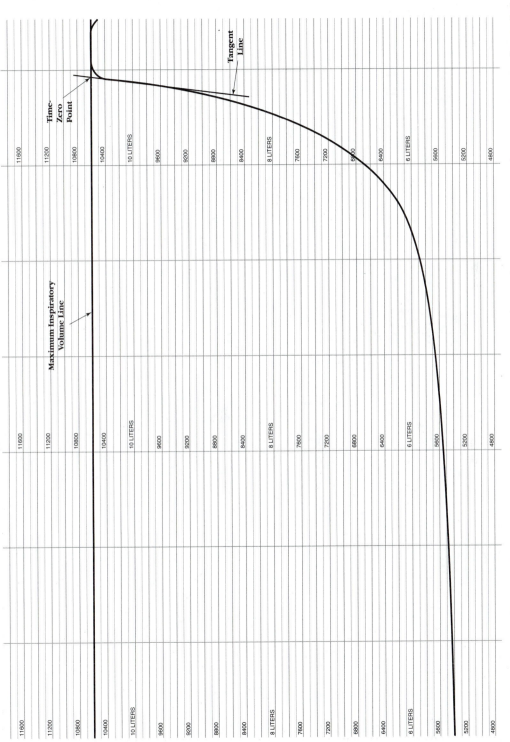

**Maximum Inspiratory Volume Line**

Time-Zero Point

Tangent Line

**Figure 2** *Example of graphic tracing for a forced vital capacity maneuver with the maximum inspiratory volume line and time-zero tangent point marked.*

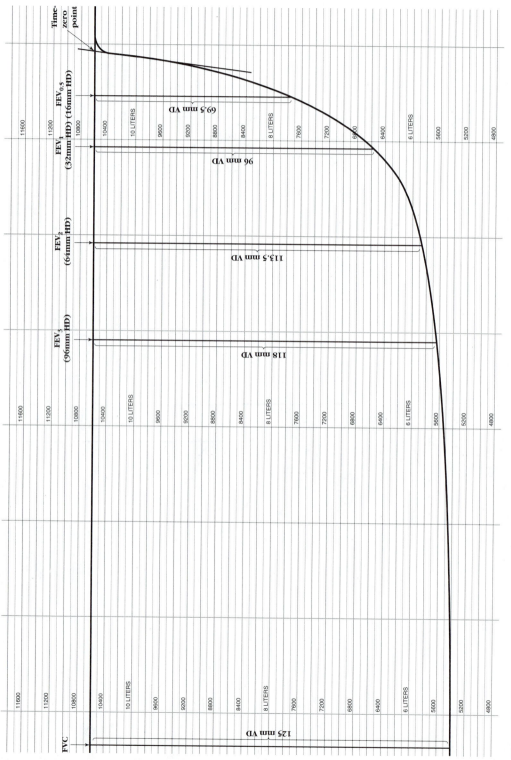

**Figure 3** *Example of a graphic tracing for a forced vital capacity maneuver with the volume determinations marked.*

strates this measurement. In the example tracing, the distance is 125 mm. Once the measurement is made, a value for FVC can be calculated by use of the equation stated earlier:

$$FVC = 125 \text{ mm} \times 0.04127 \text{ l/mm} \times 1.102$$

$$FVC = 5.685 \text{ liter}$$

## Determination of $FEV_t$ Values

The determination of values for $FEV_{0.5}$, $FEV_1$, $FEV_2$, $FEV_3$ is similar to that of a value for FVC. The difference is in how the points are selected for making the vertical distance measurements.

In order to make the measurements, the 0.5, 1, 2, and 3 second time points must be identified on the maximal inspiratory volume line. Identification is based on the fact that one second of elapsed time on the tracing is represented by 32 mm of horizontal distance. Beginning from the time-zero point,

- The 0.5 second time point is located 16 mm to the left of the time-zero point.
- The 1.0 second time point is located 32 mm to the left of the time-zero point.
- The 2.0 second time point is located 64 mm to the left of the time-zero point.
- The 3.0 second time point is located 96 mm to the left of the time-zero point.

Figure 3 demonstrates these measurements and shows the following VD values: $FEV_{0.5} = 69.5$ mm, $FEV_1 = 96$ mm, $FEV_2 = 113.5$ mm, and $FEV_3 = 118$ mm. Based on these measurements, values for the $FEV_t$ parameters can be calculated in the following way:

$$FEV_{0.5} = 69.5 \text{ mm} \times 0.04127 \text{ l/mm} \times 1.102$$

$$FEV_{0.5} = 3.161 \text{ liter}$$

$$FEV_1 = 96 \text{ mm} \times 0.04127 \text{ l/mm} \times 1.102$$

$$FEV_1 = 4.366 \text{ liter}$$

$$FEV_2 = 113.5 \text{ mm} \times 0.04127 \text{ l/mm} \times 1.102$$

$$FEV_2 = 5.162 \text{ liter}$$

$$FEV_3 = 118 \text{ mm} \times 0.04127 \text{ l/mm} \times 1.102$$

$$FEV_3 = 5.367 \text{ liter}$$

## MAKING MEASUREMENTS ON THE TRACING AND PERFORMING CALCULATIONS FOR FLOW PARAMETERS

The following flow rate parameters can be determined from a forced vital capacity volume/time curve: $FEF_{200-1200}$, $FEF_{25-75\%}$, $FEF_{78-85\%}$. Determination of flow rate parameter values is based on the principle of what a flow rate parameter represents—the amount of volume exhaled by the subject per unit of time, or

$$\text{Flow Rate} = \frac{\text{Volume Exhaled (liter)}}{\text{Time (sec)}} = \text{l/sec}$$

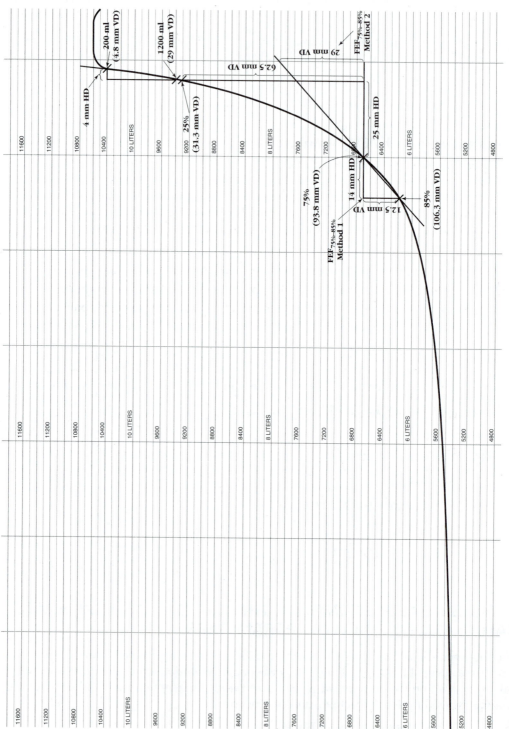

**Figure 4** *Example of graphic testing for a forced vital capacity maneuver with the flow determinations marked.*

Given the nature of the forced expiratory maneuver tracing that is used, this can also be represented as

$$\text{Flow Rate} = \frac{\text{VD in mm}}{\text{HD in mm}}$$

The key to determining flow rate values is in selecting the starting and ending points for the amount of exhaled volume that is to be used for a given parameter. For the parameters that are to be determined from this tracing, expiratory flow rates will be calculated between the following sets of exhaled volume points:

1. Between the 200 ml and 1200 ml points of exhaled volume.
2. Between the points where 25% and 75% of the subject's FVC volume was exhaled.
3. Between the points where 75% and 85% of the subject's FVC volume was exhaled.

These exhaled volume points must be identified on the forced expiratory maneuver tracing. Once the points are identified, the VD in mm (volume) and the HD in mm (time) between the points must be measured.

Once the measurements have been made, the value for flow rate is calculated by use of the following equation:

$$\text{Flow Rate} = \frac{\text{VD in mm} \times \text{BF in l/mm} \times \text{BTPS Factor}}{\text{HD in mm/32 mm/sec}}$$

Or, for the calculations for the examples in this chapter,

$$\text{Flow Rate} = \frac{\text{VD in mm} \times 0.04127 \, \text{l/mm} \times 1.102}{\text{HD in mm/32 mm/sec}}$$

where the numerator of the equation establishes a value for exhaled volume, and the denominator establishes a value for time.

## Determination of FEF$_{200-1200}$

Figure 4 demonstrates the measurements needed for making a determination of FEF$_{200-1200}$. The 200 ml and 1200 ml exhaled volume points are identified by making VD measurements from the maximum inspiratory volume line down to the tracing line. The 200 ml exhaled volume point on the tracing is located 4.8 mm down from the maximal inspiratory volume line. The 1200 ml exhaled volume point is located 29 mm down from the maximal inspiratory volume line. These volume/distance relationships are based on the bell factor being 0.04127 l/mm. All measurements are made to the nearest 0.5 mm.

The next step is for a horizontal line to be extended to the *left* from the 200 ml point and for a vertical line to be extended *up* from the 1200 ml point so that these two lines intersect. Since it is known that 200 ml and 1200 ml are at the 4.8 mm and 29 mm VD points, this means that the VD for the vertical line that was just drawn is 24.2 mm (29 mm − 4.8 mm = 24.2 mm). This makes sense because with a bell factor of 0.04127 l/mm of VD, a volume of one liter would be equal to 24.2 mm.

The HD of the horizontal line identified from the left of the 200 ml point must be measured. In Figure 4 this distance is 4 mm. Given this information, a value for $FEF_{200-1200}$ can be calculated by one of the two following methods:

**Method 1:**

$$FEF_{200-1200} = \frac{\textbf{VD in mm} \times \textbf{0.04127 l/mm} \times \textbf{1.102}}{\textbf{HD in mm/32 mm/sec}}$$

$$FEF_{200-1200} = \frac{24.2 \text{ mm} \times 0.04127 \text{ l/mm} \times 1.102}{4 \text{ mm/32 mm/sec}}$$

$$FEF_{200-1200} = \frac{1.10 \text{ liter}}{0.125 \text{ sec}}$$

$$FEF_{200-1200} = 8.8 \text{ l/sec}$$

**Method 2:**
Since the exhaled volume for the flow rate is known to be 1000 ml or 1.0 liter (1200 ml − 200 ml = 1000 ml or 1.0 liter), the following modified equation can be used:

$$FEF_{200-1200} = \frac{\textbf{1.0 liter} \times \textbf{1.102}}{\textbf{4 mm/32 mm/sec}}$$

$$FEF_{200-1200} = \frac{1.102 \text{ liter}}{0.125 \text{ sec}}$$

$$FEF_{200-1200} = 8.8 \text{ l/sec}$$

Either of these methods can work acceptably in making determinations of $FEF_{200-1200}$.

## Determination of $FEF_{25-75\%}$ and $FEF_{75-85\%}$

Figure 4 demonstrates the measurements needed for making a determination of values for $FEF_{25-75\%}$ and $FEF_{75-85\%}$. The first step in making these determinations is to identify the 25%, 75%, and 85% points on the forced exhaled volume tracing. Given that the VD for the FVC volume is 125 mm down from the maximum inspiratory volume line, the 25%, 75%, and 85% points can be identified as

25% point = .25 × 125 mm = 31.3 mm

75% point = .75 × 125 mm = 93.8 mm

85% point = .85 × 125 mm = 106.3 mm

down from the bottom of the maximum inspiratory volume line.

## Determination of $FEF_{25-75\%}$

Determination of $FEF_{25-75\%}$ is based on the following equation:

$$FEF_{25-75\%} = \frac{\textbf{VD in mm} \times \textbf{0.04127 l/mm} \times \textbf{1.102}}{\textbf{HD in mm/32 mm/sec}}$$

where the VD in the equation is equal to the VD of the 75% point minus the VD of the 25% point or

$$93.8 \text{ mm} - 31.3 \text{ mm} = 62.5 \text{ mm}$$

The HD in the equation is determined by extending a vertical line *down* from the 25% point and extending a horizontal line to the *right* of the 75% point. The length of the horizontal line from the 75% point to the vertical line down from the 25% point is the HD used in the equation. In Figure 4 this horizontal distance is 25 mm.

Given these values for VD and HD, a value for $FEF_{25\%-75\%}$ can be determined in the following way:

$$FEF_{25-75\%} = \frac{62.5 \text{ mm} \times 0.04127 \text{ l/mm} \times 1.102}{25 \text{ mm}/32 \text{ mm/sec}}$$

$$FEF_{25-75\%} = \frac{2.84 \text{ liter}}{0.781 \text{ sec}}$$

$$FEF_{25-75\%} = 3.6 \text{ l/sec}$$

## Determination of FEF$_{75-85\%}$

Determination of $FEF_{75-85\%}$ can be performed using one of two methods:

**Method 1:**

The first method is the same as the one used to determine a value for $FEF_{25-75\%}$. It is based on the following equation:

$$FEF_{75-85\%} = \frac{VD \text{ in mm} \times 0.04127 \text{ l/mm} \times 1.102}{HD \text{ in mm}/32 \text{ mm/sec}}$$

where the VD in the equation is equal the VD of the 85% point minus the VD of the 75% point, or

$$106.3 \text{ mm} - 93.8 \text{ mm} = 12.5 \text{ mm}$$

The HD in the equation is determined by extending a horizontal line to the *left* from the 75% point and extending a vertical line *up* from the 85% point. The length of the horizontal line from the 75% point to the vertical line up from the 85% point is the HD used in the equation. In Figure 4 this distance is 14 mm.

Given these values for VD and HD, a value for $FEF_{75-85\%}$ can be determined in the following way:

$$FEF_{75-85\%} = \frac{12.5 \text{ mm} \times 0.04127 \text{ l/mm} \times 1.102}{14 \text{ mm}/32 \text{ mm/sec}}$$

$$FEF_{75-85\%} = \frac{0.568 \text{ liter}}{0.438 \text{ sec}}$$

$$FEF_{75-85\%} = 1.3 \text{ l/sec}$$

**Method 2:**

The second method for determining a value for $FEF_{75-85\%}$ involves making use of the properties of the graph paper on which the tracing is made. As described earlier, since the tracing is made at a speed of 32 mm/sec, the distance between the darker vertical lines represents one second of time. The initial step in using this second method is to extend a diagonal line through the 75% and 85% points on the tracing to extend across two of the darker vertical lines. The vertical distance between the points where the diagonal crosses the two darker vertical lines can be used to calculate the volume exhaled in one second.

In Figure 4 the vertical distance between the points where the diagonal line crosses the two darker vertical lines is 29 mm. This means that the subject's expiratory effort between 75% and 85% of the FVC resulted in a tracing that demonstrated a VD of 29 mm/sec. Given this, a value for $FEF_{75-85\%}$ can be calculated by the following method:

**$FEF_{75-85\%}$ = 29 mm/sec × BF in l/mm × 1.102**

$FEF_{75-85\%}$ = 29 mm/sec × 0.04127 l/mm × 1.102

$FEF_{75-85\%}$ = 1.3 l/sec

When the subject has a significant airflow obstruction, this method can also be used to determine a value for $FEF_{25-75\%}$. Most subjects, however, have a fast enough rate of expiratory flow between the 25% and 75% points that the diagonal line would be at too great of an angle to be extended between two darker lines within the limits of the graph paper. This is true for the tracing in Figure 4.

## STUDY SECTION II

# SAMPLE CALCULATIONS FOR PULMONARY FUNCTION TESTING

With modern pulmonary function testing systems, the calculations required for making the test measurements are performed automatically by a computer. The measurement data are entered directly from the system's measurement devices to the system's computer by way of the A-D converter. The computer then performs the required calculations and displays the results of the test measurements.

Because of this degree of automation, the technologist does not have to be aware of the equations and calculations being performed by the test system's computer. In the day-to-day administration of tests, this knowledge is not absolutely necessary. For a student, however, it is useful to review examples of these calculations for the following two reasons:

- It reinforces knowledge of the types of data parameters that must be measured during a particular pulmonary function test.
- It provides examples of the value ranges that are typical for the measurement data used in making calculations for a particular pulmonary function test. For example, it reinforces the fact that the final He concentration during a closed-circuit helium dilution test to measure FRC is generally about 5%–6% instead of being a much higher value (i.e., 80%–90%).

Provided in this section is a sample calculation for each of the following types of pulmonary function tests: body plethysmography test for airway resistance, open-circuit nitrogen washout test for FRC, closed-circuit helium dilution test for FRC, body plethysmography test for $V_{TG}$, Bohr method for deadspace determination, and the single-breath procedure for $D_L CO$.

Each example will provide the data that must be measured and/or recorded during the test and the calculations that will be performed with the data. It may be helpful for you to refer to the textbook in reviewing these examples and performing the practice calculations. This will be of benefit for recognizing the symbols that are used in identifying the measured/recorded and calculated values. The corresponding chapter for each calculation is provided.

# BODY PLETHYSMOGRAPHY TEST FOR $R_{AW}$, $G_{AW}$, AND $SG_{AW}$

(Chapter 2 of the textbook)

## MEASURED/RECORDED PARAMETERS

|  | Angle | Tangent |
|---|---|---|
| $P_{Mo}/P_{Cab}$ Tracing = | 32.2° | 0.630 |
| Tan $\angle$ $\dot{V}/P_{Cab}$ = | 70.1° | 2.762 |

$P_{Mo}$ Cal = 10 cm $H_2O$/cm        $R_{Sys}$ = 0.25 cm $H_2O$/l/sec

$\dot{V}_{Cal}$ = 1 l/sec/cm $H_2O$

Additional parameters:

$W_{Sub}$ = 78 kg

$P_{Atm}$ = 748 mm Hg        $V_{Cal}$ = 30 ml/cm

NOTE: With $R_{aw}$, calculation is based on a single tangent measurement. An average value for $R_{aw}$ is determined by making separate calculations for $R_{aw}$ and averaging the calculated $R_{aw}$ values.

## CALCULATIONS

The equation used for making the calculation is

$$R_{aw} = \left[ \left( \frac{\text{Tan} \angle P_{Mo}/P_{Cab}}{\text{Tan} \angle \dot{V}/P_{Cab}} \right) \times \left( \frac{P_{Mo}\text{Cal}}{\dot{V} \text{ Cal}} \right) \right] - R_{sys}$$

Inserting the required data values:

$$R_{aw} = \left[ \left( \frac{0.630}{2.762} \right) \times \left( \frac{10 \text{cmH}_2\text{O/cm}}{1 \text{ l/sec/cm}} \right) \right] - 0.25 \text{ cm } H_2O/l/sec$$

Solving the equation requires the following steps:

$R_{aw}$ = [(.228) × (10 cm $H_2O$/l/sec)] − 0.25 cm $H_2O$/l/sec

$R_{aw}$ = 2.28 cm $H_2O$/l/sec − 0.25 cm $H_2O$/l/sec

$R_{aw}$ = 2.03 cm $H_2O$/l/sec

A value for airway conductance is calculated by use of the following equation:

$$G_{aw} = \frac{1}{R_{aw}}$$

Inserting the required data values and solving the calculation:

$$G_{aw} = \frac{1}{2.03 \text{ cm } H_2O/l/\text{sec}}$$

$$G_{aw} = .49 \text{ l/sec/cm } H_2O$$

The data presented for this example can be used to determine a value for specific conductance. This is done by dividing the value for $G_{aw}$ just calculated by the lung volume ($V_L$) at which the measurements were made:

$$SG_{aw} = \frac{G_{aw}}{V_L}$$

A value for $V_L$ is determined by using the values of the measured/recorded parameters in the equation that will be presented later in this section for determining $V_{TG}$. The difference is that only a single value for the tangent of the $P_{Mo}/P_{Cab}$ recording is available from the performance of the $R_{aw}$ testing procedure. Using the parameter values in this example, the value for $V_L$ as calculated by the $V_{TG}$ equation is 3812 ml (3.812 liter). With this value for $V_L$, the calculation for $SG_{aw}$ is as follows:

$$SG_{aw} = \frac{.49 \text{ l/sec/cm } H_2O}{3.812 \text{ liter}}$$

$$SG_{aw} = .13 \text{ l/sec/cm } H_2O/\text{liter}$$

# OPEN-CIRCUIT NITROGEN WASHOUT TEST FOR FRC

(Chapter 4 of the textbook)

## MEASURED/RECORDED PARAMETERS

$C_{Exh}N_2 = 0.078$        $BTN_2$ Factor $= 0.04$ l/min

$V_{Exh} = 28.2$ liter ATPS        $C_{Alv}N_2 = 0.76$

$V_D = 0.825$ liter        $C_FN_2 = 0.01$

$T_{Test} = 7.5$ min        Spirometer Temperature $= 24°C$

NOTE: The BTPS conversion factor for a spirometer temperature of 24°C can be determined from the chart in Table 1.

## CALCULATIONS

The equation used for making the calculation is

$$V_{FRC} = \frac{[C_{Exh}N_2 \times (V_{Exh} + V_D)] - (BTN_2 \text{ Factor} \times T_{TEST})}{C_{ALV}N_2 - C_FN_2}$$

**TABLE 1   ATPS-to-BTPS Conversion Factors and Water Vapor Pressure**

| Gas Temperature (°C) | BTPS Conversion Factor | $P_{H_2O}$ (mm Hg) | Gas Temperature (°C) | BTPS Conversion Factor | $P_{H_2O}$ (mm Hg) |
|---|---|---|---|---|---|
| 18 | 1.112 | 15.6 | 28 | 1.057 | 28.3 |
| 19 | 1.107 | 16.5 | 29 | 1.051 | 30.0 |
| 20 | 1.102 | 17.5 | 30 | 1.045 | 31.8 |
| 21 | 1.096 | 18.7 | 31 | 1.039 | 33.7 |
| 22 | 1.091 | 19.8 | 32 | 1.032 | 35.7 |
| 23 | 1.085 | 21.1 | 33 | 1.026 | 37.7 |
| 24 | 1.080 | 22.4 | 34 | 1.020 | 39.9 |
| 25 | 1.075 | 23.8 | 35 | 1.014 | 42.2 |
| 26 | 1.068 | 23.8 | 36 | 1.007 | 44.6 |
| 27 | 1.063 | 26.7 | 37 | 1.000 | 47.0 |

Note: The conversion factors are based on a $P_{Atm}$ value of 760 mm Hg. They will be less accurate when used to make conversions at $P_{Atm}$ values other than 760 mm Hg.

Inserting the required data values:

$$V_{FRC} = \frac{[0.078 \times (28.2 \text{ liter} + 0.825 \text{ liter})] - (0.04 \text{ l/min} \times 7.5 \text{ min})}{0.76 - 0.01}$$

Solving the equation requires the following steps:

$$V_{FRC} = \frac{[0.078 \times (29.025 \text{ liter})] - (0.3 \text{ liter})}{0.75}$$

$$V_{FRC} = \frac{(2.264 \text{ liter}) - (0.3 \text{ liter})}{0.75}$$

$$V_{FRC} = \frac{1.964 \text{ liter}}{0.75}$$

$$V_{FRC} = 2.619 \text{ liter ATPS}$$

Once this value for $V_{FRC}$ is calculated, it must be converted to BTPS conditions by the following calculation:

**$V_{FRC \text{ (BTPS)}}$** = **$V_{FRC \text{ (ATPS)}}$ × BTPS Conversion Factor**

$V_{FRC \text{ (BTPS)}}$  = 2.619 liter × 1.080

$V_{FRC \text{ (BTPS)}}$  = 2.829 liter

This is the value for $V_{FRC}$ that should be reported.

# CLOSED-CIRCUIT HELIUM DILUTION TEST FOR FRC

(Chapter 4 of the textbook)

## MEASURED/RECORDED PARAMETERS

$V_{Added}He = 0.5$ liter $\qquad$ $V_{He}$ Factor $= 0.1$ liter

$C_I He = 0.089$ $\qquad$ Spirometer Temperature $= 25°C$

$C_F He = 0.053$

NOTE: The BTPS conversion factor for a spirometer temperature of 25°C can be determined from the chart in Table 1.

## CALCULATIONS

The equation used for making the calculation is

$$V_{FRC} = \left( \frac{C_I He - C_F He}{C_F HE} \times V_S \right) - V_{He}\ \text{Factor}$$

Before this calculation can be performed, a value for $V_S$ must be determined. This is done by the following equation:

$$V_S = \frac{V_{Added}He}{C_I He}$$

Inserting the required data values:

$$V_S = \frac{0.5\ \text{liter}}{.089}$$

$$V_S = 5.62\ \text{liter}$$

Therefore,

$$V_{FRC} = \left( \frac{0.089 - 0.053}{0.053} \times 5.62\ \text{liter} \right) - 0.1\ \text{liter}$$

Solving the equation requires the following steps:

$$V_{FRC} = \left( \frac{0.036}{0.053} \times 5.62\ \text{liter} \right) - 0.1\ \text{liter}$$

$$V_{FRC} = (0.679 \times 5.62\ \text{liter}) - 0.1\ \text{liter}$$

$$V_{FRC} = 3.816\ \text{liter} - 0.1\ \text{liter}$$

$$V_{FRC} = 3.716\ \text{liter ATPS}$$

Once this value for $V_{FRC}$ is calculated, it must be converted to BTPS conditions by the following calculation:

$V_{FRC\ (BTPS)} = V_{FRC\ (ATPS)} \times$ **BTPS Conversion Factor**

$V_{FRC\ (BTPS)} = 3.716$ liter $\times 1.075$

$V_{FRC\ (BTPS)} = 3.99$ liter

This is the value for $V_{FRC}$ that will be reported.

# BODY PLETHYSMOGRAPHY TEST FOR $V_{TG}$

(Chapter 4 of the textbook)

## MEASURED/RECORDED PARAMETERS

| | Angle | Tangent |
|---|---|---|
| $V_{Cab} = 530$ liter | | |
| $W_{Sub} = 85$ kg $\quad P_{Mo}/P_{Cab}$ Tracing | 35.2° | 0.705 |
| $P_{Atm} = 746$ mm Hg | 36.0° | 0.727 |
| $V_{Cal} = 30$ ml/cm | 35.8° | 0.721 |
| $P_{Mo}$ Cal $= 10$ cm $H_2O$/cm $\quad V_{MD} = 100$ ml | | |

NOTE: The $R_{aw}$ calculation demonstrated previously produced an average value for $R_{aw}$ by making separate tangent measurements and calculations. Then the three calculated $R_{aw}$ values were averaged. An average value for $V_{TG}$ is based on a single calculation that makes use of the average value for the tangents from three measurements.

## CALCULATIONS

The equation used for making the calculation is

$$V_{TG} = \left( \frac{P_{Atm} - 47 \text{ mm Hg}) \times 1.36 \text{ cm } H_2O}{\text{Mean Tracing Tangent}} \times F_{Cal} \times F_{Sub} \right) - V_{MD}$$

Before this calculation can be performed, a mean value for the tracing tangents measured in the test series must be determined. Additionally, values for $F_{Cal}$ and $F_{Sub}$ must be determined. A mean value for the tracing tangents is determined by the following equation:

$$\text{Mean Tracing Tangent} = \frac{\text{Tangent}^1 + \text{Tangent}^2 + \text{Tangent}^3}{3}$$

Inserting the required data values:

$$\text{Mean Tracing Tangent} = \frac{0.705 + 0.727 + 0.721}{3}$$

$$\text{Mean Tracing Tangent} = \frac{2.153}{3}$$

Mean Tracing Tangent = 0.718

$F_{Cal}$ is calculated by the following equation:

$$F_{Cal} = \frac{V_{Cal}}{P_{Mo}\, Cal}$$

Inserting the required data values:

$$F_{Cal} = \frac{30\ ml/cm}{10\ cm\ H_2O/cm}$$

$F_{Cal} = 3\ ml/cm\ H_2O$

$F_{Sub}$ is calculated by the following equation:

$$F_{Sub} = \frac{[V_{Cab} - (W_{Sub}/1.07\ kg/l)]}{V_{Cab}}$$

Inserting the required data values:

$$F_{Sub} = \frac{[530\ liter - (85\ kg/1.07\ kg/liter)]}{530\ l}$$

$$F_{Sub} = \frac{(530\ liter - 79.4\ liter)}{530\ l}$$

$$F_{Sub} = \frac{450.6\ liter}{530\ liter}$$

$F_{Sub} = 0.850$

Therefore,

$$V_{TG} = \left( \frac{(746\ mm\ Hg - 47\ mm\ Hg) \times 1.36\ cm\ H_2O/mm\ Hg}{0.718} \times 3\ ml/cm\ H_2O \times 0.850 \right) - 100\ ml$$

Solving the equations requires the following steps:

$$V_{TG} = \left( \frac{699\ mm\ Hg \times 1.36\ cm\ H_2O/mm\ Hg}{0.718} \times 3\ ml/cm\ H_2O \times 0.850 \right) - 100\ ml$$

$$V_{TG} = \left( \frac{950.6\ cm\ H_2O}{0.718} \times 3\ ml/cm\ H_2O \times 0.850 \right) - 100\ ml$$

$$V_{TG} = (1323\ cm\ H_2O \times 3\ ml/cm\ H_2O \times 0.850) - 100\ ml$$

$$V_{TG} = (3969\ ml \times 0.850) - 100\ ml$$

$$V_{TG} = 3374 \text{ ml} - 100 \text{ ml}$$

$$V_{TG} = 3274 \text{ ml}$$

Since the measurements for $V_{TG}$ are all made under conditions of BTPS, this is the value for $V_{TG}$ that will be reported.

# BOHR METHOD FOR DEADSPACE DETERMINATION

(Chapter 5 of the textbook)

## MEASURED/RECORDED PARAMETERS

$PaCO_2 = 43 \text{ mm Hg}$ $\qquad$ $\dot{V}_E = 8.73 \text{ l/min}$

$P\bar{E}CO_2 = 26 \text{ mm Hg}$ $\qquad$ $f = 17 \text{ breaths/min}$

## CALCULATIONS

The equation used for making the calculation is

$$V_D/V_T = \frac{PACO_2 - P\bar{E}CO_2}{PACO_2}$$

Since a value for $PaCO_2$ is going to be used as a substitute for the $PACO_2$ value in this calculation, the equation that will be used is

$$V_D/V_T = \frac{PaCO_2 - P\bar{E}CO_2}{PaCO_2}$$

Inserting the required data values:

$$V_D/V_T = \frac{43 \text{ mm Hg} - 26 \text{ mm Hg}}{43 \text{ mm Hg}}$$

$$V_D/V_T = \frac{17 \text{ mm Hg}}{43 \text{ mm Hg}}$$

$$V_D/V_T = 0.40$$

Given values for $\dot{V}_E$ and f measured during the collection of the subject's exhaled gas sample, a value for the subject's average $V_T$ can be determined. This is done by the following equation:

$$V_T = \frac{\dot{V}_E}{f}$$

Inserting the required data values:

$$V_T = \frac{8.73 \text{ l/min}}{17 \text{ breaths/min}}$$

$V_T = 0.514 \text{ l/breath}$

Once a value for the subject's $V_T$ is calculated, a value for the subject's $V_D$ can be determined by the following equation:

**$V_D = V_D/V_T \times V_T$**

Inserting the required data values:

$V_D = 0.40 \times 0.514 \text{ liter}$

$V_D = 0.206 \text{ liter}$

With values for the subject's $V_T$ and $V_D$ having been determined, a value for the subject's $\dot{V}_A\text{eff}$ can be determined. This is done by the following equation:

**$\dot{V}_A\text{eff} = f \times (V_T - V_D)$**

Inserting the required data values:

$\dot{V}_A\text{eff} = 17 \text{ breaths/min} \times (0.514 \text{ l/breath} - 0.206 \text{ l/breath})$

$\dot{V}_A\text{eff} = 17 \text{ breaths/min} \times 0.308 \text{ l/breath}$

$\dot{V}_A\text{eff} = 5.236 \text{ l/min}$

# SINGLE BREATH PROCEDURE FOR D$_L$CO

(Chapter 6 of the textbook)

## MEASURED/RECORDED PARAMETERS

$V_{VC}(\text{STPD}) = 3.5 \text{ liter}$ $\qquad$ $P_{Atm} = 746 \text{ mm Hg}$

$\text{FICO} = 0.003$ $\qquad$ $T_{Hold} = 10 \text{ seconds}$

$\text{FIHe} = 0.1$ $\qquad$ $\text{FACO}_F = 0.00127$

$\text{FEHe} = 0.073$ $\qquad$ Spirometer Temperature $= 24°C$

## CALCULATIONS

The equation used for making the calculation is:

$$D_L\text{CO-SB} = \frac{V_A(\text{STPD}) \times 60}{(P_{Atm} - 47 \text{ mm Hg})(T_{Hold})} \times \text{Ln} \frac{\text{FACO}_I}{\text{FACO}_F}$$

Before this calculation can be performed, values for $V_A$ and $FACO_I$ must be determined. A value for $V_A$ is determined by the following equation:

$$V_A(STPD) = \frac{V_{VC}(STPD)}{FEHe/FIHe}$$

Inserting the required data values:

$$V_A(STPD) = \frac{3.5 \text{ liter}}{0.073/0.1}$$

$$V_A(STPD) = \frac{3.5 \text{ liter}}{0.73}$$

$$V_A(STPD) = 4.795 \text{ liter}$$

This value for $V_A$ must be converted to milliliters. Therefore the value used for $V_A$ is 4795 ml.

$FACO_I$ is calculated by the following equation:

$$FACO_I = FICO \times \frac{FEHe}{FIHe}$$

Inserting the required data values:

$$FACO_I = 0.003 \times \frac{0.073}{0.1}$$

$$FACO_I = 0.003 \times 0.73$$

$$FACO_I = 0.00219$$

Therefore,

$$D_LCO\text{-}SB = \frac{4795 \text{ ml} \times 60 \text{ sec/min}}{(746 - 47 \text{ mm Hg})(10 \text{ sec})} \times Ln \frac{0.00219}{0.00127}$$

Solving the equation requires the following steps:

$$D_LCO\text{-}SB = \frac{287700 \text{ ml/sec/min}}{(699 \text{ mm Hg})(10 \text{ sec})} \times Ln \ 1.72$$

The chart of natural logarithms in Table 2 can be used to determine a value for Ln 1.72.

$$D_LCO\text{-}SB = \frac{287700 \text{ ml/sec/min}}{(6990 \text{ mm Hg sec})} \times 0.54232$$

$$D_LCO\text{-}SB = 41.16 \text{ ml/min/mm Hg} \times 0.54232$$

$$D_LCo\text{-}SB = 22.3 \text{ ml/min/mm Hg}$$

Once this value for $D_LCO\text{-}SB$ (ATPS) is calculated, it must be converted to STPD conditions. This can be done by the following equation:

$$D_LCO\text{-}SB_{STPD} = D_LCO\text{-}SB_{ATPS} \times \left[ \left( \frac{P_{Atm} - P_{H2O} \text{ at T}}{760 \text{ mm Hg}} \right) \times \left( \frac{273°}{273° - T} \right) \right]$$

## TABLE 2 Chart of Natural Logarithms

Using the number 1.43 as an example, first find 1.4 in the far left column. Then, at the level of 1.4, move to the right across the chart to the .03 column to find .35767, which is the natural logarithm of 1.43.

| N = | .00 | .01 | .02 | .03 | .04 | .05 | .06 | .07 | .08 | .09 |
|-----|-----|-----|-----|-----|-----|-----|-----|-----|-----|-----|
| 1.0 | 0.00000 | .00995 | .01980 | .02956 | .03922 | .04879 | .05827 | .06766 | .07696 | .08618 |
| 1.1 | .09531 | .10436 | .11333 | .12222 | .13103 | .13976 | .14842 | .15700 | .16551 | .17495 |
| 1.2 | .18232 | .19062 | .19885 | .20701 | .21511 | .22314 | .23111 | .23902 | .24686 | .25464 |
| 1.3 | .26236 | .27003 | .27763 | .28518 | .29267 | .30010 | .30784 | .31481 | .32208 | .32930 |
| 1.4 | .33647 | .34359 | .35066 | .35767 | .36464 | .37156 | .37844 | .38526 | .39204 | .39878 |
| 1.5 | .40546 | .41211 | .41871 | .42527 | .43178 | .43825 | .44469 | .45108 | .45742 | .46373 |
| 1.6 | .47000 | .47623 | .48243 | .48858 | .49470 | .50078 | .50682 | .51282 | .51879 | .52473 |
| 1.7 | .53063 | .53649 | .54232 | .54812 | .55389 | .55962 | .56531 | .57098 | .57661 | .58222 |
| 1.8 | .58779 | .59333 | .59884 | .60432 | .60977 | .61519 | .62058 | .62594 | .63127 | .63658 |
| 1.9 | .64185 | .64170 | .65233 | .65752 | .66269 | .66783 | .67294 | .67803 | .68310 | .68813 |

Inserting the required values ($P_{H_2O}$ at T can be determined from the chart of values available in Table 2):

$$D_LCO\text{-}SB_{STPD} = 22.3 \text{ ml/min/mm Hg} \times \left[\left(\frac{746 \text{ mm Hg} - 22.4 \text{ mm Hg}}{760 \text{ mm Hg}}\right) \times \left(\frac{273°}{273° - 24°}\right)\right]$$

$$D_LCO\text{-}SB_{STPD} = 22.3 \text{ ml/min/mm Hg} \times \left[\left(\frac{723.6 \text{ mm Hg}}{760 \text{ mm Hg}}\right) \times \left(\frac{273°}{249°}\right)\right]$$

$$D_LCO\text{-}SB_{STPD} = 22.3 \text{ ml/min/mm Hg} \times [(0.9521) \times (1.0963)]$$

$$D_LCO\text{-}SB_{STPD} = 22.3 \text{ ml/min/mm Hg} \times (1.0438)$$

$$D_LCO\text{-}SB_{STPD} = 23.3 \text{ ml/min/mm Hg}$$

# CASE STUDIES IN PULMONARY FUNCTION TESTING

The purpose of this chapter is to provide practice in evaluating and interpreting the results of pulmonary function tests.

## REVIEW FOR THE EVALUATION AND INTERPRETATION OF PULMONARY FUNCTION TESTS

Before beginning practice in interpreting the results of pulmonary function tests, it would be useful to review the basic steps that should be followed:

1. Evaluation of the acceptability of the test data.
2. Comparison of the subject's test results with the normal values predicted for the subject.
3. Identification of the type(s) and severity of any abnormalities that are demonstrated by the subject.

Each of these steps will now be briefly reviewed.

### EVALUATION OF THE ACCEPTABILITY OF TEST DATA

Evaluation of the acceptability of the test data is based on a careful review of the raw numerical test data and the tracings that are produced during the test. This review of the test data is useful for two reasons. First, it is a way of evaluating the function of the test equipment. Malfunction of test equipment, such as the spirometer system or gas analyzers used during the test, can be identified in this way. Numerical data that are different from what should reasonably be expected or tracings that appear to be inappropriate can indicate the presence of equipment malfunctions.

A second reason for reviewing the test data is to evaluate the subject's cooperation and effort during the test. Evaluation of the tracing from a test, especially for a FVC maneuver, can be used to identify poor subject cooperation or effort. Evaluation of the numerical test data is also useful. Are the test results reasonable for this subject given his or her recorded health history and/or previous pulmonary function test results? Chapters 2, 4, 5, and 6 of the textbook provide the criteria for the acceptability of the tests covered in those chapters.

Internal consistency of test data from a test series can be used to evaluate subject cooperation and effort. One way of doing this is to compare FVC results from a series of FVC tests. Are the subject's test values reasonably consistent from test to test? Another method is to compare the values for a parameter that is tested by different methods such as vital capacity (VC). VC values may be generated during FVC tests, lung volume determinations, $D_LCO$ tests, and plethysmography. Although the VC values determined by these different methods do not have to be identical, they should be reasonably consistent.

In today's modern computerized testing systems, the software is often capable of indicating unacceptable test data. This is especially true in regard to poor subject effort and cooperation.

## COMPARISON OF SUBJECT'S TEST RESULTS WITH PREDICTED NORMAL VALUES

Once the raw data from the test are determined to be acceptable, the subject's actual test result values should be compared against the predicted normal values for that subject. Two important points are related to this stage of the process. The first is that appropriate nomograms for predicting normal values must be chosen for the subject population typically tested by the laboratory. Nomograms that are unsuitable for the population being tested will result in incorrect normal values being predicted.

The second concern is that correct information for the subject's height, age, and gender (and possibly weight and race) be used when the normal values are determined. Any errors here will also result in incorrect normal values being predicted for the subject. Chapter 7 of the textbook discusses the use of predicted normal values.

Once the predicted normal values for the subject are determined, they can be compared against the subject's test result values. Test values that fall outside the predicted normal range for the subject indicate an abnormality for that test parameter. Chapters 2, 4, 5, 6, and 11 present information on the normal values for the pulmonary function parameters presented in each chapter. Chapter 7 describes the methods used for establishing a range of normal values for pulmonary function parameters.

The computer software used with modern testing systems will in some manner indicate where a subject's test values fall outside the predicted normal range. This feature can simplify and speed up the process of interpreting pulmonary function test results.

## IDENTIFICATION OF TYPE(S) AND SEVERITY OF ABNORMALITIES

Once abnormal values are identified in the test results for a subject, the pattern of the abnormal values can reveal the nature and severity of the subject's pulmonary dysfunction.

Generally, pulmonary disorders are categorized as being either obstructive, restrictive, or a combination of both. An obstructive pulmonary disorder is generally indicated by

- Reductions in forced expiratory and possibly inspiratory flow rates.
- Often, increases in some lung volumes. These increases typically are seen in the values for RV, FRC, and TLC.

Reduced values for $D_LCO$ and abnormalities in blood gas values may also be demonstrated with obstructive pulmonary disorders.

Restrictive pulmonary disorders present a different pattern of pulmonary function abnormalities. These include

- Reductions in lung volumes. This is most evident in the values for VC and TLC.
- Reductions in values for $D_LCO$.

Abnormalities in blood gas values may also be demonstrated.

Mixed obstructive/restrictive disorders can present a more complex combination of pulmonary function testing abnormalities. Forced expiratory flow rates may be reduced as with pure obstructive disorders. At the same time, though, the increases in lung volume typically present with obstructive disorders may not be demonstrated. In fact, the restrictive component can cause lung volumes to remain relatively normal or be reduced.

The severity of a disorder is based on the amount of abnormality that is demonstrated in the tested parameters. Chapters 2 and 4 offer guidelines on determining the severity of disorders based on the degree of abnormality in the parameters discussed in those chapters. Unfortunately, the use of such severity terms as "mild," "moderate," and "severe" is not standardized. Therefore, these terms may vary according to the laboratory that is performing the tests and/or the individual who is interpreting the tests.

# PULMONARY FUNCTION TESTING CASE STUDIES

This section of the chapter contains the case studies to be used as exercises in the interpretation of pulmonary function test results.

## PREPARATION FOR USE OF THE INTERPRETATION EXERCISE

With each of the four case studies, certain information will be presented:

- General information on the subject.
- A table for presentation of specific pulmonary function testing results for the subject.
- An interpretation of the results of the pulmonary function tests performed on the subject. This interpretation is based on the one provided by a pulmonologist at the laboratory where the tests in these case studies were originally performed.

In order to make effective use of these case studies as a learning exercise, first make your own attempt to interpret the results of the tests performed for a given case study.

In doing so, you should try to determine both the nature and the severity of any abnormalities that are demonstrated by the subject in the case study. Your process for interpreting the test results should proceed in the following manner:

1. First review the information presented on each subject. It may be useful for you to make marks and notes on the tables presenting the test data as you review the information.
2. Identify the parameters that fall outside of the normal range.
3. Finally, determine whether any test parameter abnormalities that are present demonstrate a primarily *obstructive*, *restrictive*, or *combined disorder*, and *determine the severity* of the disorder.

   Once you have performed your own interpretation, look over the interpretation presented for the case study. If you find significant differences between your interpretation and the one presented for the case study, go back and review the subject's test results in order to see why your interpretation is different.

# CASE STUDY I

## Subject Information

This subject is a 62-year-old female. She has stated that she experiences some dyspnea on hills and stairs. At the time of the test, she had the following arterial blood gas analysis results: pH of 7.45, $PaCO_2$ of 41 mm Hg, BE of +3.7 mEq/l, $PaO_2$ of 89 mm Hg, and $SaO_2$ of 94.9% on room air. Her %HbCO was 1.9%.

### PULMONARY FUNCTION TESTING REPORT

Age: 62 yrs.   Height: 63 in.   Weight: 140 lb
Gender: F   Race: Cauc.   BSA: 1.66 m$^2$

| PULMONARY MECHANICS | | Actual | Pred. | % Pred. |
|---|---|---|---|---|
| **Spirometry** | | | | |
| FVC | (liter) | 2.33 | 2.86 | 81 |
| $FEV_1$ | (liter) | 1.96 | 2.31 | 85 |
| $FEV_{1\%}$ | (%) | 84 | 81 | |
| $FEF_{25\%}$ | (l/sec) | 6.60 | 4.83 | 137 |
| $FEF_{50\%}$ | (l/sec) | 4.39 | 3.57 | 123 |
| $FEF_{75\%}$ | (l/sec) | 0.71 | 1.16 | 61 |
| $FEF_{max}$ | (l/sec) | 7.09 | 5.13 | 138 |
| $FEF_{25-75\%}$ | (l/sec) | 2.50 | 2.48 | 101 |
| $FEF_{75-85\%}$ | (l/sec) | 0.45 | | |
| FIVC | (liter) | 2.28 | 2.69 | 85 |
| $FIF_{50\%}$ | (l/sec) | 1.91 | | |
| **Plethysmography** | | | | |
| $R_{aw}$ | (cm $H_2O$/l/sec) | 1.94 | <2.00 | 86 |
| $G_{aw}$ | (l/sec/cm $H_2O$) | 0.52 | >0.50 | 104 |
| $SG_{aw}$ | (l/sec/cm $H_2O$/liter) | 0.23 | >0.21 | 110 |

**(*Continued*)**

## PULMONARY VOLUMES

**Spirometry**

| | | | | |
|---|---|---|---|---|
| SVC | (liter) | 2.29 | 2.86 | 80 |
| IC | (liter) | 1.87 | 2.13 | 88 |
| ERV | (liter) | 0.42 | 0.73 | 58 |

**Plethysmography**

| | | | | |
|---|---|---|---|---|
| TGV | (liter) | 2.30 | 2.77 | 83 |
| RV | (liter) | 1.88 | 1.98 | 95 |
| TLC | (liter) | 4.17 | 4.90 | 85 |
| RV/TLC | (%) | 45 | 40 | |

## PULMONARY DIFFUSING CAPACITY

| | | | | |
|---|---|---|---|---|
| $D_LCO$ | (ml/min/mm Hg) | 19.44 | 22.91 | 85 |
| $V_L$ | (liter) | 4.05 | 4.90 | 83 |
| $D_LCO/V_L$ (ml/min/mm Hg/liter) | | 4.80 | 7.57 | 63 |

## Practice Interpretation

*Perform your practice interpretation (nature and severity of the disorder) at this time before looking at the actual interpretation.*

## Actual Interpretation

The results of this subject's pulmonary mechanics tests are within normal limits. Her lung volumes show a normal RV and TLC and her $D_LCO$ is normal. The blood gas results demonstrate normal oxygenation without hypercapnia. The value for %HbCO is normal.

## Final Impression

The subject demonstrates normal pulmonary function.

# CASE STUDY 2

## Subject Information

This subject is a 66-year-old male. He has a 40-pack-year history of smoking (one pack per day) and quit smoking five years ago. He has a complaint of dyspnea on hills and stairs and frequent episodes of shortness of breath. He has a productive cough and a constant expiratory wheeze. No blood gas values are available for the subject.

### PULMONARY FUNCTION TESTING REPORT

Age: 66 yrs.  Height: 71 in.  Weight: 210 lb
Gender: M  Race: Cauc.  BSA: 2.15 m$^2$

| PULMONARY MECHANICS | | PRE-BRONCHODILATOR | | | POST-BRONCHODILATOR | | |
|---|---|---|---|---|---|---|---|
| | | Actual | Pred. | % Pred. | Actual | % Pred | % Change |
| **Spirometry** | | | | | | | |
| FVC | (liter) | 2.92 | 4.47 | 65 | 3.06 | 68 | 5 |
| FEV$_1$ | (liter) | 2.51 | 3.55 | 71 | 2.62 | 74 | 4 |

| PULMONARY MECHANICS | | Actual | Pred. | % Pred. | Actual | % Pred | % Change |
|---|---|---|---|---|---|---|---|
| $FEV_{1\%}$ | (%) | 86 | 79 | 86 | -1 | | |
| $FEF_{25\%}$ | (l/sec) | 8.62 | 7.53 | 114 | 10.40 | 138 | 21 |
| $FEF_{50\%}$ | (l/sec) | 5.33 | 4.40 | 121 | 4.83 | 110 | -9 |
| $FEF_{75\%}$ | (l/sec) | 1.10 | 1.34 | 82 | 1.11 | 83 | 1 |
| $FEF_{max}$ | (l/sec) | 11.55 | 8.03 | 144 | 12.54 | 156 | 9 |
| $FEF_{25-75\%}$ | (l/sec) | 3.45 | 3.53 | 98 | 3.44 | 97 | 0 |
| $FEF_{75-85\%}$ | (l/sec) | 0.69 | | | 0.69 | | |
| FIVC | (liter) | 2.90 | 4.50 | 64 | 2.43 | 54 | -16 |
| $FIF_{50\%}$ | (l/sec) | 4.00 | | | | | |
| **Plethysmography** | | | | | | | |
| $R_{aw}$ | (cm $H_2O$/l/sec) | 2.96 | <2.00 | 167 | | | |
| $G_{aw}$ | (l/sec/cm $H_2O$) | 0.34 | >0.50 | 68 | | | |
| $SG_{aw}$ | (l/sec/cm $H_2O$/liter) | 0.17 | >0.21 | 81 | | | |

| PULMONARY VOLUMES | | Actual | Pred. | % Pred. |
|---|---|---|---|---|
| **Spirometry** | | | | |
| SVC | (liter) | 3.17 | 4.47 | 71 |
| IC | (liter) | 2.30 | 3.40 | 68 |
| ERV | (liter) | 0.86 | 1.07 | 81 |
| **Plethysmography** | | | | |
| TGV | (liter) | 1.48 | 3.82 | 39 |
| RV | (liter) | 0.61 | 2.42 | 25 |
| TLC | (liter) | 3.78 | 7.22 | 52 |
| RV/TLC | (%) | 16 | 34 | |

| PULMONARY DIFFUSING CAPACITY | | | | |
|---|---|---|---|---|
| $D_LCO$ | (ml/min/mm Hg) | 14.26 | 33.68 | 42 |
| $V_L$ | (liter) | 4.21 | 7.22 | 58 |
| $D_LCO/V_L$ (ml/min/mm Hg/liter) | | 3.39 | 6.47 | 52 |

## Practice Interpretation

*Perform your practice interpretation (nature and severity of the disorder) at this time before looking at the actual interpretation.*

## Actual Interpretation

The lung volumes in this subject demonstrate a marked reduction in TLC and RV. The subject's $D_LCO$ values are markedly reduced, which is consistent with the loss of lung volume. The results of the pulmonary mechanics tests for this subject confirm the loss of lung volume without demonstrating a notable decrease in forced expiratory flow rates or increase in airway resistance. The administration of an aerosolized bronchodilator does not produce a significant change in the pulmonary mechanics values.

## Final Impression

The subject demonstrates a significant restrictive pulmonary disorder, probably of interstitial origins.

# CASE STUDY 3

## Subject Information

This subject is a 65-year-old male. He has a 45-pack-year history of smoking (one pack per day) and quit seven years ago. He has a complaint of dyspnea on hills and stairs. He has a productive cough and only rare expiratory wheezes. No blood gas values are available for this subject.

## PULMONARY FUNCTION TESTING REPORT

Age: 65 yrs.  Height: 65 in.  Weight: 162 lb
Gender: M  Race: Cauc.  BSA: 1.81 m$^2$

| | | PRE-BRONCHODILATOR | | | POST-BRONCHODILATOR | | |
|---|---|---|---|---|---|---|---|
| PULMONARY MECHANICS | | Actual | Pred. | % Pred. | Actual | % Pred | % Change |
| **Spirometry** | | | | | | | |
| FVC | (liter) | 2.29 | 3.22 | 71 | 3.38 | 105 | +48 |
| FEV$_1$ | (liter) | 1.21 | 2.57 | 47 | 1.44 | 56 | +19 |
| FEV$_{1\%}$ | (%) | 53 | 80 | | 43 | | −20 |
| FEF$_{25\%}$ | (l/sec) | 1.45 | 6.58 | 22 | 1.19 | 18 | −18 |
| FEF$_{50\%}$ | (l/sec) | 0.72 | 4.28 | 17 | 0.64 | 15 | −11 |
| FEF$_{75\%}$ | (l/sec) | 0.24 | 1.16 | 21 | 0.20 | 17 | −17 |
| FEF$_{max}$ | (l/sec) | 4.33 | 7.25 | 60 | 3.98 | 55 | −8 |
| FEF$_{25-75\%}$ | (l/sec) | 0.58 | 2.68 | 22 | 0.51 | 19 | −12 |
| FEF$_{75-85\%}$ | (l/sec) | 0.22 | | | 0.15 | | −32 |
| PULMONARY MECHANICS | | Actual | Pred. | % Pred. | Actual | % Pred | % Change |
| FIVC | (liter) | 0.09 | 3.60 | 2 | 2.90 | 81 | 3122 |
| FIF$_{50\%}$ | (l/sec) | | | | 2.81 | | |
| **Plethysmography** | | | | | | | |
| R$_{aw}$ | (cm H$_2$O/l/sec) | 3.29 | <2.00 | 150 | | | |
| G$_{aw}$ | (l/sec/cm H$_2$O) | 0.30 | >0.50 | 60 | | | |
| SG$_{aw}$ | (l/sec/cm H$_2$O/liter) | 0.05 | >0.21 | 24 | | | |
| PULMONARY VOLUMES | | | | | | | |
| **Spirometry** | | | | | | | |
| SVC | (liter) | 2.96 | 3.22 | 92 | | | |
| IC | (liter) | 2.31 | 2.91 | 79 | | | |
| ERV | (liter) | 0.66 | 0.30 | 220 | | | |
| **Plethysmography** | | | | | | | |
| TGV | (liter) | 5.25 | 3.09 | 170 | | | |
| RV | (liter) | 4.60 | 2.07 | 222 | | | |
| TLC | (liter) | 7.56 | 6.00 | 126 | | | |
| RV/TLC | (%) | 61 | 35 | | | | |
| PULMONARY DIFFUSING CAPACITY | | | | | | | |
| D$_L$CO | (ml/min/mm Hg) | 19.28 | 25.60 | 75 | | | |
| V$_L$ | (liter) | 5.60 | 6.00 | 93 | | | |
| D$_L$CO/V$_L$ | (ml/min/mm Hg/liter) | 3.44 | 7.29 | 47 | | | |

## Practice Interpretation

*Perform your practice interpretation (nature and severity of the disorder) at this time before looking at the actual interpretation.*

## Actual Interpretation

The results of this subject's pulmonary mechanics test demonstrate a marked obstructive impairment that shows a slight but significant improvement after administration of an aerosolized bronchodilator. His lung volumes show a marked increase in RV and TLC (TGV) consistent with hyperinflation. The $D_L CO$ is at the lower limits of normal.

## Final Impression

The subject demonstrates a severe obstructive pulmonary disorder that improves slightly with the administration of an aerosolized bronchodilator. This is consistent with either a chronic bronchitis with some bronchospastic component or bronchial asthma with incomplete reversibility. The relatively preserved $D_L CO$ is evidence somewhat against the presence of a predominately emphysematous disorder and therefore a significant attempt at bronchodilator therapy is reasonable.

# CASE STUDY 4

## Subject Information

This subject is a 31-year-old male. He has no recorded history of having smoked. He experiences dyspnea only after severe exertion. His cough is nonproductive, and he experiences frequent expiratory wheezes. At the time of the test he had the following arterial blood gas analysis results: pH of 7.44, $PaCO_2$ of 44 mm Hg, BE of +1.4 mEq/l, $PaO_2$ of 100 mm Hg, and $SaO_2$ of 96.1% on room air.

### PULMONARY FUNCTION TESTING REPORT

Age: 31 yrs.  Height: 69 in.  Weight: 180 lb
Gender: M  Race: Cauc.  BSA: 1.98 m²

| PULMONARY MECHANICS | | Actual | Pred. | % Pred. |
|---|---|---|---|---|
| **Spirometry** | | | | |
| FVC | (liter) | 4.96 | 5.09 | 97 |
| $FEV_1$ | (liter) | 4.35 | 4.23 | 103 |
| $FEV_{1\%}$ | (%) | 88 | 83 | |
| $FEF_{25\%}$ | (l/sec) | 9.65 | 8.12 | 119 |
| $FEF_{50\%}$ | (l/sec) | 5.28 | 5.54 | 95 |
| $FEF_{75\%}$ | (l/sec) | 2.38 | 2.08 | 114 |
| $FEF_{max}$ | (l/sec) | 11.35 | 8.54 | 133 |
| $FEF_{25-75\%}$ | (l/sec) | 4.91 | 4.50 | 109 |
| $FEF_{75-85\%}$ | (l/sec) | 1.82 | | |
| FIVC | (liter) | 3.63 | 5.17 | 70 |

| PULMONARY MECHANICS | | Actual | Pred. | % Pred. |
|---|---|---|---|---|
| **Plethysmography** | | | | |
| $R_{aw}$ | (cm $H_2O$/l/sec) | 1.46 | <2.00 | 69 |
| $G_{aw}$ | (l/sec/cm $H_2O$) | 0.68 | >0.50 | 136 |
| $SG_{aw}$ | (l/sec/cm $H_2O$/liter) | 0.26 | >0.21 | 124 |
| PULMONARY VOLUMES | | | | |
| **Spirometry** | | | | |
| SVC | (liter) | 4.57 | 5.09 | 90 |
| IC | (liter) | 3.59 | 3.44 | 104 |
| ERV | (liter) | 0.98 | 1.65 | 59 |
| **Plethysmography** | | | | |
| TGV | (liter) | 2.98 | 3.26 | 92 |
| RV | (liter) | 2.00 | 1.59 | 126 |
| TLC | (liter) | 6.57 | 6.70 | 98 |
| RV/TLC | (%) | 30 | 24 | |
| PULMONARY DIFFUSING CAPACITY | | | | |
| $D_LCO$ | (ml/min/mm Hg) | 29.86 | 30.99 | 96 |
| $V_L$ | (liter) | 6.09 | 6.70 | 91 |
| $D_LCO/V_L$(ml/min/mm Hg/liter) | | 4.90 | 6.75 | 73 |

METHACHOLINE CHALLENGE TEST

| | FVC (liter) | | FEV1 (liter) | | $FEV_1$% (%) | $FEF_{max}$ (l/sec) | $FEF_{25-75\%}$ (l/sec) |
|---|---|---|---|---|---|---|---|
| Predicted | 5.09 | | 4.23 | | 83 | 8.54 | 4.50 |
| | Actual | % Pred. | Actual | % Pred. | | | |
| Normal Saline | 4.83 | 95 | 4.12 | 97 | 85 | 9.60 | 4.40 |
| 0.025 (mg/ml) | 4.92 | 96 | 4.15 | 98 | 84 | 9.36 | 4.43 |
| 0.25 (mg/ml) | 5.10 | 100 | 4.31 | 101 | 84 | 9.39 | 4.56 |
| 2.5 (mg/ml) | 5.06 | 99 | 4.36 | 103 | 86 | 8.63 | 4.93 |
| 10.0 (mg/ml) | 5.01 | 98 | 4.28 | 101 | 86 | 7.93 | 4.71 |
| 25.0 (mg/ml) | 3.75 | 73 | 2.67 | 63 | 71 | 5.53 | 1.89 |
| Albuterol | 4.64 | 91 | 3.73 | 88 | 80 | 8.35 | 3.52 |

The subject developed a cough and wheezing after administration of the 25.0 mg/ml dose of methacholine.

## Practice Interpretation

*Perform your practice interpretation (nature and severity of the disorder) at this time before looking at the actual interpretation.*

## Actual Interpretation

The results of this subject's pulmonary mechanics tests are within normal limits. His lung volumes show a minimal elevation of RV but a normal TLC. The $D_LCO$ is normal. The resting arterial blood gases are within normal limits. Pulmonary mechanics values during the methacholine challenge test remained normal until the 25.0 mg/ml dose was administered. Following the administration of Albuterol, the pulmonary mechanics parameters returned to near normal values.

## Final Impression

The initial test findings were normal. Results of the methacholine test were positive and were consistent with the presence of an underlying reactive airway disorder.

# STUDY SECTION IV

# SAMPLE CALCULATIONS FOR CARDIOPULMONARY STRESS TESTING

The discussion at the beginning of Study Section II about the automation of calculations for pulmonary function testing also holds true for the calculations made for cardiopulmonary stress testing. As with the calculations for pulmonary function testing, it is useful for you to review examples of calculations for cardiopulmonary stress testing.

This chapter provides a sample calculation for each of the following types of cardiopulmonary stress testing parameters: $\dot{V}_E(BTPS)$, $\dot{V}_T$, $V_D$, $V_D/V_T$, $\dot{V}O_2$, METS, $\dot{V}CO_2$, $\dot{V}_E/VO_2$, $\dot{V}_E/\dot{V}CO_2$, R, and $O_2$pulse. The examples will provide the data that must be measured and/recorded during the test and the calculations that would be performed with the data.

It may be helpful to you to refer to the textbook in reviewing the example calculations and performing the practice calculations. This will be of benefit for recognizing the symbols used in identifying the measured/recorded and calculated values.

# EXAMPLE CALCULATIONS FOR CARDIOPULMONARY STRESS TESTING:

(Chapter 14 of the textbook)

## MEASURED/RECORDED PARAMETERS

$V_{Meas} = 18.5$ liter                $FECO_2 = 0.031$

Ambient Temperature $= 26°C$        $FICO_2 = 0.0003$

$P_{Atm} = 748$ mm Hg              $VD_{valve} = 0.020$ liter

$T_{Meas} = 60$ sec                 $Wt_{Sub} = 92$ kg

$f = 23$ breaths/min              $HR = 112$ beats/min

$$FIO_2 = 0.2093 \qquad\qquad PetCO_2 = 38 \text{ mm Hg}$$

$$FEO_2 = 0.167$$

NOTE: The BTPS conversion factor for an ambient temperature of 26° C can be determined from the chart in Appendix B.

## CALCULATIONS

### Determination of $\dot{V}_E$

The equation used for making the calculation is

$$\dot{V}_E = \frac{\dot{V}_{Meas} \times 60}{T_{Meas}} \times \textbf{BTPS conversion factor}$$

Inserting the required values:

$$\dot{V}_E = \frac{18.5 \text{ liter} \times 60 \text{ sec/min}}{60 \text{ sec}} \times 1.068$$

$$\dot{V}_E = \frac{1110 \text{ liter sec/min}}{60 \text{ sec}} \times 1.068$$

$$\dot{V}_E = 18.5 \text{ l/min} \times 1.068$$

$$\dot{V}_E = 19.8 \text{ l/m BTPS}$$

### Determination of $V_T$

The equation used for making the calculation is

$$V_T = \frac{\dot{V}_E}{f}$$

Inserting the required values:

$$V_T = \frac{19.8 \text{ l/min}}{23 \text{ breaths/min}}$$

$$V_T = 0.861 \text{ l/breath BTPS}$$

### Determination of $V_D$

The equation used for making the calculation is

$$V_D = \left( VT \times \frac{PACO_2 - PECO_2}{PACO_2} \right) - V_D \textbf{ valve}$$

Before this calculation can be performed, a value for PECO2 must be determined. This can be done by the following equation:

$$\textbf{PECO}_2 = (\textbf{P}_{Atm} - 47) \times \textbf{FECO}_2$$

where, inserting the required values,

$PECO_2 = (748 \text{ mm Hg} - 47) \times 0.031$

$PECO_2 = 701 \text{ mm Hg} \times 0.031$

$PECO_2 = 21.7 \text{ mm Hg}$

Now, given a value for $PECO_2$ and using the value for $PetCO_2$ as a substitute for the $PACO_2$ value,

$$V_D = \left(0.861 \text{ liter} \times \frac{38 \text{ mm Hg} - 21.7 \text{ mm Hg}}{38 \text{ mm Hg}}\right) - 0.020 \text{ liter}$$

$$V_D = \left(0.861 \text{ liter} \times \frac{16.3 \text{ mm Hg}}{38 \text{ mm Hg}}\right) - 0.020 \text{ liter}$$

$$V_D = (0.861 \text{ liter} \times 0.429) - 0.020 \text{ liter}$$

$$V_D = 0.369 \text{ liter} - 0.020 \text{ liter}$$

$$V_D = 0.349 \text{ liter BTPS}$$

## Determination of $V_D/V_T$

The equation used for making the calculation is

$$V_D/V_T = \frac{V_D}{V_T}$$

Inserting the required values:

$$V_D/V_T = \frac{0.349 \text{ liter}}{0.861 \text{ liter}}$$

$$V_D/V_T = 0.41$$

## Determination of $\dot{V}O_2$

The equation used for making the calculation is

$$\dot{V}O_2 = \left\{\left[\left(\frac{1 - FEO_2 - FECO_2}{1 - FIO_2}\right) \times FIO_2\right] - FEO_2\right\} \times \dot{V}_E \text{ STPD}$$

In order to make the calculation, a value for $\dot{V}_E$ STPD must be determined. This can be done by the following equation:

$$\dot{V}_E \text{ STPD} = \dot{V}_E \text{ BTPS} \times \left[\left(\frac{P_{Atm} - 47 \text{ mm Hg}}{760 \text{ mm Hg}}\right) \times 0.881\right]$$

Inserting the required values:

$$\dot{V}_E \text{ STPD} = 19.8 \text{ l/min} \times \left[\left(\frac{748 \text{ mm Hg} - 47 \text{ mm Hg}}{760 \text{ mm hg}}\right) \times 0.881\right]$$

$$\dot{V}_E \, STPD = 19.8 \, l/min \times \left[ \left( \frac{701 \, mm \, Hg}{760 \, mm \, Hg} \right) \times 0.881 \right]$$

$$\dot{V}_E \, STPD = 19.8 \, l/min \times (0.922 \times 0.881)$$

$$\dot{V}_E \, STPD = 19.8 \, l/min \times 0.812$$

$$\dot{V}_E \, STPD = 16.1 \, l/min$$

Now, given a value for $\dot{V}_E$ STPD and inserting the other required values,

$$\dot{V}O_2 = \left\{ \left[ \left( \frac{1 - 0.167 - 0.031}{1 - 0.2093} \right) \times 0.2093 \right] - 0.167 \right\} \times 16.1 \, l/min$$

$$\dot{V}O_2 = \left\{ \left[ \left( \frac{0.833 - 0.031}{0.7907} \right) \times 0.2093 \right] - 0.167 \right\} \times 16.1 \, l/min$$

$$\dot{V}O_2 = \left\{ \left[ \left( \frac{0.8020}{0.7907} \right) \times 0.2093 \right] - 0.167 \right\} \times 16.1 \, l/min$$

$$\dot{V}O_2 = [(1.014 \times 0.2093) - 0.167] \times 16.1 \, l/min$$

$$\dot{V}O_2 = (0.2122 - 0.167) \times 16.1 \, l/min$$

$$\dot{V}O_2 = 0.0452 \times 16.1 \, l/min$$

$$\dot{V}O_2 = 0.727 \, l/min \, STPD$$

## Determination of METS

The equation used for making the calculation is

$$METS = \frac{\dot{V}O_2 max}{0.0035 \, l/min/kg \times Wt_{Sub}}$$

Assuming that the value for $\dot{V}O_2$ determined previously is a value for the subject's $\dot{V}O_2$ max, and inserting the required values,

$$METS = \frac{0.727 \, l/min}{0.0035 \, l/min/kg \times 92 \, kg}$$

$$METS = \frac{0.727 \, l/min}{0.322 \, l/min}$$

$$METS = 2.26$$

## Determinations of $\dot{V}CO_2$

The equation used for making the calculation is

$$\dot{V}CO_2 = (FECO_2 - FICO_2) \times \dot{V}_E STPD$$

Inserting the required values:

$$\dot{V}CO_2 = (0.031 - 0.0003) \times 16.1 \text{ l/min}$$

$$\dot{V}CO_2 = 0.0307 \times 16.1 \text{ l/min}$$

$$\dot{V}CO_2 = 0.494 \text{ l/min STPD}$$

## Determination of $\dot{V}_E/\dot{V}O_2$

The equation used for making the calculation is

$$\dot{V}_E/\dot{V}O_2 = \frac{\dot{V}_E \text{ BTPS} - (f \times V_D\text{valve})}{\dot{V}O_2}$$

Inserting the required values:

$$\dot{V}_E/\dot{V}O_2 = \frac{19.8 \text{ l/min} - (23 \text{ breaths/min} \times 0.020 \text{ liter})}{0.727 \text{ l/min}}$$

$$\dot{V}_E/\dot{V}O_2 = \frac{19.8 \text{ l/min} - 0.46 \text{ l/min}}{0.727 \text{ l/min}}$$

$$\dot{V}_E/\dot{V}O_2 = \frac{19.34 \text{ l/min}}{0.727 \text{ l/min}}$$

$$\dot{V}_E/\dot{V}O_2 = 26.6 \text{ l/min/l/min } \dot{V}O_2$$

## Determination of $\dot{V}_E/\dot{V}CO_2$

The equation used for making the calculation is

$$\dot{V}_E/\dot{V}CO_2 = \frac{\dot{V}_E \text{ BTPS} - (f \times V_D\text{valve})}{\dot{V}O_2}$$

Inserting the required values:

$$\dot{V}_E/\dot{V}CO_2 = \frac{19.8 \text{ l/min} - (23 \text{ breaths/min} \times 0.020 \text{ liter})}{0.494 \text{ l/min}}$$

$$\dot{V}_E/\dot{V}CO_2 = \frac{19.8 \text{ l/min} - 0.46 \text{ l/min}}{0.494 \text{ l/min}}$$

$$\dot{V}_E/\dot{V}CO_2 = \frac{19.34 \text{ l/min}}{0.494 \text{ l/min}}$$

$$\dot{V}_E/\dot{V}CO_2 = 39.1 \text{ l/min/l/min } \dot{V}O_2$$

## Determination of R

The equation used for making the calculation is

$$R = \frac{\dot{V}CO_2}{\dot{V}O_2}$$

Inserting the required values:

$$R = \frac{0.494 \; l/min}{0.727 \; l/min}$$

$$R = 0.68$$

## Determination of $O_2$pulse

The equation used for making the calculation is

$$O_2\text{pulse} = \frac{\dot{V}O_2 \times 1000}{HR}$$

Inserting the required values:

$$O_2\text{pulse} = \frac{0.727 \; l/min \times 1000 \; ml/liter}{112 \; beats/min}$$

$$O_2\text{pulse} = \frac{727 \; ml/min}{112 \; beats/min}$$

$$O_2\text{pulse} = 6.49 \; ml \; O_2/beat$$

# CASE STUDIES IN CARDIOPULMONARY STRESS TESTING

The purpose of this section is to provide practice in evaluating and interpreting the results of cardiopulmonary stress tests.

## REVIEW FOR EVALUATION AND INTERPRETATION OF CARDIOPULMONARY STRESS TESTS

Before practicing the interpretation of cardiopulmonary stress tests, it will be useful to review the basic steps that should be followed:

1. Evaluation of the acceptability of the test data.
2. Comparison of the subject's test results with the normal values predicted for the subject.
3. Identification and the type(s) and severity of abnormalities that are demonstrated.

Each of these steps will now be briefly reviewed.

## EVALUATION OF ACCEPTABILITY OF TEST DATA

Evaluation of the acceptability of the test data is based on a careful review of the raw numerical test data and graphs that are produced during the test. As with pulmonary function testing, this review of the test results is useful for two reasons. First, it is a way of evaluating the function of the test equipment. Numerical data that are different from what should reasonably be expected can signal the presence of equipment malfunctions.

A second reason for reviewing the test data is to evaluate the subject's cooperation and effort during the test. Are the test results reasonable for this subject given her or his recorded health history and/or previous stress test results?

## COMPARISON OF SUBJECT'S TEST RESULTS WITH NORMAL VALUES PREDICTED

Once the raw data from the test are determined to be acceptable, the subject's actual test result values should be compared against the predicted normal values for that subject. As with pulmonary function testing, two important points are related to this stage of the process. The first is that appropriate nomograms for predicting normal values must be chosen for the subject population typically tested by the laboratory. Nomograms that are unsuitable for the population being tested will result in incorrect normal values being predicted.

The second concern is that correct information for the subject's height, age, gender, and so on, be used when the normal values are determined. Any errors here will also result in incorrect normal values being predicted for the subject. Chapter 14 of the textbook presents examples of predictive nomograms for cardiopulmonary stress testing.

Once the predicted normal values for the subject are determined, they can be compared against the subject's test result values. Test values that fall outside the predicted normal range indicate an abnormality for that test parameter.

The computer software used with most modern testing systems will in some manner indicate where a subject's test values fall outside the predicted normal range. This feature can simplify and speed up the process of interpreting cardiopulmonary stress test results.

## IDENTIFICATION OF TYPE(S) AND SEVERITY OF ABNORMALITIES

Once abnormal values are identified in the test results of a subject, the pattern of the abnormal values can reveal the nature and severity of the subject's pulmonary dysfunction. Generally, exercise testing abnormalities are categorized as being due to either poor conditioning, pulmonary disorders, or cardiovascular disorders. Table 14.5 (in Chapter 14) of the textbook provides the general patterns for the effects of abnormalities on key stress testing parameters.

The severity of a disorder is based on the amount of abnormality that is demonstrated in the subject's $\dot{V}O_2$ results. As stated in Chapter 14, a $\dot{V}O_2$max value that is 80% or more of the subject's predicted value is considered normal. A mild to moderate impairment is indicated by a $\dot{V}O_2$max value in the range of 60–80% of predicted. A severe impairment is demonstrated when a subject's $\dot{V}O_2$max value is <60% of the predicted value. Unfortunately, the use of such severity terms as "mild," "moderate," and "severe" is not standardized. Therefore, these terms may vary according to the laboratory performing the tests and/or the individual who is interpreting the tests.

## CARDIOPULMONARY STRESS TESTING CASE STUDIES

This section of the chapter contains the case studies that can be used as an exercise in the interpretation of cardiopulmonary stress test results.

# PREPARATION FOR USE OF INTERPRETATION EXERCISE

With each of the four case studies, certain information will be presented:

- General information on the subject.
- A table for presentation of specific cardiopulmonary stress testing results for the subject.
- An interpretation of the results of the stress test performed on the subject. This interpretation is based on the one performed by a pulmonologist at the laboratory where the tests in these case studies were originally performed.

In order to make effective use of the case studies as a learning exercise, first make your own attempt to interpret the results of the tests performed for a given case study. In doing so, you should try to determine both the nature and the severity of any abnormalities that are demonstrated by the subject. Your process for interpreting the test results should proceed in the following manner:

1. First review the information presented on the subject. It may be useful for you to make marks and notes on the tables presenting the test data as you review the information.
2. Identify the parameters that fall outside the subject's normal range of values.
3. Using this information, evaluate the subject's respiratory and cardiovascular responses to the exercise test.
4. Finally, determine whether any test parameter abnormalities that are present demonstrate *deconditioning*, *a pulmonary disorder*, or *a cardiovascular disorder*, and *determine the severity* of the disorder.

Once you have performed your own interpretation of the test results, look over the interpretation presented for the case study. If you find significant differences between your interpretation and the one presented, go back and review the subject's test results in order to see why your interpretation is different.

# CASE STUDY 1

## Subject Information

This subject is a 78-year-old female (Ht = 65 inches, weight = 145 lb, race = Cauc.). She has a complaint of unexplained exertional dyspnea. At the time of the test, she had the following resting arterial blood gas analysis results on room air: pH of 7.52, $PaCO_2$ of 32 mm Hg, BE of +3.4 mEq/l, $PaO_2$ of 70 mm Hg, and $SaO_2$ of 93.1%. She had pulmonary function testing values of FVC = 2.88 liter (103% of pred.), FEV1 = 2.39 liter (111% of pred.), and $FEF_{25-75\%}$ = 2.72 l/sec (103% of pred.). Based on her $FEV_1$ value, the subject's predicted MVV is 83.7 l/min.

During the stress test, her electrocardiogram demonstrated a sinus rhythm with occasional PVCs during maximum exercise with some ST depression in V4 and V5. The test was ended when the subject experienced general fatigue.

## CARDIOPULMONARY STRESS TESTING REPORT

|  | Rest | At Peak $\dot{V}O_2$ | Pred. Max. | % Pred. |
|---|---|---|---|---|
| $\dot{V}O_2$ (ml $O_2$/min) = | 246 | 1258 | 1010 | 125 |
| $\dot{V}O_2$/kg (ml $O_2$/min/kg) = | 3.7 | 19.1 | 15.4 | 125 |
| METS = | 1.1 | 19.1 |  |  |
| $\dot{V}CO_2$ (ml $CO_2$/min) = | 280 | 814 | 1212 | 67 |
| R = | 1.14 | 0.65 |  |  |
| $\dot{V}_E$ (l/min BTPS) = | 18.1 | 42.8 | 85.6 | 44 |
| $V_D/V_T$ = | 0.41 | 0.44 |  |  |
| $\dot{V}_E/\dot{V}O_2$ (l/min/ml $O_2$/min) = | 73.6 | 33.6 | 94.6 | 36 |
| $\dot{V}_E/\dot{V}CO_2$ (l/min/ml $CO_2$/min) = | 64.6 | 52.0 | 78.8 | 66 |
| $SpO_2$ (%) = | 95 | 97 |  |  |
| HR (beats/min) = | 89 | 121 | 141 | 86 |
| $O_2$pulse (ml $O_2$/beat/min) = | 2.8 | 10.4 | 7.2 | 145 |

## Practice Interpretation

*Perform your practice interpretation (pulmonary response, cardiovascular response, and severity of any disorder present) at this time before looking at the actual interpretation.*

## Actual Interpretation

*Respiratory Response.* Baseline spirometry was within normal limits, with an $FEV_1$ of 111%. The $PaO_2$ on room air showed a mild hypoxemia. There was no significant oxygen desaturation during exercise; in fact, oxygen saturation increased from a low of 92% early in the test to 96% throughout most of the remainder of the test (including during maximum activity). Ventilation reached only 44% of the maximum predicted value, reflecting excellent efficiency of ventilation. The $V_D/V_T$ remained within normal limits. $\dot{V}_E$max/MVV value reached only 51% at the peak exercise level.

    *Cardiovascular Response.* The subject achieved a $\dot{V}O_2$max of 1258 ml/min, which is 125% of the predicted maximum for a person of her age and height. The resting heart rate was 112 and increased to a maximum of 121 during maximum exercise. This represents 86% of the predicted maximum heart rate. Occasional PVCs were noted during maximum exercise, and there was a 1–2 mm ST segment depression in $V_4$ and $V_5$ at maximum activity. However, the subject experienced no chest pain or pressure. $O_2$pulse was excellent, increasing to 10.4 ml $O_2$/beat with a predicted maximum value of 7.2 ml $O_2$/beat, indicating good cardiovascular performance.

## Final Impression

The subject demonstrates a study that is basically normal. This is indicated by several factors:

- A normal $\dot{V}O_2$max.
- No evidence of a ventilatory limitation to exercise (i.e., the $SpO_2$ remained normal, and the $\dot{V}_E$/MVV value increased during the test, although not quite to the predicted normal level).

- No evidence of a cardiovascular limitation to exercise (i.e, $O_2$pulse increased as would be expected during exercise, and no significantly abnormal rhythms were noted on ECG).

An etiology for the subject's symptoms of exertional dyspnea is not clear from this study. Specifically, significant interstitial lung disease is not likely, since there was an absence of hemoglobin desaturation and an excellent $\dot{V}O_2$ was demonstrated.

## CASE STUDY 2

### Subject Information

This subject is a 31-year-old female (Ht = 63 inches, weight = 110 lb, race = Cauc.). She has a complaint of recurrent pneumothoraces and shortness of breath. At the time of the test, she had the following resting arterial blood gas analysis results on room air: pH of 7.42, $PaCO_2$ of 35 mm Hg, BE of −1.0 mEq/l, $PaO_2$ of 105 mm Hg, and $SaO_2$ of 93.7%. She had pulmonary function testing values of FVC = 3.08 liter (92% of pred.), $FEV_1$ = 2.70 liter (94% of pred.), and $FEF_{25-75\%}$ = 2.86 l/sec (84% of pred.). Based on her $FEV_1$ value, the subject's predicted MVV is 94.5 l/min.

During the stress test, the electrocardiogram demonstrated a sinus rhythm throughout the test without rhythm abnormalities. The test was ended when the subject experienced leg cramps and general fatigue.

### CARDIOPULMONARY STRESS TESTING REPORT

|  | Rest | At Peak $\dot{V}O_2$ | Pred. Max. | % Pred. |
|---|---|---|---|---|
| $\dot{V}O_2$ (ml $O_2$/min) = | 270 | 1189 | 1623 | 70 |
| $\dot{V}O_2$/kg (ml $O_2$/min/kg) = | 5.4 | 22.8 | 32.5 | 70 |
| METS = | 1.5 | 6.5 |  |  |
| $\dot{V}CO_2$ (ml $CO_2$/min) = | 216 | 1522 | 1948 | 78 |
| R = | 0.80 | 1.34 |  |  |
| $\dot{V}_E$ (l/min BTPS) = | 9.9 | 60.2 | 108.0 | 56 |
| $V_D/V_T$ = | 0.28 | 0.25 |  |  |
| $\dot{V}_E/\dot{V}O_2$ (l/min/ml $O_2$/min) = | 36.7 | 52.9 | 66.5 | 79 |
| $\dot{V}_E/\dot{V}CO_2$ (l/min/ml $CO_2$/min) = | 45.8 | 39.6 | 55.4 | 71 |
| $SpO_2$ (%) = | 98.6 | 94.2 |  |  |
| HR (beats/min) = | 90 | 146 | 189 | 77 |
| $O_2$pulse (ml $O_2$/beat/min) = | 3.0 | 7.8 | 8.6 | 91 |

### Practice Interpretation

*Perform your practice interpretation (pulmonary response, cardiovascular response, and severity of any disorder present) at this time before looking at the actual interpretation.*

### Actual Interpretation

*Respiratory Response.* Baseline spirometry was within normal limits, with an $FEV_1$ of 94%. The $PaO_2$ on room air is normal. There was no significant oxygen desaturation during exercise. Ventilation reached only 56% of the maximum predicted value, reflecting an excellent efficiency of ventilation. The $V_D/V_T$ remained within normal limits. The subject's $\dot{V}_E/MVV$ reached 64% at the peak exercise level.

*Cardiovascular Response.* The subject achieved a $\dot{V}O_2$max of 1189 ml/min, which is less than normal (70% of the predicted maximum) for a person of her age and height. The resting heart rate was 90 and increased to a maximum of 146 during maximum exercise. This represents 77% of the predicted maximum heart rate. Her ECG demonstrated no evidence of ischemia. As is normally expected, sinus tachycardia occurred (146 beats/min) at her peak tolerated exercise level. $O_2$pulse remained at normal levels during the test and, along with the increases in heart rate, suggested a normal rise in cardiac output with increased graded exercise.

## Final Impression

This subject demonstrates a mild or moderate level of poor conditioning with a decreased work capacity. This is indicated by several factors:

- A less than predicted $\dot{V}O_2$max.
- No evidence of a ventilatory limitation to exercise (i.e., the $SpO_2$ remained normal, and the $\dot{V}_E/MVV$ value increased to a reasonable level during the test).
- No evidence of a cardiovascular limitation to exercise (i.e., $O_2$pulse increased as would be expected during exercise, and no abnormal rhythms were noted on ECG).

# CASE STUDY 3

## Subject Information

This subject is a 68-year-old male (Ht $= 70$ inches, weight $= 144$ lb, race $=$ Cauc.). He has a complaint of shortness of breath with limited exertion. At the time of the test, he had the following resting arterial blood gas analysis results on room air: pH of 7.42, $PaCO_2$ of 41 mm Hg, BE of 2.1 mEq/l, $PaO_2$ of 69 mm Hg, and $SaO_2$ of 92.3%. He had pulmonary function testing values of FVC $= 2.39$ liter (55% of pred.), $FEV_1 = 0.80$ liter (23% of pred.), and $FEF_{25-75\%} = 0.25$ l/sec (7% of pred.). Based on his $FEV_1$ value, the subject's predicted MVV is 28 l/min.

During the stress test, the electrocardiogram demonstrated a sinus rhythm throughout the test with neither ST segment depression nor evidence of an arrhythmia. The test was ended when the subject experienced shortness of breath.

### CARDIOPULMONARY STRESS TESTING REPORT

|  | Rest | At Peak $\dot{V}O_2$ | Pred. Max. | % Pred. |
|---|---|---|---|---|
| $\dot{V}O_2$ (ml $O_2$/min) = | 240 | 620 | 1782 | 35 |
| $\dot{V}O_2$/kg (ml $O_2$/min/kg) = | 3.7 | 9.5 | 27.3 | 35 |
| METS = | 1.0 | 2.7 | | |
| $\dot{V}CO_2$ (ml $CO_2$/min) = | 213 | 517 | 2139 | 24 |
| R = | 0.89 | 0.83 | | |
| $\dot{V}_E$ (l/min BTPS) = | 14.4 | 23.1 | 32 | 72 |
| $V_D/V_T$ = | 0.47 | 0.39 | | |

|  | Rest | At Peak $\dot{V}O_2$ | Pred. Max. | % Pred. |
|---|---|---|---|---|
| $\dot{V}_E/\dot{V}O_2$ (l/min/ml $O_2$/min) = | 59.8 | 37.3 | 18.0 | 208 |
| $\dot{V}_E/\dot{V}CO_2$ (l/min/ml $CO_2$/min) = | 67.2 | 44.7 | 15.0 | 298 |
| $SpO_2$ (%) = | 93.7 | 83.3 |  |  |
| HR (beats/min) = | 109 | 135 | 157 | 86 |
| $O_2$pulse (ml $O_2$/beat/min) = | 2.2 | 4.6 | 11.4 | 41 |

## Practice Interpretation

*Perform your practice interpretation (pulmonary response, cardiovascular response, and severity of any disorder present) at this time before looking at the actual interpretation.*

## Actual Interpretation

*Respiratory Response.* Baseline spirometry shows a severe obstructive ventilatory impairment, with an $FEV_1$ of only 23% of predicted. The resting arterial blood gas values demonstrate moderate hypoxemia without hypercapnia. During exercise, there was a significant hemoglobin desaturation that accompanied the development of dyspnea. The subject's $\dot{V}_E/MVV$ reached 83% at the peak exercise level.

*Cardiovascular Response.* The subject achieved a $\dot{V}O_2$max of 620 ml/min, which is less than normal (86% of the predicted maximum) for a person of his age and height. His increase in heart rate was reasonable for the maximum exercise workload achieved. His ECG demonstrated no evidence of abnormality, even at peak work load. The subject's $O_2$pulse did not increase significantly during the test, but this was probably due to the low maximum workload that was achieved before the test was ended.

## Final Impression

This subject demonstrates a severe exercise limitation that is due to a respiratory impairment. This is indicated by several factors:

- A less than predicted $\dot{V}O_2$max.
- Evidence of a ventilatory limitation to exercise (i.e., significant hemoglobin desaturation and a greater-than-normal increase in the $\dot{V}_E/MVV$ value during exercise).
- No evidence of a cardiovascular limitation to exercise (i.e., despite the $O_2$pulse value remaining low during the test, the heart rate responded reasonably, and no abnormal rhythms were noted on ECG).

## CASE STUDY 4

## Subject Information

This subject is a 77-year-old female (Ht = 63 inches, weight = 97 lb, race = Cauc.). She has a complaint of shortness of breath with exertion. At the time of the test, she had the following resting arterial blood gas analysis results on room air: pH of 7.50, $PaCO_2$ of 28 mm Hg, BE of $-0.4$ mEq/l, $PaO_2$ of 109 mm Hg, and $SaO_2$ of 96.3%. She had pulmonary function testing values of FVC = 2.92 liter (112% of pred.), $FEV_1$ = 1.86 liter (23% of pred.), and $FEF_{25-75\%}$ = 0.75 l/sec (37% of pred.). Based on her $FEV_1$ values, the subject's predicted MVV is 65.1 l/min.

The resting electrocardiogram demonstrated atrial fibrillation, a marked right-axis shift, and minor nonspecific T-wave changes. With exercise during the test, an ST segment depression of more than 1 mm, with straightening, occurred in the anterior lateral precordial leads. In 85% of cases this indicates cardiac ischemia. The test was ended when the subject experienced shortness of breath and general fatigue.

## CARDIOPULMONARY STRESS TESTING REPORT

|  | Rest | At Peak $\dot{V}O_2$ | Pred. Max. | % Pred. |
|---|---|---|---|---|
| $\dot{V}O_2$ (ml $O_2$/min) = | 266 | 482 | 841 | 57 |
| $\dot{V}O_2$/kg (ml $O_2$/min/kg) = | 6.0 | 11.0 | 19.1 | 57 |
| METS = | 1.7 | 3.1 |  |  |
| $\dot{V}CO_2$ (ml $CO_2$/min) = | 169 | 386 | 1009 | 38 |
| R = | 0.63 | 0.80 |  |  |
| $\dot{V}_E$ (l/min BTPS) = | 10.9 | 18.7 | 74.4 | 25 |
| $V_D/V_T$ = | 0.39 | 0.30 |  |  |
| $\dot{V}_E/\dot{V}O_2$ (l/min/ml $O_2$/min) = | 40.9 | 38.8 | 88.5 | 44 |
| $\dot{V}E/\dot{V}CO_2$ (l/min/ml $CO_2$/min) = | 64.6 | 48.6 | 73.7 | 66 |
| $SpO_2$ (%) = | 93.3 | 95.6 |  |  |
| HR (beats/min) = | 105 | 123 | 143 | 86 |
| $O_2$pulse (ml $O_2$/beat/min) = | 2.5 | 3.9 | 5.9 | 67 |

## Practice Interpretation

*Perform your practice interpretation (pulmonary response, cardiovascular response, and severity of any disorder present) at this time before looking at the actual interpretation.*

## Actual Interpretation

*Respiratory Response.* Baseline spirometry shows a very mild obstructive ventilatory impairment, with an $FEF_{25-75\%}$ of only 37% of predicted. The resting arterial blood gases do not demonstrate abnormalities in either oxygenation or ventilation. During exercise, there was no hemoglobin desaturation. The subject's $\dot{V}_E$/MVV remained low (29%), even at the peak exercise level. This indicates that even at a maximum workload she still had a considerable ventilatory reserve.

*Cardiovascular Response.* The subject achieved a $\dot{V}O_2$max of 482 ml/min, which is significantly less than normal (57% of the predicted maximum) for a person of her age and height. Her heart rate increased predictably during exercise, but her ECG demonstrated significant abnormalities during the test. The subject's $O_2$pulse did not increase as predicted during the test.

## Final Impression

This subject demonstrates a severe exercise limitation that is due to a cardiovascular impairment. This is indicated by several factors:

- A less than predicted $\dot{V}O_2$max.

- No evidence of a ventilatory limitation to exercise (i.e., no hemoglobin desaturation and a significantly less than normal increase in the VE/MVV value during exercise).
- Evidence of a cardiovascular limitation to exercise (i.e., a significantly reduced $O_2$pulse value during the test and the development of significant ECG abnormalities).

# APPENDIX A

# SYMBOLS AND ABBREVIATIONS

## BASIC UNITS OF MEASURE

| | |
|---|---|
| cm $H_2O$ | Centimeters of water pressure |
| °C | Degrees of temperature in centigrade |
| ft | Foot |
| gm% | Gram percent (number of grams per 100 grams of total weight) |
| in. | Inch |
| kcal | Kilocalorie |
| kg | Kilograms |
| liter | Liters |
| ml | Milliliters |
| min | Minutes |
| mM | Millimole |
| mm Hg | Millimeters of mercury pressure |
| mph | Miles per hour |
| sec | Seconds |
| m | Meters |
| vol% | Volume percent (number of ml of a substance per 100 ml of total volume) |
| beats/min | Heartbeats per minute |
| breaths/min | Breaths per minute |
| l/min | Liters per minute |
| l/sec | Liters per second |
| mEq/l | Milliequivalents per liter |
| mg/ml | Milligrams per milliliter |
| ml/min | Milliliters per minute |
| ml/kg | Milliliters per kilogram |

## BASIC MEASUREMENT SYMBOLS

ATPS    A volume of gas is at atmospheric environmental temperature, pressure, and is 100% saturated with water vapor

BTPS     A volume of gas is at body temperature ($37°C$), ambient environmental pressure, and is 100% saturated with water vapor

STPD     A volume of gas is at standard temperature ($0.0°C$), pressure (760 mm Hg), and 0.0% saturated with water vapor

A     Age

BSA     Body surface area

f     Frequency (often breaths per minute, breathing frequency or respiratory rate)

Ht     Height

Hz     Hertz

T     Temperature

P     Pressure or partial pressure

$P_A$     Pressure of air in the alveoli or partial pressure of a gas in alveolar air

$P_{Atm}$     Pressure of the ambient atmosphere

$P_{eso}$     Intraesophageal pressure

$P_{H2O}$     Partial pressure of water vapor

$P_L$     Transpulmonary pressure

$P_{pl}$     Intrapleural pressure

$P_{TL}$     Transthoracic/pulmonary pressure

R     Resistance

V     Volume

$V_L$     Lung volume

$\dot{V}$     Flow rate, ventilation, or minute ventilation

Wt     Weight

# GAS AND BLOOD GAS ANALYSIS SYMBOLS

$CaO_2$     Content of oxygen in arterial blood

$C(a-\bar{v})O_2$     Oxygen content difference between arterial and mixed venous blood

$C\bar{v}O_2$     Content of oxygen in mixed venous blood

$FCO_2$     Fraction of carbon dioxide in a gas mixture

$FACO_2$     Fraction of carbon dioxide in alveolar air

$FAN_2$     Fraction of nitrogen in alveolar air

FECO     Fraction of carbon monoxide in exhaled air

FEHe     Fraction of helium in exhaled air

$FEN_2$     Fraction of nitrogen in exhaled air

$FECO_2$     Fraction of carbon dioxide in exhaled air

$F\bar{E}CO_2$     Mean fraction of carbon dioxide in exhaled air

$FetCO_2$     Fraction of carbon dioxide in end-tidal exhaled air

$F\bar{E}N_2$     Mean fraction of nitrogen in exhaled air

$FEO_2$     Fraction of oxygen in exhaled air

$FetO_2$     Fraction of oxygen in end-tidal exhaled air

FICO     Fraction of carbon monoxide in inspired air

| | |
|---|---|
| $FICO_2$ | Fraction of inspired carbon dioxide |
| $FIHe$ | Fraction of helium in inspired air |
| $FEO_2$ | Fraction of oxygen in exhaled air |
| $FIO_2$ | Fraction of oxygen in inspired air |
| $HCO_3^-$ | Bicarbonate ion or plasma bicarbonate concentration |
| $O_2ER$ | Oxygen extraction ratio |
| $PCO_2$ | Partial pressure of carbon dioxide |
| $PO_2$ | Partial pressure of oxygen in a gas mixture |
| $PACO$ | Partial pressure of carbon monoxide in alveoli air |
| $PACO_2$ | Partial pressure of carbon dioxide in alveolar air |
| $PAO_2$ | Partial pressure of oxygen in alveolar air |
| $PaCO_2$ | Partial pressure of carbon dioxide in arterial blood |
| $PaO_2$ | Partial pressure of oxygen in arterial blood |
| $PacO_2$ | Partial pressure of oxygen in arterialized capillary blood |
| $P(a\text{-}et)CO_2$ | Difference between the arterial and end-tidal partial pressure for carbon dioxide |
| $PcCO$ | Partial pressure of carbon monoxide in capillary blood |
| $PECO_2$ | Mean partial pressure of carbon dioxide in exhaled air |
| $PetCO$ | Partial pressure of carbon monoxide in end-tidal exhaled air |
| $PetCO_2$ | Partial pressure of carbon dioxide in end-tidal exhaled air |
| $pH$ | The negative logarithm of the hydrogen ion concentration expressed as a positive number |
| $PtcCO_2$ | Partial pressure of carbon dioxide through the skin (transcutaneous) |
| $PtcO_2$ | Partial pressure of oxygen through the skin (transcutaneous) |
| $PvCO_2$ | Partial pressure of carbon dioxide in venous blood |
| $PvO_2$ | Partial pressure of oxygen in venous blood |
| $P\bar{v}CO_2$ | Partial pressure of carbon dioxide in mixed venous blood |
| $P\bar{v}O_2$ | Partial pressure of oxygen in mixed venous blood |
| $\%HbCO$ | Percent saturation of hemoglobin with carbon monoxide |
| $\%MetHb$ | Percent of methemoglobin in the blood |
| $\dot{Q}s$ | Flow value for blood that is undergoing true right-to-left shunting. |
| $\dot{Q}_{sp}$ | Flow value for blood that is undergoing physiologic right-to-left shunting |
| $\dot{Q}_{sp}/\dot{Q}_T$ | Percent (or fraction) of blood that is undergoing physiologic right-to-left shunting |
| $\dot{Q}_{sp}/\dot{Q}_T\text{est}$ | Estimated percent (or fraction) of blood that is undergoing physiologic right-to-left shunting |
| $\dot{Q}_T$ | Flow value for cardiac output |
| $SaO_2$ | Percent saturation of hemoglobin with oxygen |
| $SpO_2$ | Percent saturation of hemoglobin with oxygen when measured by pulse oximetry |
| Total Hb | Total hemoglobin in the blood |
| $\dot{T}O_e$ | Transport rate of oxygen to the tissues |

# PULMONARY VOLUME AND VENTILATION MEASUREMENT

| | |
|---|---|
| ERV | Expiratory reserve volume |
| FRC | Functional residual capacity |
| IC | Inspiratory capacity |
| IRV | Inspiratory reserve volume |
| RV | Residual volume |
| RV/TLC% | Residual volume to total lung capacity ratio expressed as a percent |
| SVC | Slow vital capacity maneuver |
| TLC | Total lung capacity |
| VC | Vital capacity |
| $V_A$ | Alveolar volume |
| $V_D$an | Anatomic deadspace |
| $V_DA$ | Alveolar deadspace |
| $V_D$ | Physiologic deadspace |
| $V_D/V_T$ | Deadspace to tidal volume ratio |
| $V_E$ | Exhaled volume |
| $V_T$ | Tidal volume |
| $V_{TG}$ | Thoracic gas volume |
| $\dot{V}_A$eff | Effective alveolar ventilation |
| $\dot{V}_D$ | Physiologic deadspace |
| $\dot{V}_DA$ | Alveolar deadspace |
| $\dot{V}_D$an | Anatomic deadspace |
| $\dot{V}_E$ | Exhaled minute ventilation |
| $\dot{V}_I$ | Inspired minute ventilation |

# PULMONARY MECHANICS MEASUREMENT

## FORCED VITAL CAPACITY MANEUVER

| | |
|---|---|
| $FEF_{200-1200}$ (or $MEFR_{200-1200}$) | Maximum expiratory flow rate; the average expiratory flow rate between the first 0.2 and 1.2 liters of the FVC volume |
| $FEF_{25\%-75\%}$ | Maximal mid-expiratory flow; the average expiratory flow rate over the middle 50% of the FVC volume |
| $FEF_{75\%-85\%}$ | Maximum end-expiratory flow rate; the average expiratory flow rate between 75% and 85% of the FVC volume |
| $FEF_{max}$ (or PEFR) | Peak expiratory flow rate; the maximum expiratory flow rate achieved at any point during the FVC maneuver |
| $FEF_{x\%}$ | Instantaneous forced expiratory flow rate; the expiratory flow rate after a specified percent of the FVC volume has been exhaled |

| $FEV_t$ | Timed forced expiratory volume; the volume of air exhaled within a specified period of time (t) from the start of a FVC maneuver. The values that may be used for t are 0.5, 1, 2, or 3 seconds. |
|---|---|
| $FEV_{t\%}$ | Forced expiratory volume percent; the percent of the total FVC volume that was exhaled within a specified time (t) from the start of the maneuver. |
| FIVC | Forced inspiratory vital capacity; the volume of an inspiratory vital-capacity maneuver inhaled as rapidly and forcefully as possible |
| $FIF_{max}$ (or PIFR) | Peak inspiratory flow rate; the maximum inspiratory flow rate achieved at any point during the FIVC maneuver |
| $FIF_{25\%-75\%}$ | Maximal mid-inspiratory flow rate; the average inspiratory flow rate over the middle 50% of the FIVC volume |
| $FIF_{x\%}$ | Instantaneous forced inspiratory flow rate; the inspiratory flow rate at a specified point in the FIVC maneuver |
| FVC | Forced vital capacity maneuver |
| MEFV | Maximum expiratory flow/volume curve |
| MIFV | Maximum inspiratory flow/volume curve |
| MVV | Maximum voluntary ventilation |
| PEFR | Peak expiratory flow rate |
| PFEV | Partial forced expiratory volume |
| $\dot{V}_{max\ x}$ | Instantaneous forced expiratory flow rate; the expiratory flow rate at the point where a specified percent of the FVC volume remains to be exhaled. |

## LOW-DENSITY GAS SPIROMETRY

| $V_{iso\dot{V}}$ | Volume of isoflow as related to low-density spirometry |
|---|---|
| $\Delta\dot{V}_{max\ 50}$ | The change in flow rate at 50% of an FVC maneuver as related to low-density spirometry |

## AIRWAY RESISTANCE/CONDUCTANCE

| $G_{aw}$ | Airway conductance |
|---|---|
| $R_{aw}$ | Airway resistance |
| $SR_{aw}$ | Specific airway resistance |
| $SG_{aw}$ | Specific airway conductance |

## ELASTIC RECOIL/COMPLIANCE

| $C_L$ | Lung compliance |
|---|---|
| $C_T$ | Thoracic compliance |
| $C_{LT}$ | Combined lung/thoracic compliance |
| $C_{Dyn}$ | Dynamic compliance |
| $C_{St}$ | Static compliance |
| $C_{Sys}$ | System compliance |

PEEP     Positive end-expiratory pressure
$P_I$     Peak inspiratory pressure
$P_{Plat}$     Plateau pressure
$SC_{LT}$     Specific lung/thoracic compliance
SVL     System volume loss
$V_{Tact}$     Actual tidal volume
$V_{Tmeas}$     Measured tidal volume

## MAXIMUM INSPIRATORY/EXPIRATORY PRESSURES

MEP     Maximum expiratory pressure
MIP     Maximum inspiratory pressure

# PULMONARY GAS DISTRIBUTION

CC     Closing capacity
CC/%TLC     Closing capacity expressed as a percent of total lung capacity
CV     Closing volume
CV/%VC     Closing volume expressed as a percent of vital capacity
$\Delta\%N_2 750\text{--}1250$     Change in the percent of nitrogen between the 750 ml point and 1250 ml point of the exhaled volume during a single-breath nitrogen elimination test
$\Delta\%N_2/\text{liter}$     Change in the percent of nitrogen per liter of exhaled volume during a single-breath nitrogen elimination test

# DIFFUSING CAPACITY

$D_LCO$ (or $D_{LCO}$)     Diffusing capacity for carbon monoxide
FuCO     Fractional uptake of carbon monoxide
$T_{gas}$     Transfer factor for a gas
$V_{CO}$     Volume of carbon monoxide in a gas mixture

# BRONCHOPROVOCATION STUDY

CDU     Cumulative dose units
$PD_{20\%}FEV_1$     Provocative dose that produces at least a 20% change in $FEV_1$ values

# STUDY FOR EXERCISE-INDUCED ASTHMA

$EI\Delta FEV_1\%$     Exercise-induced percent change in $FEV_1$ values

# COMPUTER SYMBOLS

| | |
|---|---|
| A-D | Analog-to-digital |
| D-A | Digital-to-analog |

# EXERCISE/METABOLIC/NUTRITIONAL SYMBOLS

| | |
|---|---|
| AT | Anaerobic threshold |
| BP | Blood pressure |
| CO | Cardiac output |
| d | Flywheel diameter |
| FwR | Flywheel braking force for a cycle ergometer |
| HR | Heart rate |
| HRmax | Maximum heart rate |
| $O_2$pulse | Oxygen pulse |
| R | Respiratory exchange ratio |
| REE | Resting energy expenditure |
| RQ | Respiratory quotient |
| RQ(Car-Lip) | Respiratory quotient based on carbohydrate and lipid metabolism |
| SV | Stroke volume |
| UN | Urinary nitrogen |
| $\dot{V}CO_2$ | Carbon dioxide production |
| $\dot{V}_E$max | Maximum level of minute ventilation |
| $\dot{V}_E/\dot{V}O_2$ | Ventilatory equivalent for oxygen |
| $\dot{V}_E/\dot{V}CO_2$ | Ventilatory equivalent for carbon dioxide |
| $\dot{V}O_2$ | Oxygen consumption |
| $\dot{V}O_2$max | Maximum level of oxygen consumption |
| $\dot{V}O_2$rest | Oxygen consumption at rest |

# STATISTICAL SYMBOLS

| | |
|---|---|
| 95% CL | Ninety-five percent confidence level |
| SD | Standard deviation |

# CHEMICAL SYMBOLS

| | |
|---|---|
| Ag | Silver |
| Cl | Chloride ($Cl^-$ for a chloride ion) |
| CO | Carbon monoxide |

| | |
|---|---|
| $CO_2$ | Carbon dioxide |
| $e^-$ | Electron |
| H | Hydrogen ($H^+$ for a hydrogen ion or proton) |
| He | Helium |
| Hg | Mercury |
| I | Iodine |
| Na | Sodium ($Na^+$ for a sodium ion) |
| $N_2$ | Nitrogen |
| $O_2$ | Oxygen |
| pH | Negative logarithm of the hydrogen ion concentration expressed as a positive number |
| Tc | Technetium |
| Xe | Xenon |
| ADP | Adenosine diphosphate |
| AgCl | Silver chloride |
| ATP | Adenosine triphosphate |
| $C_6H_{12}O_6$ | Glucose |
| FAD | Flavin adenine dinucleotide |
| $HCO_3^-$ | Bicarbonate ion |
| $H_6C_3O_3$ | Lactic acid |
| $Hg_2Cl_2$ | Mercurous chloride |
| $H_2CO_3$ | Carbonic acid |
| $H_2O$ | Water |
| NAD | Nicotinamid adenine dinucleotide |
| $NaHCO_3$ | Sodium bicarbonate |

# OTHER SYMBOLS USED IN THE TEXT

| | |
|---|---|
| $C_{Alv}N_2$ | Concentration of nitrogen in alveolar air |
| $C_{Exh}N_2$ | Concentration of nitrogen in exhaled air |
| $C_FHe$ | Final concentration of helium |
| $C_FN_2$ | Final concentration of nitrogen |
| $C_1He$ | Initial concentration of helium |
| $CN_2$ | Concentration of nitrogen in an air sample |
| $D_{gas}$ (or $D_{Lgas}$) | Diffusing capacity for a gas |
| $\Delta P$ | Difference, differential, or change in pressure |
| $\Delta P_A$ | Difference, differential, or change in alveolar pressure |
| $\Delta V$ | Difference or change in volume |
| $\Delta V_A$ | Difference or change in alveolar volume |
| FACO | Fraction of carbon monoxide in alveolar air |
| $FACO_I$ | Initial fraction of carbon monoxide in alveolar air |
| $FACO_F$ | Final fraction of carbon monoxide in alveolar air |
| $F_{Cal}$ | Calibration factor |

| | |
|---|---|
| $FV_DN_2$ | Correction factor for physiologic deadspace admixture during measurement of the mean fraction of exhaled nitrogen |
| $F_{SG}$ | Fractional concentration of a gas in a sample |
| $F_{Sub}$ | Calibration factor relating to the volume displaced by a subject in a body plethysmograph cabinet |
| Ln | Natural logarithm |
| $PAgas$ | Partial pressure of a gas in alveoli air |
| $P_{Cab}$ | Pressure of air within a body plethysmograph cabinet |
| $Pcgas$ | Partial pressure of a gas in capillary blood |
| $P_{Gas}$ | Partial pressure of a test signal gas |
| $P_{pl}FRC$ | Intrapleural pressure measured at a subject's FRC level |
| $P_{pl}FRC\ 0.5$ | Intrapleural pressure measured at a subject's FRC level plus 0.5 liters of additional inspiratory volume |
| $P_{pl}insp$ | Intrapleural pressure at the end of inspiration |
| $P_{pl}exp$ | Intrapleural pressure at the end of expiration |
| $P_{Mo}$ | Pressure of air in the mouth |
| $P_{Mo}Cal$ | Calibration factor for air pressure measured at the mouth |
| $\%N_2$ | Percent of nitrogen in an air sample |
| $\%N_2Cal$ | Calibration factor for the percent of nitrogen in an air sample |
| % pred. | Percent of predicted values for a subject |
| $R_{fl}$ | Resistance to air flow |
| $R_{el}$ | Resistance to lung inflation resulting from elastic forces |
| $T_{Col}$ | Time duration for the collection of a gas volume |
| $T_{Hold}$ | Time duration for an inspiratory hold maneuver |
| $T_{Test}$ | Time duration of a test or breathing maneuver |
| $V_{added}He$ | Volume of helium added to a gas mixture |
| $V_{Cab}$ | Volume of a body plethysmograph cabinet |
| $V_{ECO}$ | Volume of exhaled carbon monoxide |
| $V_{ECO2}$ | Volume of exhaled carbon dioxide |
| $V_{Exh}$ | Volume of a subject's exhaled air |
| $V_{Exh}N_2$ | Volume of nitrogen in exhaled air |
| $V_{FRC}$ | Volume of a subject's FRC |
| $V_{gas}$ | Volume of a gas in a gas mixture |
| $V_{ICO}$ | Volume of inhaled carbon monoxide |
| $V_L$ | Volume of the lungs |
| $V_{MD}$ | Volume of deadspace produced by a mouthpiece in a breathing circuit |
| $V_S$ | Volume of gas in a volume-displacement spirometer |
| $V_{S+FRC}$ | Volume of gas in a volume-displacement spirometer added to the volume of a subject's FRC |
| $V_{Sam}$ | Volume of a collected gas sample |
| $\dot{V}\ Cal$ | Calibration factor for air flow rates |
| $W_{Sub}$ | Weight of a subject |
| $V_{VC}$ | Measured vital capacity volume |

# APPENDIX B

# VOLUME CONVERSIONS

Technologists should be aware that changes in the conditions of temperature, pressure, and water vapor pressure for a gas will affect the volume that quantity of gas will occupy. This is important where a gas volume is measured under one set of conditions but is needed for a calculation where the same quantity of gas must be represented under a different set of conditions. The different sets of conditions that may be applicable to pulmonary function testing measurements and calculations are

1. ATPD—ambient temperature-pressure dry.
2. ATPS—ambient temperature-pressure saturated.
3. BTPS—body temperature-pressure saturated.
4. STPD—standard temperature-pressure dry.

The methods used for making conversions between these different sets of conditions will be presented here. These methods can be used with equal effectiveness for converting simple gas volume values (V in liters) or for converting accumulated gas volume values that were determined over a period of time ($\dot{V}$ in l/min).

## ATPS-TO-BTPS CONVERSION

There are two methods for performing an ATPS-to-BTPS conversion:

- Calculate a conversion factor for converting a given quantity of gas from conditions of ATPS to BTPS. The calculation must include all factors that affect the volume of the gas and must always provide the correct conversion.
- Select a conversion factor from a chart of standardized factors for ATPS-to-BTPS conversion. The standardized factor that is selected in a given situation depends on the initial ambient temperature of the gas. These standardized conversion factors assume the ambient (ATPS) barometric pressure to be 760 mm Hg. Consequently, the factor will be less accurate in situations where the ATPS pressure is something other than 760 mm Hg.

Each of these methods will be illustrated here.

## CALCULATED CONVERSION

Calculated conversion is performed by using the following equation:

$$V_{BTPS} = V_{ATPS} \times \left[ \left( \frac{P_{Atm} - P_{H_2O}}{P_{Atm} - 47} \right) \times \left( \frac{310}{273 + T} \right) \right]$$

where $V_{ATPS}$ (liters) is the measured volume displayed by the spirometer, $V_{BTPS}$ (liters) is the converted volume, $P_{Atm}$ (mm Hg) is the barometric pressure at the time of the test, $P_{H_2O}$ (mm Hg) is the partial pressure of water vapor at temperature T (see Table B-1 for a chart to determine a value for $P_{H_2O}$), 47 (mm Hg) is the partial pressure of water vapor under BTPS conditions, 310 (°Kelvin) is the absolute temperature scale equivalent for body temperature, 273 (°Kelvin) is the absolute temperature scale equivalent for 0°C, and T (°C) is the ATPS temperature at the time of the volume measurement.

## STANDARDIZED CONVERSION FACTOR

The use of a standardized BTPS conversion factor is an approximate method for converting a $V_{ATPS}$ value to BTPS conditions. The following equation demonstrates how a BTPS conversion factor is used:

$$V_{BTPS} = V_{ATPS} \times \text{BTPS conversion factor}$$

where $V_{ATPS}$ (liters) is the measured volume displayed by the spirometer, and $V_{BTPS}$ (liters) is the converted volume. The BTPS conversion factor must be taken from a chart such as the one presented in Table B–1. As stated earlier, the factor is selected from the chart on the basis of the value for the ATPS temperature at the time of the volume measurement.

### TABLE B–1    ATPS-to-BTPS Conversion Factors and Water Vapor Pressure

| Gas Temperature (°C) | BTPS Conversion Factor | $P_{H_2O}$ (mm Hg) | Gas Temperature (°C) | BTPS Conversion Factor | $P_{H_2O}$ (mm Hg) |
|---|---|---|---|---|---|
| 18 | 1.112 | 15.6 | 28 | 1.057 | 28.3 |
| 19 | 1.107 | 16.5 | 29 | 1.051 | 30.0 |
| 20 | 1.102 | 17.5 | 30 | 1.045 | 31.8 |
| 21 | 1.096 | 18.7 | 31 | 1.039 | 33.7 |
| 22 | 1.091 | 19.8 | 32 | 1.032 | 35.7 |
| 23 | 1.085 | 21.1 | 33 | 1.026 | 37.7 |
| 24 | 1.080 | 22.4 | 34 | 1.020 | 39.9 |
| 25 | 1.075 | 23.8 | 35 | 1.014 | 42.2 |
| 26 | 1.068 | 25.2 | 36 | 1.007 | 44.6 |
| 27 | 1.063 | 26.7 | 37 | 1.000 | 47.0 |

Note: The conversion factors are based on a $P_{Atm}$ value of 760 mm Hg. They will be less accurate when used to make conversions at $P_{Atm}$ values other than 760 mm Hg.

# ATPS-TO-STPD CONVERSION

The following equation can be used for ATPS-to-STPD conversion:

$$V_{STPD} = V_{ATPS} \times \left[ \left( \frac{P_{Atm} - P_{H_2O}}{760} \right) \times \left( \frac{273}{273 + T} \right) \right]$$

where $V_{ATPS}$ (liters) is the volume measured by the spirometer, $V_{STPD}$ (liters) is the converted volume, $P_{Atm}$ (mm Hg) is the barometric pressure at the time of the test, $P_{H_2O}$ (mm Hg) is the partial pressure of water vapor at temperature T (see Table B–1 for a chart to determine a value for $P_{H_2O}$), 760 (mm Hg) is the barometric pressure under STPD conditions, 273 (°Kelvin) is the absolute temperature scale equivalent for 0°C, and T (°C) is the ATPS temperature at the time of the volume measurement.

# BTPS-TO-STPD CONVERSION

On some occasions it may be necessary to convert a volume from BTPS conditions to STPD. The following equation can be used for BTPS-to-STPD conversion:

$$V_{STPD} = V_{BTPS} \times \left[ \left( \frac{P_{Atm} - 47}{760} \right) \times 0.881 \right]$$

where $V_{BTPS}$ and $V_{STPD}$ are in units of liters, $P_{Atm}$ (mm Hg) is the barometric pressure at the time of the test, 47 (mm Hg) is the partial pressure of water vapor under BTPS conditions, 760 (mm Hg) is the barometric pressure under conditions of STPD, and 0.881 is a number required for the conversion.

# ATPD-TO-STPD CONVERSION

On some occasions it may be necessary to convert from conditions of ATPD to STPD. The following equation can be used for this conversion.

$$V_{STPD} = V_{ATPD} \times \left[ \left( \frac{P_{Atm} - P_{H_2O}}{760} \right) \times \left( \frac{273}{273 + T} \right) \right]$$

where $V_{ATPD}$ and $V_{STPD}$ are volumes in units of liters, $P_{Atm}$ (mm Hg) is the barometric pressure at the time of the test, 760 (mm Hg) is the barometric pressure under STPD conditions, 273 (°Kelvin) is the absolute temperature scale equivalent to 0°C, and T (°C) is the ATPD temperature at the time of the volume measurement.

# STANDARDS FOR SPIROMETER SYSTEMS

The American Thoracic Society has published minimum recommendations for the performance of spirometer systems (*Am J Respir Crit Care Med* 152:1107–1136, 1995). The specific performance standards are based on the particular test that is to be performed with the system. In some cases the standards are based on whether the testing is to be for diagnostic or monitoring purposes. All volumes stated on the standards are assumed to be at BTPS. Unless specifically stated, the precision requirements are the same as the stated accuracy requirements.

These are *minimum* standards. It would be wise, if possible, to use testing systems that have a greater measuring capacity, accuracy, and precision than is given here.

## VITAL CAPACITY (VC)

The spirometer should be able to

- Measure volumes accurately to *at least* within ±3% or 50 ml (whichever is greater).
- Measure volumes of *at least* 8 liters.
- Accumulate volumes for *at least* 30 sec.
- Measure volumes accurately at air flow rates between 0 and 14 l/sec (flow measurement must be linear within this range).

## FORCED VITAL CAPACITY (FVC)

### FOR DIAGNOSTIC PURPOSES

The spirometer should be able to

- Measure volumes accurately to *at least* within ±3% or 50 ml (whichever is greater).

- Measure volumes of *at least* 8 liters. The 8 liter range applies to newly manufactured spirometers; existing systems with a 7 liter spirometer can still be used.
- Accumulate volumes for *at least* 15 sec, although longer times are recommended.
- Measure volumes accurately at air flow rates between 0 and 14 l/sec (flow measurement must be linear within this range).

## FOR MONITORING PURPOSES

The spirometer should be able to

- Measure volumes accurately to *at least* within ±5% or 100 ml (whichever is greater).
- Have a precision of *at least* ±3% or ±50 ml, whichever is greater.
- Measure volumes up to *at least* 8 liters.
- Accumulate volumes for *at least* 15 sec.
- Measure volumes accurately at air flow rates between 0 and 14 l/sec (flow measurement must be linear within this range).

# TIMED FORCED EXPIRATORY VOLUMES (FEV$_T$)

## FOR DIAGNOSTIC PURPOSES

Standards are the same as for FVC and, additionally,

- Resistance to gas flow should be less than 1.5 cm $H_2O$/l/sec at flow rates of 14 l/sec.
- The "start of test" used to indicate the start of timing will be determined by the back-extrapolation method:
  Hand measurements—back-extrapolation from the steepest slope on the volume/time curve.
  Computer—largest average value for slope over a period of 80 msec.

## FOR MONITORING PURPOSES

Standards are the same as for FVC and, additionally,

- The spirometer should have a precision of *at least* ±3% or ±50 ml, whichever is greater.
- Resistance to gas flow should be less than 2.5 cm $H_2O$/l/sec at flow rates of 14 l/sec.
- The "start of test" used to indicate the start of timing should be the same as required for diagnostic purposes.

## PEAK EXPIRATORY FLOW RATE

### FOR DIAGNOSTIC PURPOSES

The measuring device should

- Have a frequency response that is flat (±5%) up to 12 Hz.
- Measure flow rate accurately within ±10% of reading or ± 0.3 l/sec, whichever is greater.
- Intrainstrumental precision must be less than 5% of reading or 0.150 l/sec, whichever is greater. Interdevice precision must be less than 10% or 0.300 l/sec, whichever is greater.

### FOR MONITORING PURPOSES

The measuring device should

- Have a frequency response that is flat (±5%) up to 12 Hz.
- Measure flow rate accurately within ±10% of reading or ±20 l/min, whichever is greater. This is within flow rate ranges of 60–400 l/min for children and 100–850 l/min for adults.
- Intrainstrumental precision must be less than 5% of reading or 10 l/min, whichever is greater. Interdevice precision must be less than 10% or 20 l/min, whichever is greater.

## FORCED EXPIRATORY FLOWS (FEF$_{25-75\%}$)

Standards are the same as for FVC and FEV$_t$ and, additionally,

- The accuracy of flow measurement should be *at least* ±5% or ±0.2 l/sec, whichever is greater, over a range of up to 7 l/sec.

## FLOW ($\dot{V}$)

Where flow/volume loops or other uses of flow measurements are made,

- The flow measurement accuracy at flow rates of ±14 l/sec should be within ±5% of the reading or ±0.2 l/sec, whichever is greater.

## MAXIMUM VOLUNTARY VENTILATION (MVV)

The spirometer should be able to

- Have an overall accuracy of ±10% of the reading or ±15 l/min, whichever is greater.

- Have an amplitude-frequency response that is flat within ±10% from zero to 4 Hz at flow rate inputs of up to 12 l/sec over the volume range.
- Make measurements for no less than 12 sec and no more than 15 sec and have a time-based accuracy of ±3%.
- Function with a back-pressure resistance to breathing of less than ±10 cm $H_2O$. This is for a 2 Hz sine wave gas flow input of a 2 liter volume.

# APPENDIX D

# TYPICAL PULMONARY FUNCTION VALUES

## NORMAL VALUES BASED ON THE USE OF PREDICTIVE EQUATIONS

The following values are based on the predictive equations provided in Appendix E:

### MALE SUBJECT

|  |  |  |  |
|---|---|---|---|
| Age = 25 | | Height = 177.8 cm (70 in.) | |
| Body Surface Area = 1.97 m$^2$ | | Weight = 79.5 kg (175 lb) | |
| FVC | 5.45 liter | SVC | 5.45 liter |
| FEV$_{0.5}$ | 3.41 liter | IC | 3.5 liter |
| FEV$_1$ | 4.37 liter | ERV | 2.0 liter |
| FEV$_3$ | 5.18 liter | RV | 1.8 liter |
| FEV$_1$/FVC | 85% | FRC | 3.8 liter |
| FEF$_{200-1200}$ | 8.46 l/sec | TLC | 7.2 liter* |
| PEFR | 9.71 l/sec | | 7.25 liter† |
| FEF$_{25\%}$ | 9.15 l/sec | RV/TLC | 25.3% |
| FEF$_{50\%}$ | 6.49 l/sec | D$_L$CO-SS | 24 ml CO/min/mm Hg |
| FEF$_{75\%}$ | 3.38 l/sec | D$_L$CO-SB | 33 ml CO/min/mm Hg |
| FEF$_{25\%-75\%}$ | 4.68 l/sec | | |
| FEF$_{75\%-85\%}$ | 1.54 l/sec | MIP | 130 cm H$_2$O |
| MVV | 144 l/min | MEP | 240 cm H$_2$O |

*TLC is based on a predictive equation.
†TLC is based on the predicted values for SVC + RV.

### FEMALE SUBJECT

|  |  |  |  |
|---|---|---|---|
| Age = 25 | | Height = 162.6 cm (64 in.) | |
| Body Surface Area = 1.6 m$^2$ | | Weight = 56.8 kg (125 lb) | |
| FVC | 3.91 liter | SVC | 3.91 liter |
| FEV$_{0.5}$ | 2.33 liter | IC | 2.5 liter |

| | | | |
|---|---|---|---|
| $FEV_1$ | 3.07 liter | ERV | 1.4 liter |
| $FEV_3$ | 3.48 liter | RV | 1.5 liter |
| $FEV_1/FVC$ | 87% | FRC | 2.9 liter |
| $FEF_{200-1200}$ | 5.83 l/sec | TLC | 5.2 liter* |
| PEFR | 6.43 l/sec | | 5.31 liter† |
| $FEF_{25\%}$ | 6.23 l/sec | RV/TLC | 28.3% |
| $FEF_{50\%}$ | 4.92 l/sec | $D_LCO$-SS | 21 ml CO/min/mm Hg |
| $FEF_{75\%}$ | 2.69 l/sec | $D_LCO$-SB | 22 ml CO/min/mm Hg |
| $FEF_{25\%-75\%}$ | 3.64 l/sec | | |
| $FEF_{75\%-85\%}$ | 1.39 l/sec | MIP | 90 cm $H_2O$ |
| MVV | 95 l/min | MEP | 160 cm $H_2O$ |

*TLC is based on a predictive equation.
†TLC is based on the predicted values for SVC + RV.

# GENERALLY ACCEPTED NORMAL VALUES

The following are generally accepted normal values:

| | | | |
|---|---|---|---|
| $C_L$ | 0.2 l/cm $H_2O$ | $R_{aw}$ | 1.5 cm $H_2O$/l/sec |
| $C_{LT}$ | 0.1 l/cm $H_2O$ | $SG_{aw}$ | 0.25 l/sec/cm $H_2O$ |

# EXAMPLES OF PREDICTIVE EQUATIONS FOR PULMONARY FUNCTION TESTING

## EXPLANATION FOR THE APPENDIX

This appendix provides examples of predictive equations for many of the typically measured pulmonary function parameters. This is not intended to serve as a list of recommended equations. Each laboratory must go through the process described in Chapter 7 in order to select the equations that will best serve its purposes. The equations presented here serve only as representative examples.

The format used to present these equations is not the same as that used in the original source literature. In the literature, the equations are generally presented in a more abbreviated format. For example, in the original literature, the equation for SVC for a male subject is presented in the following way:

$0.58H - 0.025A - 4.24$

The modified form for the equations was chosen for two reasons:

- To make more clear the mathematical procedure used for calculating the predicted value for a parameter.
- To create a more consistent presentation of the male and female subject versions of a given equation.

As an example of how the equations are used, here is the calculation for a predicted normal value for SVC for a 25-year-old male who is 177.8 cm (70 in.) tall.

$SVC = (0.0580 \times Ht) - (0.025 \times A) - 4.24$

$SVC = (0.0580 \times 177.8) - (0.025 \times 25) - 4.24$

$SVC = (10.3124) - (0.625) - 4.24$

$SVC = 5.45 \text{ liter}$

# PREDICTIVE EQUATIONS FOR ADULT MALE AND FEMALE SUBJECTS

Ht is height in centimeters (cm), A is age in years, and BSA is body surface area in square meters (m²).

## LUNG VOLUMES

| Parameter | Predictive Equation | Reference |
|---|---|---|
| **SVC (Same as for FVC)** | | 9 |
| Male | $(0.0580 \times Ht) - (0.025 \times A) - 4.24$ | |
| Female | $(0.0453 \times Ht) - (0.024 \times A) - 2.852$ | |
| **IC** | FVC − ERV | |
| **ERV** | FRC − RV | |
| **RV** | | 6 |
| Male | $(0.027 \times Ht) + (0.017 \times A) - 3.447$ | |
| Female | $(0.032 \times Ht) + (0.009 \times A) - 3.9$ | |
| **FRC** | | 6 |
| Male | $(0.0810 \times Ht) - (1.792 \times BSA) - 7.11$ | |
| Female | $(0.0421 \times Ht) - (0.00449 \times A) - 3.825*$ | |
| **TLC** | | 6 |
| Male | $(0.094 \times Ht) - (0.015 \times A) - 9.167$ | |
| Female | $(0.079 \times Ht) - (0.008 \times A) - 7.49$ | |
| **RV/TLC** | | 6 |
| Male | $(0.343 \times A) - 16.7$ | |
| Female | $(0.265 \times A) - 21.7$ | |

*This equation is modified to include a weight estimate as per pg. VI-3 of* Pulmonary Function Testing, *Intermountain Thoracic Society, 1975.*

## PULMONARY MECHANICS

| Parameter | Predictive Equation | Reference |
|---|---|---|
| **FVC (Same as for SVC)** | | 9 |
| Male | $(0.0580 \times Ht) - (0.025 \times A) - 4.24$ | |
| Female | $(0.0453 \times Ht) - (0.024 \times A) - 2.852$ | |

**FEV$_{0.5}$**                                                                                        7
   Male               $(0.037 \times Ht) - (0.017 \times A) - 2.746$
   Female          $(0.019 \times Ht) - (0.014 \times A) - 0.406$

**FEV$_1$**                                                                                             7
   Male               $(0.052 \times Ht) - (0.027 \times A) - 4.203$
   Female          $(0.027 \times Ht) - (0.021 \times A) - 0.794$

**FEV$_3$**                                                                                             7
   Male               $(0.063 \times Ht) - (0.031 \times A) - 5.245$
   Female          $(0.035 \times Ht) - (0.023 \times A) - 1.633$

**FEV$_1$/FVC**                                                                                         7
   Male               $103.62 - (0.087 \times Ht) - (0.140 \times A)$
   Female          $107.38 - (0.111 \times Ht) - (0.109 \times A)$

**FEF$_{200-1200}$**                                                                                    9
   Male               $(0.0429 \times Ht) - (0.047 \times A) + 2.010$
   Female          $(0.0570 \times Ht) - (0.036 \times A) - 2.532$

**PEFR**                                                                                                3
   Male               $(0.0567 \times Ht) - (0.024 \times A) + 0.225$
   Female          $(0.0354 \times Ht) - (0.018 \times A) + 1.130$

**FEF$_{25\%}$**                                                                                        7
   Male               $(0.088 \times Ht) - (0.035 \times A) - 5.618$
   Female          $(0.043 \times Ht) - (0.025 \times A) - 0.132$

**FEF$_{50\%}$**                                                                                        7
   Male               $(0.069 \times Ht) - (0.015 \times A) - 5.4$
   Female          $(0.035 \times Ht) - (0.013 \times A) - 0.444$

**FEF$_{75\%}$**                                                                                        7
   Male               $(0.044 \times Ht) - (0.012 \times A) - 4.143$
   Female          $3.042 - (0.014 \times A)$

**FEF$_{25\%-75\%}$**                                                                                   9
   Male               $(0.0185 \times Ht) - (0.045 \times A) + 2.513$
   Female          $(0.0236 \times Ht) - (0.030 \times A) + 0.551$

**FEF$_{75\%-85\%}$**                                                                                   8
   Male               $(0.0051 \times Ht) - (0.023 \times A) + 1.21$
   Female          $(0.0098 \times Ht) - (0.021 \times A) + 0.321$

**MVV**                                                                                                 3
   Male               $(1.19 \times Ht) - (0.816 \times A) - 37.9$
   Female          $(0.84 \times Ht) - (0.685 \times A) - 4.87$

**MIP**                                                                                                 2
   Male               $143 - (0.55 \times A)$
   Female          $104 - (0.51 \times A)$

**MEP**                                                                                                 2
   Male               $268 - (1.03 \times A)$
   Female          $170 - (0.53 \times A)$

## DIFFUSING CAPACITY

| Parameter | Predictive Equation | Reference |
|---|---|---|
| **D$_L$CO-SS** | | 1 |
| Male | $(0.709 \times Ht) - (0.27950 \times A) + 18.37$ | |
| Female | $(0.0677 \times Ht) - (0.25099 \times A) + 15.988$ | |
| **D$_L$CO-SB** | | 5 |
| Male | $(0.0984 \times Ht) - (0.177 \times A) + 19.93$ | |
| Female | $(0.1120 \times Ht) - (0.177 \times A) + 7.72$ | |

# PREDICTIVE EQUATIONS FOR MALE AND FEMALE CHILD SUBJECTS 5–17 YEARS OLD

Ht is height in inches, and A is age in years.

## LUNG VOLUMES

| Parameter | Predictive Equation | Reference |
|---|---|---|
| **FVC, SVC—Children 42–59 Inches Tall (107–150 cm)** | | 4 |
| Male | $(0.094 \times Ht) - 3.04$ | |
| Female | $(0.077 \times Ht) - 2.37$ | |
| **FVC, SVC—Children 60–78 Inches Tall (152–198 cm)** | | |
| Male | $(0.164 \times Ht) + (0.174 \times A) - 9.43$ | |
| Female | $(0.117 \times Ht) + (0.102 \times A) - 5.87$ | |
| **FRC** | $0.067 \times (e^{0.05334 \times H})*$ | 10 |
| **RV** | $0.033 \times (e^{0.05334 \times H})*$ | 10 |
| | where e is a constant with a value of 2.71828. | |
| **TLC** | $VC + RV$ | |
| **IC** | $TLC - FRC$ | |
| **ERV** | $VC - IC$ | |

*This same equation is used for all children 5–17 years old, with no differentiation made between height ranges.*

## PULMONARY MECHANICS

| Parameter | Predictive Equation | Reference |
|---|---|---|
| **FEV$_1$—Children 42–59 Inches Tall (107–150 cm)** | | 4 |
| Male | $(0.085 \times Ht) - 2.86$ | |
| Female | $(0.074 \times Ht) - 2.48$ | |
| **FEV$_1$—Children 60–78 Inches Tall (152–198 cm)** | | |
| Male | $(0.142 \times Ht) + (0.126 \times A) - 7.86$ | |
| Female | $(0.100 \times Ht) + (0.085 \times A) - 4.94$ | |
| **FEF$_{25\%-75\%}$—Children 42–59 Inches Tall (107–150 cm)** | | 4 |
| Male | $(0.094 \times Ht) - 2.61$ | |
| Female | $(0.087 \times Ht) - 2.39$ | |
| **FEF$_{25\%-75\%}$—Children 60–78 Inches Tall (152–198 cm)** | | |
| Male | $(0.135 \times Ht) + (0.126 \times A) - 6.50$ | |
| Female | $(0.093 \times Ht) + (0.083 \times A) - 3.50$ | |
| **PEFR—Children 42–59 Inches Tall (107–150 cm)** | | 4 |
| Male | $(0.161 \times Ht) - 5.88$ | |
| Female | $(0.130 \times Ht) - 4.51$ | |
| **PEFR—Children 60–78 Inches Tall (152–198 cm)** | | |
| Male | $(0.181 \times Ht) + (0.205 \times A) - 9.54$ | |
| Female | $(0.100 \times Ht) + (0.139 \times A) - 4.12$ | |
| **MVV—Regardless of Height** | | 4 |
| | $(3.18 \times Ht) - 134$ | |

## DIFFUSING CAPACITY

| Parameter | Predictive Equation | Reference |
|---|---|---|
| **D$_L$ CO-SB** | $(0.0693 \times Ht) - 20.13$ | 5 |

# REFERENCES

1. Bates D.V., P.T. Macklem, and R.V. Christie. *Respiratory Function in Disease.* Philadelphia: W.B. Saunders Company, 1971.
2. Black, L.F. and R.E. Hyatt. "Maximal Respiratory Pressures: Normal Values and Relationship to Age and Sex." *Am Rev Respir Dis* 99 (1969):696–702.
3. Cherniack, R.M. and M.D. Raber. "Normal Standards for Ventilatory Function Using an Automated Wedge Spirometer." *Am Rev Respir Dis* 106 (1972):38.
4. Dickman, M.L., C.D. Schmidt, and R.M. Gardner. "Spirometric Standards for Normal Children and Adolescents (Ages 5 Through 18 Years)." *Am Rev Respir Dis* 104 (1971):680.
5. Gaensler, E.A. and G.W. Wright. "Evaluation of Respiratory Impairment." *Arch Environ Health* 12 (1966):146.
6. Goldman, H.I. and M.R. Becklake. "Respiratory Function Tests: Normal Value at Median Altitude and Predictions of Normal Results." *Am Rev Respir Dis* 76 (1959):457–467.
7. Knudson, R.J., R.C. Slatin, M.D. Lebowitz, and B. Burrows. "The Maximal Expiratory Flow Volume Curve Normal Standards Variability and Effects of Age." *Am Rev Respir Dis* 113 (1976):587–600.
8. Morris, J.F., A. Koski, and J.D. Breese. "Normal Values and Evaluation of Forced End-Expiratory Flow." *Am Rev Respir Dis* 111 (1975):755–762.
9. Morris, J.F., A. Koski, and L.C. Johnson. "Spirometric Standards for Healthy Non-Smoking Adults." *Am Rev Respir Dis* 103 (1971):57–67.
10. Weng, T.R. and H. Levison. "Standards of Pulmonary Function in Children." *Am Rev Respir Dis* 99 (1969):879–894.

# APPENDIX F

# INFECTION CONTROL

## THE NEED FOR INFECTION CONTROL PRACTICES

The pulmonary function testing laboratory is not considered a major potential source of infection in the health care setting. However, contaminated laboratory equipment can be a source of infection. Contaminated equipment can result in infection being transmitted between different subjects who use the equipment and between the subjects and laboratory personnel.

Pathogens are generally spread by one of two mechanisms, airborne transfer or physical contact. Airborne contamination is a risk in the pulmonary function testing laboratory. Some breathing maneuvers, such as the one performed for an FVC test, can result in mucus, saliva, or small droplets of other material being made airborne and deposited in breathing circuits. As a result, proper equipment disinfection and infection control procedures are necessary to prevent the further spread of the infection.

In the laboratory, physical-contact infection can result from testing equipment that is poorly disinfected before reuse. It should be noted, though, that hand-carried contamination by health care workers is the number one source of infection in a hospital. Even if equipment starts out being properly disinfected, it can be contaminated by the technologist during its assembly and use. Correct handwashing procedures are essential to limiting physical-contact infection problems.

It is very important to have clear-cut infection control guidelines in a laboratory's procedure manual. The guidelines should include information on handwashing, changing and cleaning of equipment, use of protective equipment such as gloves and masks, and how to handle special problems with subjects who have infections with hepatitis B, the human immunodeficiency virus (HIV), *Pneumocystis carinii*, tuberculosis, or other significant organisms.

Following are general guidelines for infection control in the pulmonary function testing laboratory.

# GUIDELINES FOR INFECTION CONTROL PRACTICES

## HANDWASHING

A thorough handwashing procedure should be performed at the start and at the end of the work day in the laboratory. Handwashing procedures must be performed between testing sessions with subjects and before and after handling any subject-related equipment.

## BACTERIA FILTERS

One way of preventing breathing circuit contamination by the subject's breathing maneuvers is to use a bacteria filter, sometimes at the subject connection. Care must be taken in selecting a filter for use, however. Because some filters can retain excessive moisture from exhaled air, a filter may begin to produce a resistance to airflow. Although this may not be noticed significantly by the subject, it can affect some of the more sensitive measurements made by the equipment.

With some tests, the volume of breathing circuit components must be considered in the calculations. Depending on its placement in the circuit, the volume of the bacteria filter may have to be determined and included in the calculation.

## CHANGING OF EQUIPMENT BETWEEN SUBJECTS

The guidelines for changing equipment components between subjects can vary considerably between testing systems. It is important, therefore, that the equipment manufacturer's guidelines be followed. Minimally, the mouthpiece of the breathing circuit must be changed between subjects. Breathing circuit tubing and valves will often also have to be changed.

## USE OF DISPOSABLES

Where cost-effective, the use of disposable mouthpieces and other equipment can minimize the risk of contamination. This works effectively, however, only if proper handwashing is performed by the technologist before the equipment is connected to the testing system.

Nebulizers are used for the administration of tests such as bronchodilator-benefit studies and bronchoprovocation studies. Unfortunately, because they are designed to generate particulate water/medication for deposition in the subject's airways, they are a significant potential source of infection. If possible, disposable, single-use nebulizers should be used by a laboratory.

In some instances, metered-dose inhalers are used for bronchodilator-benefit studies. Disposable mouthpieces and/or disposable reservoir systems can be used to minimize the risk of contamination and infection.

## CLEANING OF EQUIPMENT

Nondisposable mouthpieces, if used, will need to be disinfected or sterilized after each use. With many systems, tubing and other nondisposable test system components will require disinfection after each test. Equipment that has undergone disinfection or sterilization must be stored correctly in sealed plastic bags.

If nondisposable nebulizer units are used they must be *sterilized* after each use. The sterilization procedure should be one that is effective in destroying pathologic organisms (i.e., vegetative organisms, tubercle bacilli, fungal spores, and some viruses).

The cleaning and maintenance needs of spirometers can differ significantly. The spirometer manufacturer's recommendations should be followed. Many primary flow measuring spirometers have the flow sensor placed near the subject connection. In this case, the sensor should be cleaned daily. Flow sensors placed more distal from the subject in a breathing circuit can be cleaned less often. Where disposable flow sensors are used, they should be used only once and then disposed of properly.

Water-sealed spirometers require a greater level of maintenance. They should be drained and refilled on a weekly basis. Once drained, they should be permitted to dry completely before being refilled. The water used for refilling should be sterile, distilled (deionized) water. Dry rolling seal and bellows-type spirometers should be maintained on a regular schedule as recommended by the manufacturer.

## USE OF PROTECTIVE BARRIERS

Gloves, or some other protective barrier, should be used by the technologist in removing the mouthpiece from a breathing circuit after it has been used. This is particularly true if a test has been performed on a subject who has a documented infection. In some instances, depending on the infectious nature of the subject, it may be appropriate for the technologist to wear a mask while in contact with the subject.

## INFECTION SURVEILLANCE

It is important to document that a laboratory's infection control practices are successful. This is done by performing regular infection surveillance procedures. These surveillance procedures include routinely culturing swab samples taken from "clean" reusable equipment and, occasionally, new disposable equipment. Infection surveillance is especially important for equipment that is likely to come in contact with a subject's mucous membranes.

# PRECAUTIONS FOR HANDLING BLOOD AND OTHER POTENTIALLY INFECTIOUS BODY FLUIDS

Precautions relating to the handling of blood and certain other body fluids have been established by the Centers for Disease Control. These precautions are built on four basic practices:

1. All blood and body fluid samples *must* be treated as if they are potentially contaminated.

2. Proper care must be taken when handling needles, lancets, scalpels, and other sharp instruments.
3. Protective barriers such as lab coats/gowns, gloves, goggles, and masks should be worn.
4. Hands and other skin surfaces potentially contaminated with the blood and/or fluids must be washed immediately and thoroughly. Disposal sinks and sites of blood spills should be cleaned well.

These precautions relate to the possible transmission of human immunovirus (HIV) and hepatitis B infections. Transmission of other pathogens may be prevented as well by use of the precautions. Table F-1 provides specific information on the precautions for handling blood and other body fluids.

---

### TABLE F–1  Guidelines for Handling Blood and Other Potentially Infectious Body Fluids

#### Fluids Requiring Use of the Universal Precautions

- Blood, amniotic fluid, cerebrospinal fluid, pericardial fluid, pleural fluid, semen, synovial fluid, and vaginal secretions.

#### Fluids Requiring Precautions Only If They Contain Blood

- Sputum, nasal secretions, sweat, tears, vomitus, urine, and feces.

#### Precautions for Handling Needles and Other Sharp Objects

- The following *should not* be done by hand:
  1. Resheathing of used needles.
  2. Removal of needles from disposable syringes.
  3. Bending or breaking of needles.
- A rubber cube or block should be used to obstruct the needle after an arterial puncture is performed.
- Sharps must be disposed of in an approved puncture-resistant container. Disposal containers should be located in all areas where sharps are likely to be used.

#### Use of Protective Barriers

- A lab coat or gown must be worn in any clinical area where there is the possibility of exposure to blood or other body fluids of concern.
- Gloves must be worn in the following situations, especially if the technologist has any cuts, scratches, raw patches, or other breaks in the skin.
  1. When drawing blood samples by any method or while working in clinical setting, such as the emergency department, where contact with free-flowing blood or other body fluids is likely.*

2. When handling blood samples for analysis in the laboratory setting.
3. When performing preventative maintenance or repair procedures on blood analysis equipment (e.g., emptying waste containers, maintenance/repair of electrodes or machine tubing, etc.).
4. In situations where hand contact may be made with the mucous membranes of a subject.

• Masks and goggles should be worn in situations where blood or other body fluids may be splashed (e.g., emergency department, arterial catheterization procedure, etc.).

---

## Cleaning of Disposal Sinks and Blood Spills

---

• A 0.5% bleach solution should be used for cleaning of sinks and spills. The solution may be made by mixing one part regular liquid bleach (5% sodium hypochlorite) with nine parts water.

---

*Gloves cannot prevent puncture injuries by sharp objects. Even with gloves, care must be taken to avoid puncturing and cutting the technologist's gloves and hands.*

# APPENDIX G

# REFERENCE SOURCES FOR TESTING STANDARDS AND GUIDELINES

The American Thoracic Society (ATS) and the American Association for Respiratory Care (AARC) both publish standards or guidelines for testing. Access to these references is available through the journals published by these organizations. Guidelines published by the AARC are also available through the Internet. Provided below is a listing of published sources for testing standards and guidelines from these organizations. Additionally, Internet addresses for other pulmonary medicine–oriented organizations are provided.

## ATS STANDARDS

The ATS publishes standards for pulmonary function testing in its journal, *American Journal of Respiratory and Critical Care Medicine*. These standards are updated and republished periodically. Listed below are the most current published standards from the ATS and the journal references that contain them:

"Standardization of Spirometry—1994 Update." *Am J Respir Crit Care Med* 152 (1995):1107–1136.

"Single-Breath Carbon Monoxide Diffusing Capacity (Transfer Factor), Recommendations for a Standard Technique—1995 Update." *Am J Respir Crit Care Med* 152 (1995):2185–2198.

"Standards for the Diagnosis and Care of Patients with Chronic Obstructive Pulmonary Disease." *Am J Respir Crit Care Med* 152 (1995):S77–S120.

"Respiratory Function Measurements in Infants: Measurement Conditions." *Am J Respir Crit Care Med* 151 (1995):2058–2064.

"Respiratory Function Measurements in Infants: Symbols, Abbreviations, and Units." *Am J Respir Crit Care Med* 151 (1995):2041–2057.

The ATS has a site on the World Wide Web. The address of this site is **http://www.thoracic.org/**. Although this site does not provide the ability to download standards on pulmonary function testing, it may still serve as a source of other useful information.

# AARC CLINICAL PRACTICE GUIDELINES

The AARC publishes guidelines to standardize the quality of respiratory care services. A number of these guidelines cover topics that relate to pulmonary function testing, blood gases, exercise testing, and indirect calorimetry.

There are two sources for these guidelines. One is the AARC's journal, *Respiratory Care*. The other is the AARC's World Wide Web site. Copies of the clinical practice guidelines can be downloaded from this site. The address for the AARC web site is **http://www.aarc.org/**. Following are the AARC clinical practice guidelines that relate to topics in this book and the journal references that contain them:

## CLINICAL PRACTICE GUIDELINES RELATING TO PULMONARY FUNCTION TESTING

AARC Clinical Practice Guideline, "Single-Breath Carbon Monoxide Diffusing Capacity." *Respir Care* 38 (1993):511–515.

AARC Clinical Practice Guideline, "Static Lung Volumes." *Respir Care* 39 (1994): 830–836.

AARC Clinical Practice Guideline, "Body Plethysmography." *Respir Care* 39 (1994): 1184–1190.

AARC Clinical Practice Guideline, "Spirometry, 1996 Update." *Respir Care* 41 (1996): 629–636.

AARC Clinical Practice Guideline, "Assessing Response to Bronchodilator Therapy at Point of Care." *Respir Care* 40 (1995):1300–1307.

AARC Clinical Practice Guideline, "Bronchial Provocation." *Respir Care* 37 (1992): 902–906.

## CLINICAL PRACTICE GUIDELINES RELATING TO PEDIATRIC PULMONARY FUNCTION TESTING

AARC Clinical Practice Guideline, "Infant/Toddler Pulmonary Function Tests." *Respir Care* 40 (1995):761–768.

## CLINICAL PRACTICE GUIDELINES RELATING TO BLOOD GASES

AARC Clinical Practice Guideline, "Pulse Oximetry." *Respir Care* 36 (1991): 1406–1409.

AARC Clinical Practice Guideline, "Sampling for Arterial Blood Gas Analysis." *Respir Care* 37 (1992):913–917.

AARC Clinical Practice Guideline, "In-Vitro pH and Blood Gas Analysis and Hemoximetry." *Respir Care* 38 (1993):505–510.

AARC Clinical Practice Guideline, "Transcutaneous Blood Gas Monitoring for Neonatal and Pediatric Patients." *Respir Care* 39 (1994):1176–1179.

AARC Clinical Practice Guideline, "Capnography/Capnometry During Mechanical Ventilation." *Respir Care* 40 (1995):1321–1324.

## CLINICAL PRACTICE GUIDELINES RELATING TO EXERCISE TESTING

AARC Clinical Practice Guideline, "Exercise Testing for Evaluation of Hypoxemia and/or Desaturation." *Respir Care* 37 (1992):907–912.

## CLINICAL PRACTICE GUIDELINES RELATING TO INDIRECT CALORIMETRY

AARC Clinical Practice Guideline, "Metabolic Measurements Using Indirect Calorimetry During Mechanical Ventilation." *Respir Care* 39 (1994):1170–1175.

# INTERNET ADDRESSES FOR OTHER PULMONARY MEDICINE-ORIENTED ORGANIZATIONS

Although these organizations do not publish standards or guidelines for testing, communication with them through Internet connections can provide access to useful professional information.

American College of Chest Physicians—**http://www.chestnet.org/**
American Lung Association—**http://www.lungusa.org/**
Centers for Disease Control—**http://www.cdc.gov/**
Food and Drug Administration—**http://www.fda.gov/**
National Institute of Occupational Safety and Health—**http://www.cdc.gov/niosh/**
Occupational Safety and Health Administration—**http://www.osha.gov/**
American Academy of Allergy, Asthma, and Immunology—**http://www.aaaai.org/**
American Association for Cardiovascular and Pulmonary Rehabilitation—**http://www.jhbmc.jhu.edu/aacvpu/**

# BIBLIOGRAPHY

American Association for Respiratory Care. AARC Clinical Practice Guideline, "Pulse Oximetry." *Respir Care* 36 (1991):1406–1409.

American Association for Respiratory Care. AARC Clinical Practice Guideline, "Broncial Provocation." *Respir Care* 37 (1992):902–906.

American Association for Respiratory Care. AARC Clinical Practice Guideline, "Exercise Testing for Evaluation of Hypoxemia and/or Desaturation." *Respir Care* 37 (1992):907–912.

American Association for Respiratory Care. AARC Clinical Practice Guideline, "Sampling for Arterial Blood Gas Analysis." *Respir Care* 37 (1992):913–917.

American Association for Respiratory Care. AARC Clinical Practice Guideline, "In-Vitro pH and Blood Gas Analysis and Hemoximetry." *Respir Care* 38 (1993):505–510.

American Association for Respiratory Care. AARC Clinical Practice Guideline, "Single-Breath Carbon Monoxide Diffusing Capacity." *Respir Care* 38 (1993):511–515.

American Association for Respiratory Care. AARC Clinical Practice Guideline, "Static Lung Volumes." *Respir Care* 39 (1994):830–836.

American Association for Respiratory Care. AARC Clinical Practice Guideline, "Metabolic Measurements Using Indirect Calorimetry During Mechanical Ventilation." *Respir Care* 39 (1994):1170–1175.

American Association for Respiratory Care. AARC Clinical Practice Guideline, "Transcutaneous Blood Gas Monitoring for Neonatal and Pediatric Patients." *Respir Care* 39 (1994):1176–1179.

American Association for Respiratory Care. AARC Clinical Practice Guideline, "Body Plethysmography." *Respir Care* 39 (1994):1184–1190.

American Association for Respiratory Care. AARC Clinical Practice Guideline, "Infant/Toddler Pulmonary Function Tests." *Respir Care* 40 (1995):761–768.

American Association for Respiratory Care. AARC Clinical Practice Guideline, "Assessing Response to Bronchodilator Therapy at Point of Care." *Respir Care* 40 (1995):1300–1307.

American Association for Respiratory Care. AARC Clinical Practice Guideline, "Capnography/Capnometry During Mechanical Ventilation." *Respir Care* 40 (1995):1321–1324.

American Association for Respiratory Care. AARC Clinical Practice Guideline, "Spirometry, 1996 Update." *Respir Care* 41 (1996):629–636.

American College of Sports Medicine. *Guidelines for Graded Exercise Testing and Exercise Prescription.* Philadelphia: Lea & Febiger, 1980.

Apelgren, K.N., J.L. Rombeau, P.L. Twomey, and R.A. Miller. "Comparison of Nutritional Indices and Outcomes in Critically Ill Patients." *Crit Care Med* 10(5) (1982):305–307.

Askanazi, J., S.H. Rosenbaum, A.I. Hyman, P.A. Silverberg, J. Milic-Emili, and J.M. Kinney. "Respiratory Changes Induced by the Large Glucose Loads of Total Parenteral Nutrition." *JAMA* 243(14) (1980):1444–1447.

Ayers, L.N., B.J. Whipp, and I. Ziment. *A Guide to the Interpretation of Pulmonary Function Tests.* New York: Roerig, 1978.

Bageant, R.A. "Oxygen Analyzers." *Respir Care* 21(5) (1976):410–416.

Ballard, R.D., P.L. Kelly, and R.J. Martin. "Estimates of Ventilation from Inductance Plethysmography in Sleeping Asthmatic Patients." *Chest* 92(1) (1988):128–133.

Barnes, T.A. *Respiratory Care Practice.* Chicago: Year Book Medical Publisher, Inc., 1988.

Bates D.V., P.T. Macklem, and R.V. Christie. *Respiratory Function in Disease.* Philadelphia: W.B. Saunders Company, 1971.

Bergner, E.C. *The Physiology of Adequate Perfusion.* St. Louis: The C.V. Mosby Company, 1979.

Black, L.F. and R.E. Hyatt. "Maximal Respiratory Pressures: Normal Values and Relationship to Age and Sex." *Am Rev Respir Dis* 99 (1969):696–702.

Browning J.A., S.E. Linberg, S.Z. Turney, and P. Chodoff. "The Effects of a Fluctuating $FIO_2$ on Metabolic Measurements in Mechanically Ventilated Patients." *Crit Care Med* 10(2) (1982):82–85.

Burrows, B. "Pulmonary Diffusion and Alveolar-Capillary Block." *Medical Clinics of North America* 51(2) (1967):427–438.

Burrows, B., R.D. Knudson, and L.J. Kettel. *Respiratory Insufficiency.* Chicago: Year Book Medical Publishers, Inc., 1975.

Burton, G.G. and J.E. Hodgkin. *Respiratory Care Practice: A Guide to Clinical Practice.* 3d ed. Philadelphia: J.B. Lippincott Company, 1991.

Cherniack, R.M. *Pulmonary Function Testing.* Philadelphia: W.B. Saunders Company, 1977.

Cherniack, R.M. and L. Cherniack. *Respiration in Health and Disease.* 3d ed. Philadelphia: W.B. Saunders Company, 1983.

Cherniack, R.M. and M.D. Raber. "Normal Standards for Ventilatory Function Using an Automated Wedge Spirometer." *Am Rev Respir Dis* 106 (1972):38.

Clausen, J. *Pulmonary Function Testing Guidelines and Controversies: Equipment, Methods, and Normal Values.* Orlando: Grune & Stratton, Inc., 1982.

Coates, A.L., K.J. Desmond, D. Demizio, P. Allen, and P.H. Beaudry. "Sources of Error in Flow-Volume Curves: Effect of Expired Volume Measured at the Mouth vs. Measured in a Body Plethysmograph." *Chest* 94(5) (1988):976–982.

Coates, J.E. *Lung Function: Assessment and Application in Medicine.* 2d ed. Philadelphia: F.A. Davis Company, 1968.

"Computer Guidelines for Pulmonary Laboratories." *Am Rev Respir Dis* 136 (1987):628–629.

Comroe, J.H. *Physiology of Respiration: An Introductory Text.* Chicago: Year Book Medical Publishers, Inc., 1965.

Comroe, J.H., R.E. Forster, A.B. Dubois, W.A. Briscoe, and E. Carlsen. *The Lung: Clinical Physiology and Pulmonary Function Tests*. Chicago: Year Book Medical Publishers, Inc., 1962.

Coultas, D.B., C.A. Howard, B.J. Skipper, and J.M. Samet. "Spirometric Prediction Equations for Hispanic Children and Adults in New Mexico." *Am Rev Respir Dis* 138 (1988):1386–1392.

Crapo, R.O., A.H. Morris, and R.M. Gardner. "Reference Spirometric Values Using Techniques and Equipment That Meet ATS Recommendations." *Am Rev Respir Dis* 123 (1981):659–664.

Dantzker, D. *Cardiopulmonary Critical Care*. 2d ed. Philadelphia: W.B. Saunders Company, 1991.

Dejours, P. *Respiration*. New York: Oxford Press 1966.

Des Jardins, T.R. *Clinical Manifestations of Respiratory Disease.* Chicago: Year Book Medical Publishers, Inc., 1984.

Des Jardins, T.R. *Cardiopulmonary Anatomy and Physiology: Essentials for Respiratory Care*. Albany: Delmar Publisher, Inc., 1988.

Dickman, M.L., C.D. Schmidt, and R.M. Gardner. "Spirometric Standards for Normal Children and Adolescents (Ages 5 Through 18 Years)." *Am Rev Respir Dis* 104 (1971):680.

*Dorland's Illustrated Medical Dictionary*. 25th ed. Philadelphia: W.B. Saunders Company, 1974.

"Evaluation of Impairment/Disability Secondary to Respiratory Disease." *Am Rev Respir Dis* 126 (1982):945–951.

Farzan, S. *A Concise Handbook of Respiratory Diseases*. 3d ed. Norwalk: Appleton & Lange, 1992.

Ferris, B.G. (Principle Investigator). "Epidemiology Standardization Project." *Am Rev Respir Dis* 118 (1978):55–88.

Filley, F.G. *Acid-Base and Blood Gas Regulation*. Philadelphia: Lea & Febiger, 1972.

Fishman, A.P. *Assessment of Pulmonary Function*. New York: McGraw-Hill Book Company, 1980.

Frye, M., R. DiBenedetto, D. Lain, and K. Morgan. "Single Arterial Puncture vs. Arterial Cannula for Arterial Gas Analysis After Exercise: Change in Arterial Oxygen Tension Over Time." *Chest* 93(2) (1988):294–298.

Gaensler, E.A. and G.W. Wright. "Evaluation of Respiratory Impairment." *Arch Environ Health* 12 (1966):146–189.

Gieseke, T., G. Gurushanthaiah, and F.L. Glauser. "Effects of Carbohydrates on Carbon Dioxide Excretion in Patients with Airway Disease." *Chest* 71(1) (1977):55–58.

Goldman, H.I. and M.R. Becklake. "Respiratory Function Tests: Normal Value at Median Altitude and Predictions of Normal Results." *Am Rev Respir Dis* 76 (1959):457–467.

Green, J.F. *Fundamental Cardiovascular and Pulmonary Physiology*. Philadelphia: Lea & Febiger, 1987.

Guyton, A.C. *Basic Human Physiology: Normal Function and Mechanisms of Disease*. Philadelphia: W.B. Saunders Company, 1971.

Harris, W.H. and J.S. Levey. *The New Columbia Encyclopedia.* New York: Columbia University Press, 1975.

Hathirat, S., A.D. Renzetti, and M. Mitchell. "Measurement of the Total Lung Capacity by Helium Dilution in a Constant Volume System." *Am Rev Respir Dis* 102 (1970):760–770.

Hess, D. "Capnometry and Capnography: Technical Aspects, Physiologic Aspects and Clinical Application." *Resp Care* 35(6) (1990):557–576.

Hess, D. "Measurement of Maximal Inspiratory Pressure: A Call for Standardization." *Respir Care* 34 (1989):857–859.

Hyatt, R.E. and L.F. Black. "The Flow-Volume Curve: A Current Perspective." *Am Rev Respir Dis* 107 (1973):191–193.

Jensen, J.T. *Physics for the Health Sciences.* Philadelphia: J.B. Lippincott Company, 1976.

Jones, N.L. "Exercise Testing in Pulmonary Evaluation: Rationale, Methods and the Normal Respiratory Response to Exercise." *N Engl J Med* 293(11) (1975):541–44.

Jones, N.L., E.J. Campbell, R.H.T. Edwards, and D.G. Robertson. *Clinical Exercise Testing.* Philadelphia: W.B. Saunders Company, 1975.

Kapp, M.C., E.N. Schachter, G.J. Beck, L.R. Maunder, and T.J. Witek. "The Shape of the Maximum Expiratory Flow Volume Curve." *Chest* 94(4) (1988):799–806.

Kavanah, P. *Brief Review in Chemistry.* New York: Cebco Standard Publishing Company, 1972.

Knudson, R.J., R.C. Slatin, M.D. Lebowitz, and B. Burrows. "The Maximal Expiratory Flow Volume Curve Normal Standards Variability and Effects of Age." *Am Rev Respir Dis* 113 (1976):587–600.

Kory, R.C., R. Callahan, H.G. Boren, and J.C. Syner. "The Veterans Administration-Army Cooperative Study of Pulmonary Function." *Am J Med* 30 (1961):243–258.

Lane, L.E. and J.F. Walker. *Clinical Arterial Blood Gas Analysis.* St. Louis: The C.V. Mosby Company, 1987.

Larka L. and D.M. Greenbaum. "Effectiveness of Intensive Nutritional Regimes in Patients Who Fail to Wean from Mechanical Ventilation." *Crit Care Med* 10(5) (1982):297–300.

Lodrup Carlsen, K., P. Magnus, and K. Carlsen. "Lung Function by Tidal Breathing in Awake Healthy Newborn Infants." *Eur Respir J* 7 (1994):1660–1668.

MacNamara, J., F.J. Prime, and J.D. Sinclair. "An Assessment of the Steady-State Carbon Monoxide Method of Estimating Pulmonary Diffusing Capacity." *Thorax* 14 (1959):166–175.

Manahan, S.E. *Quantitative Chemical Analysis.* Monterey: Brooks/Cole Publishing Company, 1986.

Marcus, E.B., A.S. Buist, J.D. Curb, C.J. MacLean, D.M. Reed, L.R. Johnson, and K. Yano. "Correlates of $FEV_1$ and Prevalence of Pulmonary Conditions in Japanese-American Men." *Am Rev Respir Dis* 138 (1988):1398–1404.

Martin, D.E. and J.W. Youtsey. *Respiratory Anatomy and Physiology.* St. Louis: The C.V. Mosby Company, 1988.

Martin, T., J. Zeballos, and I. Weisman. "Gas Exchange During Maximal Upper Extremity Exercise." *Chest* 99 (1991):420–425.

McArdle, W. *Exercise Physiology: Energy, Nutrition, and Human Performance.* Philadelphia: Lea & Febiger, 1991.

McElvaney, G., S. Blackie, N.J. Morrison, P.G. Wilcox, M.S. Fairbarn, and R.L. Pardy. "Maximum Static Respiratory Pressures in the Normal Elderly." *Am Rev Respir Dis* 139 (1989):277–281.

McPherson, S.P. and C.B. Spearman. *Respiratory Therapy Equipment.* 3d ed. St. Louis: The C.V. Mosby Company, 1985.

Mitchell, R.S. and T.L. Petty. *Synopsis of Clinical Pulmonary Disease.* 3d ed. St. Louis: The C.V. Mosby Company, 1982.

Moran, R.F. "Assessment of Quality Control of Blood Gas/pH Analyzer Performance." *Resp Care* 26(6) (1981):538–546.

Morris, J.F., A. Koski, and J.D. Breese. "Normal Values and Evaluation of Forced End-Expiratory Flow." *Am Rev Respir Dis* 111 (1975):755–762.

Morris, J.F., A. Koski, and L.C. Johnson. "Spirometric Standards for Healthy Non-Smoking Adults." *Am Rev Respir Dis* 103 (1971):57–67.

Morris, J.F., A. Koski, W.P. Temple, A. Claremont, and D.R. Thomas. "Fifteen-Year Interval Spirometric Evaluation of the Oregon Predictive Equations." *Chest* 92(1) (1988):123–127.

Murray, J.F. *The Normal Lung: The Basis for Diagnosis and Treatment of Pulmonary Disease.* Philadelphia: W.B. Saunders Company, 1976.

Nave, C.R. and B.C. Nave. *Physics for the Health Sciences.* Philadelphia: W.B. Saunders Company, 1985.

Neukirch, F., R. Chansin, R. Liard, M. Levallois, and P. Leproux. "Spirometry and Maximal Expiratory Flow-Volume Curve Reference Standards for Polynesian, European, and Chinese Teenagers." *Chest* 94(4) (1988):792–798.

Ogilvie, C.M., R.E. Forster, W.S. Blakemore, and J.W. Morton. "A Standardized Breath Holding Technique for the Clinical Measurement of the Diffusing Capacity of the Lung for Carbon Monoxide." *J Clin Invest* 36 (1957):1–17.

"Quality Assurance in Pulmonary Function Laboratories." *Am Rev Respir Dis* 136 (1987):625–627.

"Respiratory Function Measurements in Infants: Measurement Conditions." *Am J Respir Crit Care Med* 151 (1995):2058–2064.

"Respiratory Function Measurements in Infants: Symbols, Abbreviations, and Units." *Am J Respir Crit Care Med* 151 (1995):2041–2057.

Rosendorff, C. *Clinical Cardiovascular and Pulmonary Physiology.* New York: Raven Press, 1983.

Rosenthal, R.R., B.L. Laube, D.B. Hood, and P.S. Norman. "Analysis of Refractory Period after Exercise and Eucapnic Voluntary Hyperventilation Challenge." *Am Rev Respir Dis* 141 (1990):368–372.

Ruppel, G. *Manual of Pulmonary Function Testing.* 6th ed. St. Louis: The C.V. Mosby Company, 1994.

Saltzman, H.A. and J.V. Salzano. "Effects of Carbohydrate Metabolism upon Respiratory Gas Exchange in Normal Men." *J Appl Sci* 30(2) (1971):228–231.

Schwartz, J.D., S.A. Katz, R.W. Fegley, and M.S. Tockman. "Analysis of Spirometric Data from a National Sample of Healthy 6– to 24–Year-Olds (NHANES II)." *Am Rev Respir Dis* 138 (1988):1405–1414.

Schwartz, J.D., S.A. Katz, R.W. Fegley, and M.S. Tockman. "Sex and Race Difference in the Development of Lung Function." *Am Rev Respir Dis* 138 (1988):1415–1421.

Shane, J.G. *Programming for Microcomputers, Apple II Basic.* Boston: Houghton Mifflin Company, 1983.

Shapiro, B.A., R.A. Harrison, R.D. Cane, and R. Kozlowski-Templin. *Clinical Application of Blood Gases.* 4th ed. Chicago: Year Book Medical Publishers, 1989.

Sienko, J.M. and R.A. Plane. *Chemistry.* New York: McGraw-Hill Book Company, 1971.

"Single-Breath Carbon Monoxide Diffusing Capacity (Transfer Factor), Recommendations for a Standard Technique—1995 Update." *Am J Respir Crit Care Med* 152 (1995):2185–2198.

Skoog, D.A. and D.A. West. *Fundamentals in Analytical Chemistry.* 4th ed. Philadelphia: Saunders College Publishing, 1982.

Slonim, N.B. and L.H. Hamilton. *Respiratory Physiology.* St. Louis: The C.V. Mosby Company, 1987.

"Standards for the Diagnosis and Care of Patients with Chronic Obstructive Pulmonary Disease." *Am J Respir Crit Care Med* 152 (1995):S77–S120.

"Standization of Spirometry—1994 Update." *Am J Respir Crit Care Med* 152 (1995):1107–1136.

Steen, D. "The Guts Behind the Glory." *PC World* 11(2) (1988):91–98.

Tilley, D.E. and W. Thumm. *Physics for College Students: With Applications to the Life Sciences.* Menlo Park: Cummings Publishing Company, 1974.

Tortora, G.J. and N.P. Anagnostakos. *Principles of Anatomy and Physiology.* New York: Harper & Row, 1984.

Villee, C.A. and V.G. Dethier. *Biological Principles and Processes.* Philadelphia: W.B. Saunders Company, 1971.

Wanger, J. *Pulmonary Function Testing: A Practical Approach.* 2d ed. Baltimore: Williams & Wilkins, 1996.

Warren, R.H. and S.H. Alderson. "The Accuracy of Respiratory Inductive Plethysmography in Measuring Breathing Patterns of Sedated Piglets Receiving Controlled Mechanical Ventilation." *Respir Care* 33(10) (1988):846–851.

Wasserman, K., J.E. Hansen, D.Y. Sue, and B.J. Whipp. *Principles of Exercise Testing and Interpretation.* Philadelphia: Lea & Febiger, 1987.

Weng, T.R. and H. Levison. "Standards of Pulmonary Function in Children." *Am Rev Respir Dis* 99 (1969):879–894.

West, J.B. *Respiratory Physiology: The Essentials.* Baltimore: Williams & Wilkins, 1985.

Whitman, R.A. *Body Plethysmography.* Dallas: The American Association for Respiratory Care, 1978.

Wilkes, D.L., M. Revow, M.H. Bryan, and S.J. England. "Evaluation of Respiratory Inductive Plethysmography in Infants Weighing Less Than 1,500 Grams." *Am Rev Respir Dis* 136 (1987):416–419.

Wilkins, R.L., R.L. Sheldon, and S.J. Krider. *Clinical Assessment in Respiratory Care.* St. Louis: The C.V. Mosby Company, 1985.

Williams, F.H. and H.Z. Bencowitz. "Differences in Plethysmographic Lung Volumes: Effects of Linked vs. Unlinked Spirometry." *Chest* 95(1) (1989):117–123.

Wilson, A.F. *Pulmonary Function Testing: Indications and Interpretations.* Orlando: Grune & Stratton, Inc., 1985.

Wine, R.L. *Statistics for Scientists and Engineers.* Englewood Cliffs, NJ: Prentice-Hall, Inc., 1964.

Withers, R.T., M.A. Bourdon, and A. Crockett. "Lung Volume Standards for Healthy Male Lifetime Nonsmokers." *Chest* 92(1) (1988):91–97.

Wojciechowski, W.V. and W.B. Davis. *Respiratory Care Sciences: An Integrated Approach.* New York: John Wiley & Sons, 1985.

*The Wright Respirometer: Instruction and Training Manual.* Cleveland: The Harris Calorific Company.

# GLOSSARY

**absorption atelectasis**—alveolar collapse that results from alveolar gas absorption into the pulmonary capillaries. It is more likely to occur in subjects who are breathing high concentrations of oxygen or have airway obstruction to the affected alveoli.

**acid**—a substance in solution that, to some degree, undergoes a dissociation to release a proton ($H^+$). The resulting increase in $H^+$ concentration in the solution is what makes the solution more acid (reduces the pH value). An example of this is hydrochloric acid (HCl), where

$$HCl \longleftrightarrow H^+ + Cl^-$$

**acidotic**—a condition in which the blood has a higher than normal free $H^+$ concentration and is therefore more acid than normal (i.e., the pH is less than 7.35).

**adsorption**—the attraction and attachment of one substance to the surface of another. It can be used as a physical filtration or substance-trapping mechanism.

**A-D (analog/digital) converter**—a device that converts a DC analog electrical signal to the form of digital data that can be managed by a computer. This permits the computer to use the electrical data signal from a measuring device.

**albumin**—a protein compound normally found within human blood.

**alphanumeric**—the use of alphabet letters and/or numerals to present data that are written or displayed.

**alternating current**—an electrical current that undergoes changes in either direction or polarity.

**ammeter**—a device containing a galvanometer that is designed for measuring the amount of electrical current flow in a circuit.

**analog electrical signal**—an electrical current, used as a signal, that varies continuously, without break over a range of values. Often the signal range developed by pulmonary function testing equipment is between −5 and +5 volts.

**anemia**—the presence of less than normal values for hematocrit and/or hemoglobin.

**anemometer**—an instrument for measuring the velocity of an airstream.

**anode**—the pole in an electrochemical cell that attracts negatively charged ions.

**ARDS**—acute (or adult) respiratory distress syndrome.

**arterialized capillary blood**—tissue capillary blood that is made to have blood gas values similar to arterial blood. Arterialization is accomplished by heating the tissue site, which causes arteriolar dilation and increases tissue capillary perfusion (hyperemia).

**arteriolar constriction**—arterioles are the last arterial vessels through which blood passes before entering the tissue capillary beds. Contraction of the smooth muscle tissue in the walls of arterioles causes constriction of the vessels. The use of varying degrees of constriction is the basis for controlling the rate of blood flow to a particular tissue capillary bed.

**ATPS**—indicates that a volume of gas is at ambient (room) temperature and pressure and is 100% saturated with water vapor.

**blood gas**—the partial pressure values for gases dissolved in the blood. Most often measured are partial pressures of oxygen and carbon dioxide. Though not partial pressure values, the values for pH, bicarbonate ion concentration, and base excess are often also reported with blood gas results.

**Briggs adapter**—a T-shaped airway connector that has a straight body with a 22 mm OD breathing circuit connection at each end and a 15 mm ID patient connection that is perpendicular to the center of the body of the adapter.

**BTPS**—indicates that a volume of gas is at body temperature (37°C), ambient (room) pressure, and 100% saturated with water vapor.

**buffering system**—a chemical reaction system that acts to control the number of free protons ($H^+$) in a solution (e.g., blood). The purpose of this system is to maintain acid/base stability (a stable pH value) in the solution.

**bulk flow**—a process involving the net movement of *all* the molecules within a fluid or gas system. Movement is caused by an "upstream" to "downstream" (high-to-low) *pressure difference* within the fluid or gas system that affects all of the molecules equally. This causes the net movement of all the molecules in the fluid or gas to be toward the same direction at the same time (e.g., water molecules flowing together down a stream).

**capacity**—the maximum value possible for a given set of conditions.

**capnogram**—a tracing that demonstrates exhaled $PCO_2$ values as measured over a period of time.

**capnography**—the display of a continuous tracing or a series of individual tracings that represent exhaled $PCO_2$ values measured over a period of time; the display of a capnogram.

**capnometry**—the display of numerical $PCO_2$ values.

**carboxyhemoglobinemia**—the presence of carboxyhemoglobin values that are greater than normal (greater than 2% of total hemoglobin).

**cardiac decompensation**—the inability of the heart to maintain adequate circulation of blood.

**cathode**—the pole in an electrochemical cell that attracts positively charged ions.

**Charles' law**—a gas law expressed as $P = T/V$, which indicates that if pressures remain constant, gas volumes change directly with changes in gas temperature. For example, a decrease in gas temperature results in a corresponding decrease in gas volume.

**closed-circuit spirometry**—method of spirometry in which the subject places the mouthpiece in her or his mouth before any breathing maneuvers are performed.

**coefficient of variation**—an expression of the standard deviation as a percentage of the mean value for the population. It is calculated by dividing the standard deviation value by the mean value:

$$\text{Coefficient of Variation} = \frac{\text{Standard Deviation}}{\text{Mean Value}}$$

**95% confidence limit (or interval)**—the range of predicted values that contain 95% of the population with normal pulmonary function. If a measured value falls outside of this range, there is only a 5% chance that it is a normal value that is falsely being identified as abnormal. For pulmonary function parameters that require only a low normal value range, the 95% confidence limit is set at 1.65 standard deviations below the predicted mean normal value. For parameters that require both a high and a low normal range, a range of 1.96 standard deviations above and below the predicted mean value is used.

**contact (salt) bridge**—a liquid junction between two electrochemical half-cells. It includes a semipermeable membrane that allows the diffusion of ions from half-cell to half-cell without an exchange of liquid.

**content**—the actual value present at a given time. The value may be less than or equal to the capacity for the same given situation.

**cytoplasm**—a thick, semitransparent, elastic fluid that is surrounded by the outer membrane of a cell but is outside the cell's nucleus. It is composed of 75%–90% water, with the remainder of the composition being components such as proteins, carbohydrates, lipids, and inorganic substances.

**D-A (digital/analog) converter**—A device that converts the digital data signal from a computer into a DC analog electrical signal that can be used to control the function of a measuring system's components. This permits the computer to use the electrical data signal from a measuring device.

**DC analog electrical signal**—a direct current electrical signal generated by a sensing mechanism. The electrical signal increases or decreases in direct proportion to the measured physical changes in a system.

**DC electrical current**—an electrical signal in the form of a direct current (as opposed to an alternating electrical current).

**dermis**—The thicker layer of the skin just below the surface layer (epidermis). It consists of dense, vascular connective tissue.

**dessicant**—a substance with the property of attracting and absorbing moisture from air or other substances.

**diatomaceous earth**—a substance that consists of the skeletal remains of microorganisms called diatoms. It has the ability of being able to adsorb some substances.

**diffusion**—a process that can involve the net movement of *a single type* of atom, ion, or molecule within a fluid or gas system. Movement is caused by a high-to-low *concentration difference* for that substance within the fluid or gas system. Other types of substances in the system will be unaffected. The fluid or gas system itself may or may not be undergoing bulk flow movement at the time that diffusion is occurring (e.g., during breathing, movement of oxygen molecules from within the alveolus, where it has a high concentration, through the alveolocapillary membrane, to the pulmonary capillaries, where it has a lesser concentration).

**digital electronic signal**—A discrete, noncontinuous electrical signal that can only have one of two possible values. For example, the signal may only have a value of either −5 or +5 volts. No other value in between −5 and +5 is possible.

**disability**—an *administrative* or *legal* judgment of an individual's ability to perform certain tasks, generally work-related. Disability is often caused by a physical impairment.

**Douglas bag**—a large plastic bag (approximately 22 liters) designed for the collection of exhaled air.

**electrical potential**—the electrical pressure or force available in a circuit to drive a current flow.

**end-tidal sampling**—the sampling of exhaled air late in a subject's expiration. This represents an attempt to perform analysis on gas assumed to be directly from the alveoli as opposed to deadspace gas.

**enteral**—within, by way of, or pertaining to the small intestine. With feeding or nutrition, it refers to feeding methods that permit foodstuffs to enter and pass through the small intestine. These could be normal feedings by mouth or support feedings by nasogastric tube, gastric tube, or jejunostomy tube.

**enzyme**—a protein capable of participating in and, as a result, accelerating the progress of a physiologic chemical reaction. Most enzymes are specific to a given chemical reaction.

**epidemiologic studies**—studies for evaluating the relationships of various factors that determine the frequency and distribution of diseases within a human community.

**ergometer** or **dynamometer**—a device for measuring or regulating the force of muscular contraction.

**flywheel**—a heavy wheel (often metal) that, because of its inertia, resists sudden changes in rotational speed.

**gain**—the degree of increase in an analog signal's value, based on the amount of amplication the signal receives in processing.

**galvanometer**—a sensitive measuring instrument designed to provide a response to the effects of an electrical current.

**gender**—an individual's category as assigned on the basis of physical and physiologic sex characteristics (i.e., either male or female).

**homeostasis**—the tendency for physiologic parameters to be maintained within stable limits that best support continued well-being. A tendency for an organism to maintain a stable physiologic state (e.g., maintenance of a stable, normal body temperature).

**homogenous**—something is homogenous when the substances that compose it are uniformly distributed within its volume.

**hygroscopic**—the property of a substance to readily take up and retain moisture.

**hypercapnia**—the presence of $PCO_2$ values that are greater than normal (greater than 45 mm Hg).

**hypercapnia**—an arterial $PCO_2$ greater than the upper limits of normal.

**hyperoxia**—an arterial $PO_2$ greater than the upper limits of normal.

**hyperventilation**—an increase in ventilation that results in hypocapnia.

**hypocapnia**—an arterial $PCO_2$ less than the lower limits of normal (less than 35 mm Hg).

**hypoventilation**—a decrease in ventilation that results in hypercapnia.

**hypoxemia**—an arterial $PO_2$ less than the lower limits of normal.

**Hz (Hertz)**—a unit of frequency equal to one cycle per second (60 Hz indicates a frequency of 60 cycles per second).

**impairment**—a state that results from an anatomic or functional abnormality. The abnormality is one where *medical evaluation* identifies a *measurable*, clinically significant change in body function

**inductance**—the result of an alternating current passing through a coiled wire. The current produces a magnetic field around the wire that in turn impedes the passage of an electrical current through the wire.

**inertia**—the tendency of an object at rest to stay at rest or a body in motion to stay in motion.

**intermittent positive pressure breathing (IPPB)**—a form of inhalation therapy where a mechanical device is used to apply positive pressure to patient's airways during inspiration in order to increase the volume of the patient's inspiratory efforts.

**interstitial fluid**—fluid contained within the interstitial space. This is fluid within the body that is not contained either within the body's cells or within the blood vessels. The concentration of substances within the interstitial fluid is virtually identical to that of the plasma of blood. The only exception is the greater concentration of protein molecules in the plasma.

**interstitial space**—the physiologic compartment that lies between the vasculature (blood vessels) and the cells. Substances that pass from the blood into the cells (or the reverse) must pass through the interstitial space.

**intubated**—having had an artificial airway introduced into the trachea for the purpose of airway management and supporting ventilation.

**in vitro**—the occurrence of a biologic process within an artificial environment, that is, outside a living body.

**in vivo**—the occurrence of a biologic process within a living body.

**iodine**—a nonmetallic element with an atomic weight of 126.904; symbol I.

**isothermal**—the property of maintaining a constant temperature.

**Korotkoff sounds**—the term used for the sounds hearing during auscultation for measurement of blood pressure by use of the cuff method.

**lactate**—a term that refers to lactic acid.

**laminar air flow**—air flow where all of the molecules in the gas stream are moving forward together in straight, parallel lines (as opposed to the chaotic, disorganized movement of gas molecules during turbulent air flow).

**lancet**—a small, pointed, two-edged surgical knife.

**light-emitting diode (LED)**—miniature, elongated electron tubes. When stimulated by an electrical current, LEDs emit light like a tiny fluorescent bulb.

**linear measurements**—where measured values are equal to actual values when compared over a range of measurements.

**liquid crystal display (LCD)**—a display using a special liquid compound that can organize and change its ability to reflect light when subjected to an electrical current or a change in temperature.

**mean value (arithmetic mean)**—the average value of a population (or series) of numbers. It is determined by adding the series of numerical values ($X_1$, $X_2$, $X_3$, etc.) and then dividing the sum by the number of values (N) that were added:

$$\text{Mean Value} = \frac{(X_1 + X_2 + X_3 + \cdots + X_N)}{N}$$

**metered-dose inhaler (MDI)**—a type of self-propelled nebulizer that is designed to administer individual puffs of a concentrated form of a medication.

**methacholine chloride**—a drug that has the capability of producing a parasympathomimetic response, including the triggering of bronchospasm.

**methemoglobinemia**—the presence of methemoglobin values that are greater than normal (greater than 1.5% of total hemoglobin).

**metronome**—an electronic or mechanical instrument that uses a pulselike sound or light to indicate a regular tempo or rhythm. Metronomes are commonly used in music.

**mitochondria**—small spherical- to rod-shaped organelles found within cells (singular—mitochondrion).

**mixed venous blood**—blood sampled from the pulmonary artery.

**mole**—a quantity of a substance that contains $6.02 \times 10^{23}$ atoms, ions, or molecules of that substance. The weight of one mole of a substance is equal to the molecular weight of that substance.

**morbidity**—the condition of having or being affected by a disease; the rate at which this occurs within a population.

**mortality**—death; the rate at which death occurs within a population.

**neurocirculatory asthenia**—a disorder that can occur in soldiers in active war service (and possibly in civilians). It is characterized by a symptom complex that includes breathlessness, a sense of fatigue, precordial chest pain, and palpitation.

**nonlinear measurements**—where measured values begin to show a variance from actual values when compared over a range of measurements.

**nonvolatile acid**—an acid that represents either normal dietary acids (primarily the result of protein digestion and metabolism) or lactic and keto acids that are produced as a result of abnormal metabolic pathways.

**normal (Gaussian) distribution**—a distribution for a population of numbers where the majority of numbers have values relatively close to the mean value for the population. This produces what is referred to as a *bell-shaped distribution* when the values are plotted on a graph.

**open-circuit spirometry**—method of spirometry in which the subject takes a full inspiration before placing the mouthpiece into his or her mouth to perform a test.

**organelle**—membrane-bound, organized living substances present within nearly all cells. Organelles participate in a variety of different cellular functions.

**oxygen content**—the total volume of oxygen contained within a given volume of blood. It includes both the oxygen dissolved in the plasma and the oxygen that is attached to hemoglobin in the red blood cells. (Units = vol% or ml $O_2$/100 ml blood.)

**pack years**—a specification of an individual's cigarette-smoking history that is described in the following way: Pack Years = Number of Packs Smoked per Day × Number of Years Smoked.

**parasympatholytic**—a physiologic response that is the opposite of one that normally results from stimula-

tion of the parasympathetic division of the autonomic nervous system.

**parasympathomimetic**—a physiologic response that is the same as one that normally results from stimulation of the parasympathetic division of the autonomic nervous system.

**peristalsis**—a wave of muscle contraction progressing in one direction down the length of a hollow organ or tubular structure.

**P$_{H_2O}$**—the partial pressure of water vapor at body temperature and 100% saturation (BTPS), 47 mm Hg.

**pinna**—the soft-tissue, outer shell of the ear that projects from the side of the head.

**planimeter**—an instrument designed for measuring the area of surfaces.

**pneumotachometer**—an instrument for measuring the velocity of respired air.

**polycythemia**—an increase in total red blood cell mass.

**potentiometer**—an electromechanical device that changes its electrical voltage output in response to physical movement.

**proprioceptors**—sensory nerve receptors within muscles and tendons that provide information to the central nervous system regarding the position and movement of body parts.

**pulmonary function screening**—administration of basic pulmonary function testing for a large population of subjects to identify certain characteristics or disorders.

**ramp study**—a cardiopulmonary stress test in which there is a gradual, continuous increase in the subject's workload throughout the test. This increase in workload continues up to the maximum level tolerated by the subject. A ramp study differs from a *progressive graded test* in which workload levels are increased in a series of stages (steps) and a workload level is maintained for a short period of time before there is an increase to the next workload level.

**real-time recordings**—test tracings that are produced directly and at the same time as the breathing maneuver is being performed by the subject.

**regression equation**—an equation that is able to make a prediction or correlation based upon a set of statistical relationships. For example, a regression equation for predicting the normal value for a slow vital capacity in male subjects is SVC = [(0.148)(height)] − [(0.025)(age)] − 4.24.

**resection**—excision of a portion of an organ or other anatomic structure.

**scintiphotographs**—photographs made to record a scintiscan.

**scintiscan**—a display of the radiation emitted from a radioisotope. It is used to reveal the varying concentrations of the isotope within an organ system.

**sedentary**—a condition of being habitually physically inactive.

**sensitivity**—the degree to which a device is sensitive or responsive to a change in input.

**shunting**—a condition in pulmonary gas exchange units where perfusion is present in excess of available ventilation or when no ventilation exists.

**skeletal muscle**—striated muscle tissue that is attached to bone and that typically crosses at least one joint. Striations are bandlike structures visible in the muscle tissue when it is examined under a microscope. Skeletal muscle is normally under voluntary (conscious) control from the central nervous system and is generally used to perform movement of body parts.

**small-volume nebulizer (SVN)**—a nebulizer of small volume, generally holding up to 10–15 ml of solution. It is usually powered by a continuous flow of air or oxygen in the range of 5–10 l/min.

**smooth muscle**—nonstriated muscle tissue that is not attached to bone and is usually under involuntary (unconscious) control by the central nervous system. Smooth muscle tissue is generally contained within organ systems (e.g., within the walls of the gastrointestinal tract).

**soda lime**—a compound of calcium hydroxide that includes sodium or potassium hydroxide or both. It is used to adsorb carbon dioxide from air.

**software**—any programs designed to control various aspects of a computer's operation.

**spirogram**—a tracing or graph of air volume movements into and out of the lung.

**standard deviation**—the average amount by which the numbers in a population (or series) vary from the mean value (MV) for the number series. It is determined in the following way, where the final value is expressed as a positive number.

$$\text{Standard Deviation} = \sqrt{\frac{[(X_1 - MV)^2 + (X_2 - MV)^2 + (X_3 - MV)^2 + \cdots + (X_N - MV)^2]}{N}}$$

**STPD**—the abbreviation to describe a gas that is at standard temperature (0°C) and pressure (760 mm Hg) and that has a water vapor pressure of 0.0 mm Hg.

**subject**—the patient or individual who is the recipient of a pulmonary function test.

**surgical risk**—a judgment of the likelihood that, given a patient's presurgical condition, the patient may experience either morbidity or mortality as a result of undergoing a surgical procedure.

**sympathomimetic**—a physiologic response that is the same as one that normally results from stimulation of the sympathetic division of the autonomic nervous system.

**syncopal episode**—a temporary loss of consciousness due to cerebral ischemia; fainting.

**Swan-Ganz catheter**—a multi-lumen cardiovascular catheter that can be used in the critical care setting. The catheter permits measurement of cardiovascular values such as central venous pressure, pulmonary artery pressure, approximations of left atrial pressure (pulmonary capillary wedge pressure), and cardiac output (by means of a thermodilution method).

**tangent of an angle**—the function of an angle on a graph that is equal to its Y-axis value divided by its X-axis value.

**technetium**—a metallic, radioactive, synthetic chemical element with an atomic weight of 99; symbol Tc.

**thermodilution cardiac output determination**—a procedure in which, through use of a pulmonary artery catheter (Swan-Ganz type), a bolus of isotonic saline (approximately 10 ml) at a known temperature (e.g., 0°C) is injected into the right atrium. A distal temperature sensory in the catheter's tip (in the pulmonary artery) measures the rate of blood temperature change that occurs after the injection. The rate of temperature change is interpreted by computer as an indicator of cardiac output (i.e., a fast rate of cooling and the rewarming of blood at the sensor would indicate a greater rate of cardiac output). The computer gives a numerical value for cardiac output and, if given a value for the subject's body surface area, can provide a value for cardiac index.

**Tissot spirometer**—a water-sealed spirometer with a volume of approximately 100 liters. It was designed for collecting and measuring large volumes of exhaled air.

**tissue resistance to ventilation**—the work or pressure required to displace involved body tissues during ventilation.

**tonometer**—a device that allows the operator to expose a blood sample to controlled quantities of one or more gases. The purpose is to establish specific gas partial pressures within the gas sample.

**ultrasonic**—sound frequencies in a range beyond human hearing (greater than 20,000 cycles per second).

**Valsalva maneuver**—a forceful expiratory maneuver against a closed glottis.

**ventilatory failure**—a ventilatory disorder that results in a subject's $PaCO_2$ increasing to greater than or equal to 50 mm Hg.

**volatile acid**—an acid capable of chemically changing between the gaseous and liquid states. Carbon dioxide, with its ability to combined with water in the blood to form carbonic acid, is an example of a volatile acid, ($CO_2 + H_2O \longleftrightarrow H_2CO_3$).

**voltmeter**—a device containing a galvanometer that is designed for measuring the electrical potential in a circuit.

**watt**—a unit of measure for power that is equal to 6.12 KPM/min, where

a. KPM standards for kilopond-meters. One KPM is equal to the work of moving a mass of 1 kg vertically upward against gravity for a distance of one meter (1 m).

b. KPM/min is the number of KPMs of power that are used per minute of work.

c. 100 watts of power approximately equals 600 KPM/min.

**workload**—the work output being performed by a group of muscles per minute of work. Units of watts or kilopond-meters (KPM) are used to measure workload.

**xenon**—a chemically unreactive gaseous element with an atomic weight of 131.30; symbol Xe.

# INDEX

Page numbers with *f* indicate figures; page numbers with *t* indicate tables.